SRERE, PAUL A
MICROENVIRONMENTS AND METABOLIC
000330056

000330056

KU-405-547

QH604.3.S77

WITHDRAWN FROM STOCK
The University of Liverpool

22 AF

- 9 NOV 1987

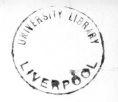

Microenvironments
and
Metabolic Compartmentation

Edited by

Paul A. Srere

Ronald W. Estabrook

Veterans Administration Hospital
and
Department of Biochemistry
Southwestern Medical School
University of Texas Health Science Center
Dallas, Texas

ACADEMIC PRESS   NEW YORK SAN FRANCISCO LONDON   1978

A Subsidiary of Harcourt Brace Jovanovich, Publishers

COPYRIGHT © 1978, BY ACADEMIC PRESS, INC.
ALL RIGHTS RESERVED.
NO PART OF THIS PUBLICATION MAY BE REPRODUCED OR
TRANSMITTED IN ANY FORM OR BY ANY MEANS, ELECTRONIC
OR MECHANICAL, INCLUDING PHOTOCOPY, RECORDING, OR ANY
INFORMATION STORAGE AND RETRIEVAL SYSTEM, WITHOUT
PERMISSION IN WRITING FROM THE PUBLISHER.

ACADEMIC PRESS, INC.
111 Fifth Avenue, New York, New York 10003

United Kingdom Edition published by
ACADEMIC PRESS, INC. (LONDON) LTD.
24/28 Oval Road, London NW1 7DX

Library of Congress Cataloging in Publication Data

Main entry under title:

Microenvironments and metabolic compartmentation.

Proceedings of a Virginia Lazenby O'Hara bio-
chemistry symposium held Jan. 16–17, 1978, in
Dallas, and organized by the Dept. of Biochemistry,
University of Texas Health Science Center.
Includes index.
1. Cell compartmentation—Congresses.
2. Cell organelles—Congresses. I. Srere,
Paul A. II. Estabrook, Ronald W. III. Uni-
versity of Texas Health Science Center at Dallas.
Dept. of Biochemistry.
QH604.3.M53   574.8'76   78-16858
ISBN 0-12-660550-5

PRINTED IN THE UNITED STATES OF AMERICA

Table of Contents

650458

Metabolic Pools

Multienzymic Systems

Microenvironmental Aspects

List of Participants

Sarah Ben-Or, Hebrew University, Hadassah Medical School, Israel

Samuel P. Bessman, Department of Pharmacology, University of Southern California, School of Medicine, Los Angeles, California 90033

James B. Blair, Department of Biochemistry, West Virginia University Medical Center, Morgantown, West Virginia 26506

Günter Blobel, The Rockefeller University, New York, New York 10021

Jacob J. Blum, Department of Physiology and Pharmacology, Duke University Medical Center, Durham, North Carolina 27706

Arthur Bollon, Department of Biochemistry, The University of Texas Health Science Center at Dallas, Dallas, Texas 75235

Barry Bowman, Department of Human Genetics, Yale University, Medical School, New Haven, Connecticut 06510

Michael Brown, Center for Genetic Disease, The University of Texas Health Science Center at Dallas, Dallas, Texas 75235

Ronald A. Butow, Department of Biochemistry, The University of Texas Health Science Center at Dallas, Dallas, Texas 75235

Britton Chance, Department of Biophysics and Physical Biochemistry, The University of Pennsylvania, School of Medicine, Johnson Research Foundation, Philadelphia, Pennsylvania 19174

Jane-Jane Chen, Department of Biochemistry, University of Southern California, School of Medicine, Los Angeles, California 90033

Jack E. Davis, Department of Biochemistry, Indiana University School of Medicine, Indianapolis, Indiana 46202

Rowland H. Davis, Department of Developmental and Cell Biology, University of California, Irvine, School of Biological Sciences, Irvine, California 92717

Christian deDuve, Department of Biochemistry, The Rockefeller University, New York, New York 10021

J. A. DeMoss, Department of Biochemistry, University of Texas Medical School, Houston, Texas 77025

John Dietschy, Department of Internal Medicine, The University of Texas Health Science Center at Dallas, Dallas Texas 75235

Ronald W. Estabrook, Department of Biochemistry, The University of Texas Health Science Center at Dallas, Dallas, Texas 75235

Johannes Everse, Department of Biochemistry, Texas Tech University, School of Medicine, Lubbock, Texas 79409

Kathleen Everse, Department of Biochemistry, Texas Tech University, School of Medicine, Lubbock, Texas 79409

Leonard A. Fahien, Department of Pharmacology, The University of Wisconsin Medical Center, Madison, Wisconsin, 53706

Mary B. Finkelstein, Department of Biochemistry, The University of Texas Health Science Center, Dallas, Texas 75235

Daniel Foster, Department of Internal Medicine, The University of Texas Health Science Center at Dallas, Texas 75235

Frank H. Gaertner, Department of Biology, The University of Tennessee, Oak Ridge National Laboratory, Oak Ridge, Tennessee 37830

Charles W. Garner, Department of Biochemistry, Texas Tech University, Lubbock, Texas 79409

Paul Geiger, Department of Pharmacology, University of Southern California, School of Medicine, Los Angeles, California 90033

David M. Gibson, Department of Biochemistry, Indiana University, School of Medicine, Indianapolis, Indiana 46202

Joseph Goldstein, Center for Genetic Disease, The University of Texas Health Science Center at Dallas, Dallas, Texas 75235

Robert Guynn, Department of Psychiatry, University of Texas Medical School, Houston, Texas 77030

Laura A. Halper, Department of Biochemistry, The University of Texas Health Science Center at Dallas, Dallas, Texas 75235

Robert A. Harris Department of Biochemistry, Indiana University, School of Medicine, Indianapolis, Indiana 46202

Mary Ellen Jones, Department of Biochemistry, University of Southern California, School of Medicine, Los Angeles, California 90033

Vasudev Joshi, Marrs McLean Department of Biochemistry, Baylor College of Medicine, Texas Medical Center, Houston, Texas 77030

Joseph Katz, Department of Biochemistry, Cedars-Sinai Medical Center, Los Angeles, California 90048

Hans Krebs, Nuffield Department of Clinical Medicine, Metabolic Research Laboratory, Radcliffe Infirmary, Oxford, England

Fritz Lipmann, The Rockefeller University, New York, New York 10021

John Lowenstein, Department of Biochemistry, Brandeis University, Waltham, Massachusetts 02154

Franz Matschinsky, Department of Pharmacology, Washington University, School of Medicine, St. Louis, Missouri 43110

J. Denis McGarry, Department of Internal Medicine, The University of Texas Health Science Center at Dallas, Dallas, Texas 75235

Howard E. Morgan, Department of Physiology, The Milton S. Hershey Medical Center, The Pennsylvania State University, Hershey, Pennsylvania 17033

Vivian Moses, Department of Microbiology, Queen Mary College University of London, London, England

James R. Neely, Department of Physiology, The Milton S. Hershey Medical Center, The Pennsylvania State University, Hershey, Pennsylvania 17033

David O'Keeffe, Department of Biochemistry, The University of Texas Health Science Center at Dallas, Dallas, Texas 75235

Merle Olson, Department of Biochemistry, The University of Texas Health Science Center, San Antonio, Texas 78284

Joseph A. Ontko, Cardiovascular Research Program, Oklahoma Medical Research Foundation, Oklahoma City, Oklahoma 73104

James R. Paterniti, Department of Biochemistry, Mount Sinai School of Medicine, New York, New York 10029

John W. Pelley, Department of Biochemistry, Texas Tech University, School of Medicine, Lubbock, Texas 79409

Julian A. Peterson, Department of Biochemistry, The University of Texas Health Science Center at Dallas, Dallas, Texas 75235

Luisa Raijman, Department of Biochemistry, University of Southern California, School of Medicine, Los Angeles, California 90033

Lester J. Reed, Department of Chemistry, Clayton Foundation Biochemical Institute, The University of Texas at Austin, Austin, Texas 78712

John Reeves, Department of Physiology, The University of Texas Health Science Center at Dallas, Dallas, Texas 75235

Thomas Roche, Department of Biochemistry, Kansas State University, Manhattan, Kansas 66506

Robert Rognstad, Department of Research-Biochemistry, Cedars-Sinai Medical Center, Los Angeles, California 90048

Charles C. Sprague, President, The University of Texas Health Science Center at Dallas, Dallas, Texas 75235

Paul A. Srere, Veterans Administration Hospital and Department of Biochemistry, The University of Texas Health Science Center at Dallas, Dallas, Texas 75235

James K. Stoops, Marrs McLean Department of Biochemistry, Baylor College of Medicine, Texas Medical Center, Houston, Texas 77030

Thomas W. Traut, Department of Biochemistry, University of Southern California, School of Medicine, Los Angeles, California 90033

Richard L. Veech, Laboratory of Metabolism, National Institute of Alcohol, Abuse and Alcoholism, St. Elizabeths Hospital, Washington, D.C. 20032

James R. Weisiger, Director, Extramural Metabolism Program, National Institute of Arthritis Metabolism and Digestive Disease, National Institute of Health, Bethesda, Maryland 20014

Richard L. Weiss, Department of Chemistry, University of California, Los Angeles, Los Angeles, California 90024

G. Rickey Welch, Department of Biochemistry, University of Texas Medical School, Houston, Texas 77025

Jurgen Werringloer, Department of Biochemistry, The University of Texas Health Science Center at Dallas, Dallas, Texas 75235

John R. Williamson, Johnson Research Foundation, University of Pennsylvania, Philadelphia, Pennsylvania 19104

Jeanie McMillin Wood, Department of Medicine and Biochemistry, Baylor College of Medicine, Houston, Texas 77030

Preface

There are many easily recognized forms of biological compartmentation.

(1) In the biosphere each life form is a separate compartment (composed of a set of complex biological compartments). The interaction between these compartments is referred to as the study of ecology.

(2) In each multicellular species the carrying out of special functions by differentiated cells is another example of compartmentation.

(3) Within individual cells compartmentation is achieved with organelles (nuclei, mitochondria, chloroplasts, lysosomes, peroxisomes, vacuoles) separated from each other by enclosing membranes. Even prokaryotic cells, at one time thought to be devoid of organelles, have minimally the separate regions of cytosol and periplasmic space.

(4) In the absence of membrane-limited organelle compartmentation, functional separation exists by means of isolatable, stable complexes of enzymes.

(5) Finally, it seems probable that compartmentation exists even in the absence of membranes and stable enzyme complexes. In this last case the compartment may be the microenvironment in a region of weakly interacting proteins, or the microenvironment near a surface due to unstirred water layers or due to a proposed water structure in the cell. Indeed, certain nonbiological catalytic systems in homogeneous solution have been shown to become an oscillating structure as a result of cyclical changing microenvironments.

In the symposium held January 16–17, 1978, in Dallas, the following subjects were considered: (1) Compartmentalization due to the existence of organelles and spaces separated by membranes; (2) the regulatory significance of metabolic pools; (3) compartmentalization due to multienzyme complexes; and (4) microenvironmental effects due to enzyme association or unstirred layer effects. Research on compartmentation can not be as easily compartmented as the concepts and natural overlaps exist between the results presented in a single chapter and the content of other chapters in this book. For that reason we have included the Discussions that followed the presentations so that the reader can see those interacting subjects as well as those areas in which the evidence presented for compartmentation is not universally accepted.

The editors are indebted to the distinguished group of scientists that consented to travel to Dallas, Texas, and participate in this Symposium. Regretably Fitzi Lynen and Klaus Mosbach were unable to be present but did submit manuscripts that are included in this volume. The success of a symposium depends not only on the participants but also on those behind the scene who ensure the smooth running of such a meeting. In particular we cite Mrs. Marie Rotondi, Mrs. Marty Parkey, Ms. Barbara Lewis, and a large cadre of enthusiastic graduate students in the Department of Biochemistry for their dedication and boundless energy in working to fulfill all the many tasks that required attention. The generosity of financial support from the Virginia Lazenby O'Hara Research Fund of the Southwestern Medical Foundation, for the Department of Biochemistry, Southwestern Medical School, made possible the bringing together of the leaders in research on this important topic of microenvironments in biological systems. The scientific presentations, as summarized in this book, were stimulating, provocative, and of the highest quality. The complexity of the subject and the current state of the art in carrying out investigations in this area of science illustrates that much has been learned but much more remains to be mastered.

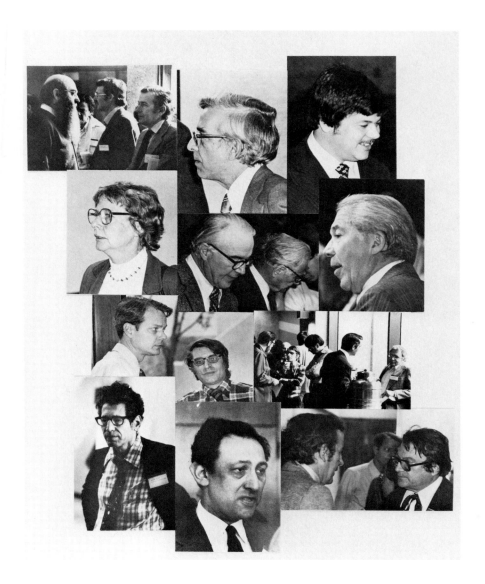

From top, left to right: Paul Srere, Thomas Traut, John Lowenstein, Lester Reed, Michael Brown, Mary Ellen Jones, Britton Chance, Hans Krebs, Christian deDuve, Richard Veech, John Williamson, Rowland Davis, John Williamson, Denis McGarry, Jack DeMoss, Jacob Blum, Vivian Moses, John Lowenstein, Richard Veech, Samuel Bessman.

Microenvironments
and
Metabolic Compartmentation

ORGANELLAR COMPARTMENTS

REGULATION OF THE CONCENTRATION OF LOW MOLECULAR CONSTITUENTS IN COMPARTMENTS

Hans A. Krebs[1]

Metabolic Research Laboratory
Nuffield Department of Clinical Medicine
Radcliffe Infirmary
Oxford, U.K.

In this contribution I will attempt to analyse some of the factors which make up compartmentation by regulating the chemical composition of compartments. In a general sense, compartmentation means sub-division of an organism, or an organ, or of a cell, into areas which differ qualitatively or quantitatively in respect to their chemical constituents. It is the chemical composition which determines the functional potential and functional characteristics of a compartment. The most characteristic constituents of compartments are high molecular substances, especially proteins, and among these enzymes. The molecules making up membranes also contribute to the characteristics.

The constituents with which I will concern myself, however, are the low molecular substances such as amino acids, nucleotides, co-enzymes, glucose, lactate, intermediary metabolites and inorganic ions. These low molecular compounds occur in all tissues and in all compartments, but there are large and characteristic quantitative differences between compartments, for example between blood plasma and the cytosol of vertebrate

[1]Supported by a grant from the Medical Research Council, U.K. and NIH grant AM 11748-07 MET.

Copyright © 1978 by Academic Press, Inc.
All right of reproduction in any form reserved.
ISBN 0-12-660550-5

cells. This leads to the question of the mechanisms which regulate the concentrations of cell constituents in different compartments and thereby determine their low-molecular environment. I will illustrate some of the mechanisms by an analysis of a few selected examples which demonstrate general principles.

A useful starting point is the fact that some substances are in near-thermodynamic equilibrium within a compartment. This means that the concentration of some cell constituents are determined by the concentration of other substances. For example the concentration of pyruvate, at a fixed redox state of the cytoplasmic NAD couple, depends on the concentration of lactate. In recent years a number of major equilibrium systems have become known. Since Dr. Veech's contribution deals extensively with the fundamentals of near-equilibrium, i.e. readily reversible, systems, I can limit my discussion to a few special aspects.

One important reversible system is represented by stages of the respiratory chain and associated reactions. This system involves the adenine nucleotides in the cytosol and the NAD couple in the mitochondrial matrix. That some steps of the respiratory chain and of oxidative phosphorylation are reversible has been known since about 1961, thanks to the work of Chance and Hollinger (1) and of Klingenberg and Schollmeyer (2). Reversibility between the mitochondrial NAD couple and the adenine nucleotides indicates that in principle equilibrium can exist between the redox couples of the respiratory chain, the NAD couple and the adenine nucleotides. More recently Wilson and his collaborators (3) have shown that near-equilibrium can exist between the cytoplasmic phosphorylation state of the adenine nucleotides, the matrix NAD couple and cytochrome c, not only in isolated mitochondria but also in intact isolated hepatocytes. The overall reaction of this complex system is formulated by the equation

$$NADH + 2 \text{ cytochrome } c^{3+} + 2ADP + 2Pi$$
$$= NAD^+ + 2 \text{ cytochrome } c^{2+} + 2ATP$$

The equilibrium constant of this reaction is
defined by the equation

$$K = \frac{[NAD^+]}{[NADH]} \times \frac{[\text{cytochrome } c^{2+}]^2}{[\text{cytochrome } c^{3+}]^2} \times \frac{[ATP]^2}{[ADP]^2[Pi]^2}$$

I must emphasize that the NAD couple in this
equation refers to that of the mitochondria, whereas the adenine nucleotide system refers to the
cytosol. If this overall system is at near-
equilibrium, then all intermediary stages must also
be at near-equilibrium, including the translocator
for the ADP and ATP across the mitochondrial membrane.

Electron transport is known to be controlled by
coupling with phosphorylation, that is by feedback
control involving, above all, the availability of
ADP. Electron transport comes to a stop when ADP
has reached a relatively low concentration and when
the phosphorylation state has reached a certain
value which cannot be precisely predicted or formulated. One reason for this uncertainty is that the
relevant molecular species are the magnesium
complexes, the concentrations of which cannot be
accurately ascertained though in the liver at least
they are probably very near to the total ADP and
total ATP. In addition to the magnesium complexes
and free adenine nucleotides there are present also
adenine nucleotides bound to enzymes.

It follows from the existence of a near-
equilibrium that the mitochondrial redox state of
the NAD couple is controlled by the cytoplasmic
phosphorylation state of the adenine nucleotides.
Once the redox state is fixed the mass action
ratios in the β-hydroxybutyrate dehydrogenase
system and glutamate dehydrogenase system in the
liver are also fixed. I must stress that the
ratios and not the absolute concentrations are
fixed. I must also make it clear that we do not
know whether this applies to <u>all</u> animal tissues.
It is probably true generally, but cannot be easily
demonstrated. It can be readily shown in tissues
where the capacities of β-hydroxybutyrate dehydrogenase and glutamate dehydrogenase are very high.

The mitochondrial NAD couple is not the only
redox system at near-equilibrium with the cytosolic
adenine nucleotide system. There is also near-

equilibrium between the cytosolic adenine nucleotides and the cytosolic pyridine nucleotides (4)(5).
This is brought about by the combined action of
glyceraldehyde phosphate dehydrogenase and
3-phosphoglycerate kinase which promote the following reaction

$$GAP + NAD^+ + ADP + Pi \rightleftharpoons 3PG + NADH + ATP$$

The capacity of these two enzymes in the liver and
many other tissues is very high. The ready reversibility in the <u>liver</u> is indicated by the fact that
glycolysis and gluconeogenesis both occur in the
liver (and many other tissues) at rapid rates,
depending on the physiological situation. The
ready reversal indicates that the system must be
poised at near-equilibrium under many conditions.
The equilibrium relation is defined by the equation

$$\frac{[NAD^+]}{[NADH]} = K \times \frac{[3PG]}{[GAP]} \times \frac{[ATP]}{[ADP] \times [Pi]}$$

The redox state of other readily reversible cytosolic dehydrogenases, e.g. malate dehydrogenase and
glycerophosphate dehydrogenase, are likewise controlled in this way by the cytosolic phosphorylation state of the adenine nucleotides.
    These considerations show how the well-
established differences between the cytosolic and
mitochondrial redox states can be controlled by one
and the same cellular property - a master regulator
- the cytosolic phosphorylation state. But the
redox state is a matter of ratios of concentrations
and the question of how absolute concentrations are
controlled remains unanswered.
    There are many other equilibrium systems in
animal tissues. To quote a few examples: alanine,
aspartate or creatine phosphate can be formed or
removed only by equilibrium reactions. There is no
other way by which the formation or removal of
these three substances is determined. Hence any
concentration changes depend on disturbances of the
equilibrium position. Some of the components of
the equilibrium systems can be changed by nonequilibrium reaction: oxoglutarate or oxaloacetate
can react through the tricarboxylic acid cycle.
Glutamate can be removed by dehydrogenation. ATP
can be consumed by many energy-requiring processes.

In these systems, I emphasize, mass-action ratios but not absolute concentrations are controlled by equilibria.

If, then, equilibrium relations do not control absolute concentrations, what kinds of other factors are responsible for fixing and maintaining absolute concentrations? The various factors may be classified into a few groups. One is the rate of entry and the rate of outflux into and out of a compartment. The complexity of these systems may be illustrated by the example of blood plasma. There is the entry of substances from many tissues into the plasma, in the form of metabolites discharged by the tissue, or of substances absorbed from the gut and transferred to the plasma or re-absorbed by the renal tubules. There is the outflow from the plasma by glomerular filtration and the uptake of substances by tissues. In principle, the situation is the same in every other compartment, including those at subcellular level, but blood plasma in one respect is simpler than cells in that plasma neither uses nor produces substances whereas cells modify intracellular concentrations by producing and by utilising metabolites.

Thus absolute concentrations represent the result of steady states and the investigation of the regulation of concentrations must be directed towards the factors which control addition to, and removal from, a compartment. Some aspects of this complex problem may be illustrated by a discussion of the factors which maintain the plasma lactate concentration between about 0.5 and 1 mM.

Lactate is produced by many organs in small quantities, and in major amounts by blood cells and the working muscle. The major sites of lactate removal are the liver and kidney cortex which convert lactate to glucose and the organs which can oxidise lactate, e.g. brain, muscle, heart, in fact all tissues which possess lactate dehydrogenase and an active pyruvate dehydrogenase.

On addition of lactate to the isolated perfused liver or isolated hepatocytes the concentration of lactate in the medium falls well below 0.5 mM. This means that the liver alone does not regulate the plasma lactate concentration. A plausible explanation for the fact that higher concentrations are maintained is the assumption that steady state

concentrations result from the balance between
lactate shedding by blood cells and other tissues
and lactate uptake, especially by the liver.   Both
lactate oxidation and lactate conversion to glucose
depend on lactate dehydrogenase - the first step of
gluconeogenesis and complete degradation.   The K_m
of lactate dehydrogenase in the liver is rather
high (1.7 *x* 10^{-2} M in ox liver) which implies that
the rate of lactate uptake by the liver is relatively low at concentrations below 1 mM.   This high
K_m value illustrates the general principle that K_m
values can be of major importance in preventing
the complete removal of metabolites from tissues and
the circulation (6).

   This principle is forcefully demonstrated by
some of the enzymes bringing about the degradation
of the essential amino acids, in particular of the
branched-chain amino acids.   These can be removed
only by transaminations.   The K_m **values** of the
amino transferases are high which safeguards the
preservation of these substances that cannot be
synthesised by the mammalian body (7).

   Lactate is a special case from the point of
view of compartmentation in that it enters and
leaves very readily.   There seem to be no permeability barriers, nor is there a pump.   In other
cases the factors concerned with the regulation of
concentrations include a selective permeability of
membranes, transport facilitated by translocators
or by carriers, energy-driven pumps and membrane
potentials.   As I cannot discuss all these aspects
I will limit myself to one aspect, the regulation
of the concentration of glucose in one compartment,
the blood plasma.   This illustrates an important
feature, control of metabolite concentration by
feedback.

   The glucose concentration of mammalian plasma
is kept at about 5 mM, the main regulatory instrument being feedback control by insulin and glucagon.
The release of these hormones from the pancreas
depends i.a. on the plasma concentration of glucose.
Above a critical concentration glucose causes
insulin release and an inhibition of glucagon
secretion.   When the plasma glucose concentration
is low and insulin is not required for the promotion of glucose entry into muscle and several other
tissues, the insulin concentration in the plasma
remains low.   At the same time the inhibition of

glucagon secretion by glucose diminishes with the
fall of plasma glucose and the glucagon concentration increases. This leads to a release of glucose
from the glycogen stores of the liver, as well as
to increased rates of gluconeogenesis. True, this
is not the whole story of plasma glucose control.
Other factors include the rate of utilisation by
the tissues and the influx from the gut. Moreover,
the secretion of the pancreatic hormones is not
only affected by glucose, but also by amino acids,
fatty acids, ketone bodies, the nervous system and
other hormones such as somatostatin. However,
normally the central factor in the "fine" control
appears to be the feedback control of insulin and
glucagon release by plasma glucose.

I suspect that feedback control of the concentration of cell constituents is widespread and of
different kinds. Another example is the sodium-
potassium-ATP dependent pump. The operation of
this pump depends on the concentrations of intracellular sodium and extracellular potassium. The
pump is activated when intracellular sodium rises
above about 15 mM and it stops when intracellular
potassium is about 110 mM. Thus the pump is
subject to feedback inhibition by potassium, the K_i
being clearly definable. In the steady state the
rate of exchange of intracellular potassium with
extracellular potassium is determined by the leakage of potassium from the cell and the concomitant
entry of sodium into the cell. The pump then makes
good the leaking (8).

The compartmentation of cells into some
organelles like nucleus and lysosomes may be
readily understood on the straightforward basis of
the function of these organelles, but the physiological significance of the mitochondrial matrix as
a special compartment is not immediately obvious.
True, oxidative phosphorylation, i.e. energy trans-
duction, requires membranes on which the catalysts

are assembled in fixed positions but, one may ask,
why could such a membrane not be floating freely in
the cytosol? Why is there a matrix separated from
the cytosol by a membrane with very limited and
very effectively controlled permeability characteristics?

The environment which the matrix provides
differs in respect to the concentrations of many
low molecular metabolites as has been clearly
brought to light by the ingenious technique of
Zuurendonk and Tager (9) which permits a separation
for analysis of the whole mitochondrion and the
rest of the cell. This technique is based on the
experience that digitonin disrupts the outer cell
membrane much more rapidly than the mitochondrial
membranes. Much the same separation is achieved by
the more recent cavitation technique of Tischler
and Williamson (10). Although the interpretation
of the data obtained involves calculations based on
a number of somewhat arbitrary assumptions, there
can be no doubt that the concentrations of some
important low molecular substances in the matrix
are very different from that of the cytosol. The
main uncertainties in the calculation arise from
the sub-compartmentation of mitochondria into
matrix and inter-membrane space.

Outstanding features among the differences
between matrix and cytosol are those concerning the
redox state of the pyridine nucleotides and phosphorylation state of the adenine nucleotides (Table 1).

The values are representative. They vary with
the physiological state. The redox state of the
cytosol is more oxidised by a factor of about 100
than that for the mitochondrial matrix (i.e. the
redox potential is more positive by 0.06 V). The
phosphorylation potential in terms of Kcal is
greater by 2 Kcal in the matrix than in the cytosol
(11.3 against 13.2 Kcal).

It would appear that the redox state of the
cytosolic NAD couple is best suited for the occurrence of the two redox reactions of glycolysis,
those catalysed by lactate- and glyceraldehyde
dehydrogenase. These involve the NAD couple in
opposite directions and their redox state must
therefore be so adjusted as to suit both directions.
At the matrix redox state the [lactate]/[pyruvate]
at equilibrium would be about 1,000, against 10 in
the cytosol, and the equilibrium concentration of

TABLE I.

The values for the NAD couple are based on measurements of redox couples in freeze-clamped rat liver by Williamson et al. (11). The values for the phosphorylation potential are those of Akerboom et al. (12). They are based on measurements on hepatocytes treated for the separation of cytosol and mitochondria with digitonin by the method of Zuurendonk and Tager. The "cavitation" method of Tischler et al. gives similar results. The latter technique breaks the plasma membrane of hepatocytes by squirting the cells through a narrow capillary. The redox potential between the cytosolic NAD couple and cytochrome a_3 is taken to be 0.85 V and that between mitochondrial NAD couple and cyto-chrome a_3 to be 0.91 V.

	Matrix	Cytosol
$\dfrac{\text{Free [NAD]}}{\text{Free [NADH]}}$	8	800
$\dfrac{\text{[ATP]}}{\text{[ADP][Pi]}}$	110	2670
Redox potential of NAD couple (V)	-0.293	-0.233
Phosphorylation potential (Kcal)	11.3	13.2
Energy available between NADH and cytochrome a_3 (Kcal)	42	39

pyruvate would be exceedingly low, 10^{-3} instead of 10^{-1} mM. Considering the key position of pyruvate in carbohydrate metabolism one can imagine that such low concentration would not suit the functions of pyruvate, those catalysed by pyruvate dehydrogenase and pyruvate carboxylase.

Analogously the redox state as well as the phosphorylation potential of the matrix may be advantageous for certain reactions involving ATP. The synthesis of cytoplasmic ATP (which is energised in the matrix) requires about 13 Kcal per mol. This figure depends on whether Burton's value of 8.4 Kcal (13) or that of Rosing and Slater of 7.0 (14) is used for the calculation of the free energy of hydrolysis of ATP under standard conditions of pH 7.0; it also depends on the concentrations of the relevant species of ATP, ADP and PPi used in the calculations. As Table 1 indicates, the respiratory chain between the mitochondrial NAD couple and cytochrome a_3 makes available 42 Kcal or 14 Kcal for the synthesis of one mol of ATP. About 9 Kcal, set free when electrons are transferred from cytochrome a_3 to molecular oxygen, are wasted. Thus the gap between the calculated available free energy and the calculated required free energy is small. At the redox state of the cytosolic NAD couple the free energy made available by the transfer of the electrons from NADH to cytochrome a_3 would be about 3 Kcal less, i.e. 1 Kcal less for each mol of ATP to be synthesised. This difference may be critical, and the fact that the mitochondrial matrix NAD couple is more reduced may from the functional point of view be one of the major advantages of compartmentation.

Thus the fission of ATP to ADP and Pi supplies energy parcels of different magnitude in the cytosol and the mitochondrial matrix. A parcel of still another size is provided in the cytosol when ATP is split into AMP and PPi because the concentrations of AMP and especially of PPi are considerably lower than those of ADP and Pi, that of AMP may be two to four times lower and that of PPi as much as 100 times lower. This would add up to 3.5 Kcal to the free energy release by the fission of ATP to AMP and PPi. This type of fission occurs especially when fatty acids and amino acids are converted into their Co-A derivatives, presumably because the free energy requirement of the synthesis of the Co-A esters demands more energy than the hydrolysis of the terminal phosphate bond of ATP can supply.

Another functionally important difference, often discussed (15), may be a pH difference between matrix and cytosol, though this is small. Gradients

of pH are postulated in connection with hypotheses
of oxidative phosphorylation, but these are at the
microcompartmentation level - a level not readily
accessible to direct experimental tests. The postulated pH gradients occur within the inner membrane and do not apply to the matrix as a whole.
The concentrations of bicarbonate and CO_2 are very
similar in the matrix and in the cytosol; hence the
pH gradient cannot be large.

The matrix may also provide an advantageous
environment from the point of view of economy of
energy expenditure in connection with reactions
requiring ATP. There are reactions where on
account of stoichiometry one molecule of ADP is
required per molecule of substrate reacting. At
the same time the energy required is less than that
liberated on hydrolysis of one pyrophosphate bond
at the cytosolic phosphorylation potential. Thus
the formation of oxaloacetate from pyruvate
requires under standard conditions 6.5 Kcal and
less in vivo because of the low steady state concentration of oxaloacetate. In the matrix the
wastage of energy is less than it would be in the
cytosol. The fact that synthesis of carbamoyl
phosphate, the first step of urea synthesis in the
liver, occurs in the mitochondrial matrix rather
than in the cytosol, may be looked upon from the
same point of view. This reaction requires 2 ATP
per molecule of carbamoyl phosphate synthesised.
presumably for the stoichiometric rather than
energetic reasons. The energy required should be
much less than the energy yield of the hydrolysis
of 2 ATP at the cytosolic phosphorylation potential.

It is difficult as yet to propose an explanation for the compartmentation between the cytosol
and mitochondrial matrix of some intermediary
stages of gluconeogenesis. The formation of
oxaloacetate from pyruvate and bicarbonate, catalysed by pyruvate carboxylase, occurs almost
exclusively in the matrix in all species, whereas
the next step, the formation of phosphoenolpyruvate
from oxaloacetate, occurs in some species in the
matrix and in others in the cytosol (16). Perhaps
these species-differences are related to species-
specific physiological circumstances but the nature
of these species-differences is still obscure.

SUMMARY

An attempt is made to analyse the factors which determine the concentrations of low molecular constituents of compartments. These factors include the permeability characteristics of membranes, equilibrium relations (which control the ratios of the concentrations of a number of metabolites) and feedback control of transport (operating for example in the regulation of the concentration K in the cytosol and of glucose in the blood plasma).

The physiological significance of the compartmentation between mitochondrial matrix and cytosol in hepatic metabolism, with special reference to the differences in the redox state of the NAD couple and the phosphorylation state of the adenine nucleotides (the ratio $[ATP]/[ADP][Pi]$), is discussed.

REFERENCES

1. Chance, B. and Hollunger, G., J. Biol. Chem. 236:1577 (1961).
2. Klingenberg, M. and Schollmeyer, P., Biochem. Z. 335:243 (1961).
3. Wilson, D.F., Stubbs, M., Veech, R.L., Erecinska, M. and Krebs, H.A., Biochem. J. 140: 57 (1974).
4. Krebs, H.A. and Veech, R.L., in: "Pyridine Nucleotide-Dependent Dehydrogenases" (H. Sund, ed.), p. 413, Springer-Verlag Berlin, Heidelberg, New York (1970).
5. Veech, R.L., This volume.
6. Cleland, W.W., Ann. Rev. Biochem. 36:77 (1967).
7. Krebs, H.A., Adv. Enz. Reg. 10:397 (1972).
8. Cotterrell, D. and Whittam, R., J. Physiol. London 214:509 (1972).
9. Zuurendonk, P.F. and Tager, J.M., Biochim. Biophys. Acta 333:393 (1974).
10. Tischler, M.E., Hecht, P. and Williamson, J.R., Arch. Biochem. Biophys. 181:278 (1977).
11. Williamson, D.H., Lund, P. and Krebs, H.A., Biochem. J. 103:514 (1967).

12. Akerboom, T.P.M., Bookelman, H., Zuurendonk, P.F., van der Meer, R. and Tager, J.M., In Press in Eur. J. Biochem. (1978).
13. Burton, K., Nature 181:1594 (1958).
14. Rosing, J. and Slater, E.C., Biochim. Biophys. Acta 267:275 (1972).
15. Boyer, P.D., Chance, B., Ernster, L., Mitchell, P., Racker, E. and Slater, E.C., Ann. Rev. Biochem. 46:955 (1977).
16. Söling, H.-D. and Kleineke, J., in: "Gluconeo-genesis: Its Regulation in Mammalian Species" (R.W. Hanson and M.A. Mehlman, eds.), p. 369, John Wiley & Sons New York, London, Sydney, Toronto (1976).

REGULATION OF COENZYME POTENTIAL BY
NEAR EQUILIBRIUM REACTIONS

Richard L. Veech

Laboratory of Metabolism
National Institute of Alcohol Abuse and Alcoholism
St. Elizabeths Hospital
Washington, D.C.

I. INTRODUCTION

The purpose of this presentation is to review the evidence
that a number of intracellular reactions are in near-equilibrium.
This work is a continuation of that carried on by Krebs and his
collaborators. I will concentrate on those near-equilibrium
reactions which use common co-enzyme pools.

The implication of this presentation is, therefore, that the
co-factors and substrates of a great number of cellular reactions equilibrate with one another. It is further implied that
many of interactions can be explained simply in conformity with
the laws of solution thermodynamics and kinetics and that no
special forces need be involved. This is not to deny the existence of microenvironments such as the glycogen particle, the
surface of fatty acid synthase and others.

It is an attempt to state a position clearly. "But," as
Bacon has well pointed out, "truth is more likely to come out of
error if it is clear and definite, than out of confusion and my
experience teaches me that it is better to hold a well understood and intelligible opinion, even if it should turn out to
be wrong, than to be content with a muddle-headed mixture of
conflicting views, sometimes called impartiality, and often no
better than no opinion at all. But, at the same time there
must never be the least hesitation in giving up a position the
moment it is shown to be untenable." (1).

Copyright © 1978 by Academic Press, Inc.
All right of reproduction in any form reserved.
ISBN 0-12-660550-5

I hope to review the evidence for some of the equilibrium reactions which use common co-factors. I also hope to correct some mistakes we have made in our previous work. The evidence I will present is of three types: 1) values of apparent equilibrium constants measured <u>in vitro</u>; 2) activities of enzymes measured <u>in vitro</u>; 3) measurements of the metabolite contents of living tissue which have been rapidly frozen. The conclusions drawn from this type of evidence differ in some particulars from the view derived from <u>in vitro</u> studies using isolated mitochondria, isolated enzymes or, in some cases, isolated cells. If I understand the purpose of this symposium, however, one aim will be to understand the origins of these divergent conclusions, why these different conclusions are arrived at, and how they relate to the methods from which the data were obtained.

I will begin with a brief survey of the major reactions thought to be near-equilibrium <u>in vivo</u>, followed by a short discussion of some of the major criticisms of this type of analysis.

II. THE FREE $[NAD^+]/[NADH]$ AND $[NADP^+]/[NADPH]$ COUPLES

The first attempt to measure free pyridine nucleotides in cells by measurement of the ratios of their metabolites was done in yeast by Holtzer, Schultz and Lynen in 1956 (2). This attempt was necessary because it had long been recognized that the pyridine nucleotides bind to dehydrogenases as well as non-specifically to other cell constituents. Direct measurement of these nucleotides in tissue, therefore, fail to differentiate between bound and free nucleotides and give no information on the distribution of nucleotides between the cell compartments which is known to be uneven (3). The problem was first put on a firm basis in mammalian tissue when in 1959 Hohorst, Kruetz and Bucher (4) proposed that three enzymes with high activity relative to their normal flux in liver, namely lactate dehydrogenase, malate dehydrogenase and α-glycerophosphate dehydrogenase, catalyse near-equilibrium reactions with the cytoplasmic free NAD^+ and NADH. They further proposed that the measured cell content of their substrates, lactate/pyruvate, malate/oxaloacetate and α-glycerophosphate/dihydroxyacetone-phosphate could give an accurate indication of the redox state of the cytoplasmic NAD-couple. This was based on the assumption that the percent of bound non-nucleotide substrate was relatively low and would not produce a significant error.

Even though malate dehydrogenase is present both in liver cytoplasm and mitochondrial matrix, it was assumed that because mitochondria make up about 20% of liver cell volume and the mitochondrial matrix space somewhat less (5), the measured contents represented mainly cytoplasmic contents. Formally stated, the contention was that:

(1) $\dfrac{[NAD_c^+]}{[NADH_c]} = \dfrac{measured\ [pyruvate]}{measured\ [lactate]} \times \dfrac{[H^+]}{K_{LDH}}$

(2) " $= \dfrac{measured\ [oxaloacetate]}{measured\ [malate]} \times \dfrac{[H^+]}{K_{MDH}}$

(3) " $= \dfrac{measured\ [dihydroxyacetone]}{measured\ [\alpha\text{-glycerophosphate}]} \times \dfrac{[H^+]}{K_{\alpha GPDH}}$

This contention has been empirically verified in many labs. Further, the agreement between couples has been taken to indicate that compartmentation of these metabolites within mitochondrial matrix was not great *in vivo* although it was recognized that their concentration in mitochondrial matrix could be less than in cytoplasm without being discernable. This view has been increasingly challenged in recent times as a result of studies using mitochondria cell fractions rich in mitochondria. These methods will be discussed later in the symposium. It is sufficient to say here that it was recognized quite early that some metabolites would have to be compartmented between mitochondrial and cytoplasmic space (3). The question was then, and still is now, which metabolites are severely compartmented or bound *in vivo* and how accurately do mitochondria isolated from hepatocytes in 30 seconds reflect *in vivo* conditions. In other words, the question is how good are these newer methods?

Shortly after the papers defining the concepts for obtaining the free cytoplasmic [NAD$^+$]/[NADH] the technique for freeze-clamping was described (6). This method allows the analysis of tissue without significant post-mortal changes. Freeze-clamping and simple methods of enzymatic analysis are the basic tools of the studies to be discussed.

In 1967, Williamson, Lund and Krebs (7) published the paper which in retrospect is the most amazing and consistently controversial one in this series. In it they showed that the free mitochondrial [NAD$^+$]/[NADH] calculated for rat liver from the measured tissue contents of the reactants of β-hydroxybutyrate dehydrogenase, which is attached to the inner mitochondrial membrane, and glutamate dehydrogenase, which is located within the mitochondrial matrix, give the same value of 7 to 10 for

TABLE 1. Calculation of Free Mitochondrial [NAD]/[NADH] Ratios in Rat Liver From the Measured Tissue Contents of the Reactants of the β-Hydroxybutyrate and Glutamate Dehydrogenase Reactions

The pH was assumed to be 7. Values are given as μmoles/g ± S.E.M. The number of observations is in parentheses.

	Glutamate	α-Ketoglutarate	NH_4^+	Acetoacetate	β-Hydroxybutyrate	$[NAD^+_m]/[NADH_m]$ from HBDH	from GLDH
			μmoles/g ± S.E.M				
Fed Liver (7)	2.41 ±0.29	0.145 ±0.013	0.47 ±0.15	0.055 ±0.020	0.144 ±0.048	7.8	7.3
Starved liver (23)	2.64 ±0.65	0.086 ±0.032	0.56 ±0.25	0.55 ±0.24	1.79 ±0.83	5.6	4.7
Alloxan-diabetic (12) liver	0.96 ±0.31	0.045 ±0.008	0.86 ±0.22	3.75 ±2.08	7.73 ±3.26	9.6	10.8

From Williamson, Lund and Krebs (1967) (7)

	Gluta-mate	α-Ketoglu-tarate	NH$_4^+$	Aceto-acetate	β-Hydroxy-butyrate	[NAD^+_m]/[NADH$_m$] from HBDH	[NAD^+_m]/[NADH$_m$] from GLDH
			μmoles/g ± S.E.M.				
Control liver (5)	2.35 ±0.73	0.16 ±0.02	0.71 ±0.27	0.053 ±0.020	0.105 ±0.043	10.2	12.9
2 min. ischemic (5)	2.84 ±0.57	0.068 ±0.002	0.77 ±0.22	0.028 ±0.010	0.187 ±0.028	3.0	4.7
5 min. ischemic (5)	2.65 ±0.61	0.041 ±0.001	0.69 ±0.26	0.026 ±0.015	0.201 ±0.010	2.6	2.8

From Brosnan, Krebs and Williamson (1970) (8)

the mitochondrial [NAD$^+$]/[NADH] ratio according to the equations:

(4) $\dfrac{[\text{NAD}^+{}_m]}{[\overline{\text{NADH}}_m]} = \dfrac{\text{measured } [\alpha\text{-ketoglutarate}][\text{NH}_4{}^+]}{\text{measured } [\text{glutamate}]} \times \dfrac{[\text{H}^+]}{\text{K}_{\text{GLDH}}}$

(5) $\dfrac{[\text{NAD}^+{}_m]}{[\overline{\text{NADH}}_m]} = \dfrac{\text{measured } [\text{acetoacetate}]}{\text{measured } [\beta\text{-hydroxybutyrate}]} \times \dfrac{[\text{H}^+]}{\text{K}_{\text{HBDH}}}$

The question has arisen concerning the agreement between these values. What follows is a compilation of values calculated for rat liver in different dietary conditions and during a period of relatively rapid change such as ischemia. (See Table 1 .

The calculated mitochondrial redox state changes in a predictable way during starvation and during ischemia, yet the agreement between the two couples remained within a factor of 1.6. That agreement is, in my opinion, quite good and it established that a free mitochondrial [NAD$^+$]/[NADH] can be calculated.

Similar calculations were attempted in freeze-clamped rat kidney (9) where the free mitochondrial [NAD$^+$]/[NADH] was 7.8 from the measured reactants of the HBDH reaction and 7.2 from those of the GLDH reaction in the fed animal. In the starved rat the HBDH reaction gave 2.9 and the GLDH reaction gave 5.1. The agreement was therefore considered to be good here also, although the situation in kidney is more complex because of the differences in redox state between cortex and medulla as well as a gradient between cellular and urinary NH$_4{}^+$ which had to be considered. It is not possible to check the agreement between the two couples in brain (10) because of the high gradient between blood and brain ketone bodies.

In 1966, this was essentially where matters stood. The cytoplasmic redox state calculated from the metabolite couples defined by Bucher and his co-workers gave an [NAD$_c$]/[NADH$_c$] of 200 to 1500 in liver depending on conditions and the mitochondrial [NAD$^+$]/[NADH] estimated by the couples defined by Krebs and his co-workers gave values of 2-12. The question naturally arose as to whether the free [NADP$^+$]/[NADPH] ratio could be estimated using similar principles.

The hepatic activities of potentially useful NADP-linked enzymes are as follows:

TABLE 2.   Activity of NADP-Linked Cytoplasmic Enzymes

Measurements were made at 25°, pH 7.4 under optimal conditions (11). Values are μmoles/min/g wet weight ± S.E.M. The number of observations is given in parentheses.

Isocitrate dehydrogenase	22.4 ± 0.88	(6)
Glutathione reductase (12)	7.0	
6-Phosphogluconate dehydrogenase	2.8 ± 0.16	(3)
Glucose 6-phosphate dehydrogenase	1.4 ± 0.11	(8)
Malic enzyme	1.27 ± 0.12	(4)

Like malate dehydrogenase, NADP linked isocitrate dehydrogenase exists in both cytoplasm and mitochondria, but with rat liver only about 20% of the activity is in the mitochondria (13). Therefore this enzyme would appear to be the most active NADP linked enzyme in liver cytoplasm. Glutathione reductase is the next most likely candidate,but in practice it is not possible to determine accurately the amounts of oxidized glutathione in animal tissue due to the peroxidative oxidation of reduced glutathione during deproteinization (14). The activity of glutamate dehydrogenase is well over 100 I.U./g in rat liver, but it is confined to mitochondrial matrix, and in vitro shows no nucleotide specificity.

After measurement of the requisite equilibrium constants in vitro and the necessary tissue metabolite levels,the results were as follows in liver, brain and heart from three different laboratories. (See Table 3).

The free cytoplasmic $[NADP^+]/[NADPH]$ ratio calculated from the measured substrate contents of these three reactions agree within a factor of two. The values reported here from heart and brain were obtained with no preconceived notion of what should be found in these ratios. This agreement in three enzymes and three tissues was taken to show that the free cytoplasmic $[NADP^+]/[NADPH]$ ratio in cytoplasm is approximately 0.01 to 0.002. Later work showed that the $[NADP^+]/[NADPH]$ ratio is extremely sensitive in liver to many hormonal effects. For example, glucagon lowers this ratio within 3 minutes while the $[NAD_c]/[NADH_c]$ is unaffected (19).

TABLE 3. Summary of Values of Free $[NADP^+]/[NADPH]$ Ratios in Cytoplasm

The tissue CO_2 was measured to be 1.16 μmoles/g wet weight of liver based on measurement of hepatic venous blood and assumed to be the same in brain and heart. The measured metabolite values are taken from the sources indicated in the references. For values of equilibrium constants see Table 4.

	$\dfrac{[NADP^+]}{[NADPH]}$ from $\dfrac{[\alpha KG][CO_2]}{[isocitrate]} \times \dfrac{1}{K_{ICDH}}$	$\dfrac{[NADP^+]}{[NADPH]}$ from $\dfrac{[pyruvate][CO_2]}{[malate]} \times \dfrac{1}{K_{M.E.}}$	$\dfrac{[NADP^+]}{[NADPH]}$ from $\dfrac{[ribulose\text{-}5\text{-}P][CO_2]}{[6\text{-}phosphogluconate]} \times \dfrac{1}{K_{6PGDH}}$
Rat Liver (15)			
Fed (12)	0.0101 ± 0.0018	0.0118 ± 0.0019	---
Starved (8)	0.0044 ± 0.0003	0.0019 ± 0.0003	---
High Sucrose (8)	0.0087 ± 0.0014	0.0091 ± 0.0025	---

	$\dfrac{[NADP^+]}{[NADPH]}$ from $\dfrac{[\alpha KG][CO_2]}{[isocitrate]} \times \dfrac{1}{K_{ICDH}}$	$\dfrac{[NADP^+]}{[NADPH]}$ from $\dfrac{[pyruvate][CO_2]}{[malate]} \times \dfrac{1}{K_{M.E.}}$	$\dfrac{[NADP^+]}{[NADPH]}$ from $\dfrac{[ribulose\text{-}5\text{-}P][CO_2]}{[6\text{-}phosphogluconate]} \times \dfrac{1}{K_{6PGDH}}$
Rat Heart (16)			
Fed	0.0036	0.0082	----
Starved	0.0025	0.0040	----
Mouse Brain (17,18)			
Fed	0.007	0.008	0.005

TABLE 4. Values of Apparent Equilibrium Constants of Dehydrogenase Reactions Catalyzing Near Equilibrium Reactions In Vivo

Values of these constants are defined at 38°C, ionic strength 0.25 and measured in vitro near pH 7.0.

Cytoplasmic NAD-Linked Dehydrogenases

Enzyme Reaction	Definition	Value	Reference
Lactate dehydrogenase	$K_{LDH} = \dfrac{[\Sigma pyruvate][NADH][H^+]}{[\Sigma lactate][NAD^+]} =$	$1.11 \times 10^{-11} M$	(7)
Malate dehydrogenase	$K_{MDH} = \dfrac{[\Sigma oxaloacetate][NADH][H^+]}{[\Sigma malate][NAD^+]} =$	$2.86 \times 10^{-12} M$	(20)
α-Glycerophosphate dehydrogenase	$K_{\alpha GPDH} = \dfrac{[\Sigma dihydroxyacetone-P][NADH][H^+]}{[\alpha-glycerophosphate][NAD^+]} =$	$1.35 \times 10^{-11} M$	(21)

TABLE 4. (Continued)

Cytoplasmic NADP-Linked Dehydrogenases

Enzyme Reaction	Definition	Value	Reference
Isocitrate dehydrogenase	$K_{ICDH} = \dfrac{[\Sigma\alpha\text{-ketoglutarate}][CO_2] \text{ x}[NADPH]}{[\Sigma\text{isocitrate}][NADP^+]} =$	1.17M	(22)
6-Phosphogluconate dehydrogenase	$K_{6PGDH} = \dfrac{[\Sigma\text{ribulose-5-P}][CO_2][NADPH]}{[\Sigma\text{6-phosphogluconate}][NADP^+]} =$	0.172M	(23)
Malic Enzyme	$K_{M.E.} = \dfrac{[\Sigma\text{pyruvate}][CO_2][NADPH]}{[\Sigma\text{malate}][NADP^+]} =$	0.0344	(14)

Mitochondrial NAD-Linked Dehydrogenases

Enzyme Reaction	Definition	Value	Reference
β-Hydroxybutyrate dehydrogenase	$K_{HBDH} = \dfrac{[\Sigma\text{acetoacetate}][NADH][H^+]}{[\Sigma\beta\text{-hydroxybutyrate}][NAD^+]} =$	4.93×10^{-9}M	(7)
Glutamate dehydrogenase	$K_{GLDH} = \dfrac{[\alpha\text{-ketoglutarate}] \ [NH_4^+][NADH][H^+]}{[\text{glutamate}][NAD^+]} =$	3.87×10^{-13}M^2	(24)

A consideration of the metabolites involved in determining
the redox states of the cytoplasm and mitochondria led to
another interesting idea, namely that the redox state of the
pyridine nucleotides were linked by certain common metabolites.
Thus,changes in one redox state would be transferred to another
but not without the possibility of change due to change in
metabolites. This was,then, a massive system of redox states
that communicated to each other through common intermediates.
As Dr. P. A. Srere once put it, "In this system everything
controls everything else".

The following is a list of some of the near-equilibrium
dehydrogenase reactions and their equilibrium constants. (See
Table 4.)

It is obvious from these values that equilibrium constants
for the cytoplasmic NADP-linked reactions differ by orders of
magnitude from those for cytoplasmic NAD-linked reactions. At
an intracellular pH of 7 the value of cytoplasmic NAD linked
reaction is between 10^{-4} and 10^{-5} while the NADP-linked
reactions have equilibrium constants of 0.03 to 1.2. This
difference in equilibrium constants accounts for the fact that
the cytoplasmic NADP-system is a low potential system, about
-0.40V, used for reductive synthesis in cytoplasm while the NAD
system is a much more positive system operating at around -0.20V.
The cytoplasmic NAD system is therefore capable of accepting
hydrogen transfered from substrates. This is a functional
form of compartmentation resulting from the nucleotide specificity of the enzymes themselves. For this reason removal of
hydrogen can be occuring from degradation of substrates via the
high potential NAD-linked dehydrogenases at the same time
reductive syntheses can be going on in the same compartment via
the more negative potential--NADP system.

Another obvious conclusion to be derived from this list of
equilibrium constants is that these reactions are not independent but are linked to one another through common metabolites.
Since α-ketoglutarate, pyruvate and malate are reactants in
more than one system, changes in any one system must have effects
on the other. These linkages and interrelationships have been
discussed earlier (25). It is worth re-emphasizing, however,
that in an extensive and linked system of near-equilibrium
reactions, changes in one part of the system must inevitably
affect the other parts of the system as well. In a meeting
focusing on microenvironments it should be remembered that a
large portion of the cell's activities appears to be described
by simple laws of classical thermodynamics and kinetics.

Finally, these equilibrium constants, in addition to those
presented later, indicate the importance of small inorganic ions
such as CO_2 and NH_4^+, Pi, PPi and Mg^{2+} in controlling intermediary metabolism. This list of equilibrium constants shows
that the NADP-linked reactions are not only insensitive to

changes in $[H^+]$ ion concentration but are instead sensitive to $[CO_2]$ while the NAD-linked reactions are sensitive to $[H^+]$. As an example, changes in CO_2 and its base partner HCO_3^- have very important, rapid and direct effects not only on the steady state levels of many metabolites, but also on the redox states. (See Table 5, Page 14.)

It would be expected that the $[NADP_c^+]/[NADPH_c]$ would change with CO_2 but it might not be immediately obvious that the $[NAD_c^+]/[NADH_c]$ would rise. The $[NAD_m]/[NADH_m]$ falls under the influence of increasing CO_2.

TABLE 6. Brain Redox States After CO_2

Condition	n	Cytoplasmic $\dfrac{[NAD^+]}{[NADH][H^+]}$	Mitochondrial $\dfrac{[NAD^+]}{[NADH][H^+]}$
Control	10	515 ± 34	1.38 ± 0.08
Exposure to:			
20% CO_2 for 2.5 min.	6	616 ± 56	0.654 ± 0.37
20% CO_2 for 5 min.	8	660 ± 44	0.569 ± 0.053
20% CO_2 for 10 min.	6	645 ± 40	0.480 ± 0.038
20% CO_2 for 60 min.	6	555 ± 33	1.14 ± 0.12

Redox states (±S.E.M.) for cytoplasm and mitochondria have been calculated from the data contained in Table 3. For details, see reference (26).

The concentration of CO_2 in all organs *in vivo* is set by the brain. Because CO_2 is rapidly diffusible, its concentration can change quickly and thus affect many metabolic pathways.

In spite of these widespread effects on metabolite levels and on the kinetics of certain mitochondrial translocases (27), CO_2 is often ignored in many *in vitro* studies of mitochondria. I suggest that some of the problems that will be discussed in this meeting will be attempts to reconcile data, from simpler *in vitro* systems to the more complex *in vivo*, which result from a failure to consider the effects of CO_2, and assuming Tris at pH 7.4 with 10 mM EDTA is comparable to the *in vivo* situation.

The inorganic ion which was not initially considered along with CO_2, NH_4^+ and Pi which should have been at that time, was free $[Mg^{2+}]$. Many divalent metals have significant catalytic effects on metabolism, but, with the possible exception of calcium in the mitochondrial matrix (28), only magnesium is present in cells in sufficient quantities to significantly influence the type of near-equilibrium analysis presented here.

TABLE 5. The Effect of 10 and 30% CO_2 Exposure on Brain Metabolite Concentration After 5 Minutes

Metabolite	Control (21)	10% CO_2 (8)	30% CO_2 (8)
Glucose	1.54 ± 0.05	2.83 ± 0.10†	4.16 ± 0.10†
Glucose 6-phosphate	0.180 ± 0.005	0.188 ± 0.005	0.280 ± 0.003†
Fructose 1-6-diphosphate	0.0131 ± 0.0004	0.0120 ± 0.009	0.0084 ± 0.0009†
Dihydroxyacetone phosphate	0.0164 ± 0.0009	0.0122 ± 0.0009†	0.0070 ± 0.0005†
α-Glycerophosphate	0.103 ± 0.004	0.064 ± 0.007†	0.056 ± 0.003†
Pyruvate	0.0890 ± 0.0020	0.0463 ± 0.0031†	0.0296 ± 0.0019†
Lactate	1.36 ± 0.04	0.641 ± 0.054†	0.407 ± 0.028†
Citrate	0.298 ± 0.008	0.225 ± 0.009†	0.170 ± 0.011†
α-Oxoglutarate	0.209 ± 0.004	0.102 ± 0.008†	0.0579 ± 0.0015†
Malate	0.300 ± 0.008	0.159 ± 0.010†	0.115 ± 0.007†
Glutamate	11.7 ± 0.16	10.3 ± 0.19†	8.80 ± 0.14†
Aspartate	2.96 ± 0.04	3.76 ± 0.11†	4.48 ± 0.10†
NH_4^+	0.275 ± 0.025	0.339 ± 0.035	0.304 ± 0.030
ATP	2.48 ± 0.05	2.48 ± 0.08	2.52 ± 0.04
ADP	0.591 ± 0.015	0.563 ± 0.014	0.545 ± 0.020
AMP	0.0577 ± 0.0028	0.0558 ± 0.0032	0.0566 ± 0.0044
Creatine phosphate	3.94 ± 0.05	3.62 ± 0.12*	2.55 ± 0.12†
HCO_3^-	10.5 ± 0.5	13.3 ± 0.6	18.1 ± 0.3†
pH	7.1	7.0	6.6

All values are means (±S.E.M.) with the number of observations indicated in parentheses. The symbols * and † indicate statistical significance at the 5 and 1% levels respectively. For other details see reference (26).

III. THE PHOSPHORYLATION STATES

While total tissue magnesium had been known for some time, estimates of free intracellular $[Mg^{2+}]$ were rather late in developing and yielded estimated values of 0.15 mM in red cell (30) and between 0.6 to 1.3 mM in rat brain, kidney and liver (31). While not all apparent equilibrium constants are sensitive to changes in free $[Mg^{2+}]$ to an extent larger than could be explained on the basis of ionic strength effects, some are extremely sensitive (32). Among such sensitive reactions are many kinases where the Mg-binding constants of the various substrates can be very different.

Prior to recognizing the importance of free $[Mg^{2+}]$ in the quantitative aspects of this problem, it had been recognized that the free cytoplasmic $[NAD_c^+]/[NADH_c]$ could be linked to the cytoplasmic phosphorylation state of $[ATP_c]/[ADP_c][Pi_c]$ ratio through the combined glyceraldehyde-3-phosphate dehydrogenase, 3-phosphoglycerate kinase reaction (25). Furthermore, the activities of the glyceraldehyde-3-phosphate dehydrogenase and 3-phosphoglycerate kinase are both extremely high relative to the flux through glycolysis or gluconeogenesis. Finally, the requirement that the liver must reverse the net flux through this system in switching from glycolysis to gluconeogenesis necessitates that this reaction system operate near equilibrium in vivo. The relationship:

$$(6) \quad \frac{[NAD_c^+]}{[NADH_c]} = \frac{1}{K_{G+G}} \frac{[3PG]}{[GAP]} \times \frac{[ATP]}{[ADP][HPO_4^{2-}]}$$

was postulated as the link between the adenine and the pyridine nucleotide systems.

A value for K_{G+G} of 59 M^{-1} was found (29). This value differed from the value of 250 M^{-1} calculated by Burton (33) but this degree of variation was not too surprising at that time because of the methods used in the experiments on which those calculations were based.

Flurometric assays suitable for measurement of glyceraldehyde-3-phosphate in tissue were developed and all the required components were measured. Using the value for K_{G+G} determined above, the measured ratio of $[ATP_c]/[ADP_c][Pi_c]$ was essentially the same as the calculated $[ATP_c]/[ADP_c][Pi_c]$ in seven different dietary conditions, differing at most by a factor of 1.8. It was felt that this indicated near-equilibrium between the cytoplasmic $[ATP_c]/[ADP_c] \times [Pi]$ and the $[NAD_c^+]/[NADH_c]$ in rat liver. As I hope to demonstrate later, this is probably still the case, but the problem is that the value of K_{G+G} is not 59 M^{-1} at pH 7.0 as I originally determined it to be, but rather 1830 M^{-1} at 1 mM free $[Mg^{2+}]$, ionic strength 0.25, 38°C (40). The major error had been in failing to consider the effects of free $[Mg^{2+}]$ on this constant measured in vitro.

The answer to whether the glyceraldehyde-3-phosphate dehydrogenase-3-phosphoglycerate kinase system in fact is in near-equilibrium with the pyridine nucleotide system in vivo can, I think, be satisfactorily demonstrated in three tissues: red cell, muscle and brain. The situation in liver is more complex because of the lack of any cytoplasmic kinase with an activity comparable to 3-phosphoglycerate kinase. Pyruvate kinase has the activity in vitro but apparently not in vivo since the measured ratio of its metabolites are 10^5 away from equilibrium. Muscle and brain however, contain the very active creatine kinase with activities of 1400 and 600 μmoles/min/g at 38° respectively. Furthermore, like lactate, creatine phosphate must be formed and disposed of by the same reaction. Creatine kinase in vivo rapidly phosphorylates and dephosphory- lates creatine phosphate in order to maintain cellular ATP levels (34 & 35). This enzyme can therefore be utilized to evaluate the cytoplasmic ATP/ADP ratio in muscle and brain and the value obtained can be compared with that from comparison made to the value obtained using the glyceraldehyde-3-phosphate dehydrogenase-3-phosphoglycerate kinase system.

Another kinase with a high activity which has long been thought to be in near-equilibrium is adenylate kinase or myo- kinase (36). In most tissues myokinase is mainly located in mitochondria (37) between the inner and outer mitochondrial membranes (38, 39). It does however have about 20% of its activity in cytoplasm in rat liver. Its distribution in brain is at present unclear, but it is assumed to be similar to liver.

The equilibrium constants of the myokinase reaction, the creatine phosphokinase (41) reaction and the glyceraldehyde- 3-phosphate dehydrogenase-3-phosphoglycerate kinase reactions (40) were therefore redetermined taking care to include the appropriate free $[Mg^{2+}]$. (See Table 7).

The appropriate metabolites were measured to evaluate these constants in four tissues. The values of these metabolites are given in Table 8: red cell, brain, muscle and liver. In addition, the intracellular pH was found to be 7.2 in all four tissues from measurement of tissue $[HCO_3^-]$, of 20 mM, and estimated intracellular pCO_2 of 50 mM Hg and the Henderson- Hesselbach equation. This value agreed with earlier reports by Krebs (43) using CO_2/HCO_3 in liver and with other reports using DMO (44) where the liver pH was reported a 7.22 and 7.23 respectively.

Calculations of the value of K_{MYK}, K_{G+G} and K_{CPK} were then made from these measured values. (See Table 9). In red cells perfect near-equilibrium reigned. K_{MYK} was expected to be 0.744 and was found to be 0.784 ± 0.037. K_{G+G}/K_{LDH} was expected to be $0.67 \times 10^{+7}$ and was found to be $0.699 \times 10^{+7}M^{-1} \pm 0.085 \times 10^{+7}M^{-1}$. This agreement therefore confirms the earlier reports by Minikami (45) that near-equilibrium exists in the red cell at the glyceraldehyde-3-phosphate dehydrogenase-3-phosphoglycerate kinase system.

In brain and muscle the value of K_{G+G}/K_{LDH} expected at equilibrium was $1.65 \times 10^{+7}M^{-1}$ while the values found using whole tissue metabolites were respectively $0.033 \times 10^{+7}M^{-1}$ and $0.052 \times 10^{+7}M^{-1}$, both significantly removed from equilibrium. In the case of K_{CK} a value of $1.66 \times 10^{+9}M^{-1}$ was expected, but in brain and muscle values of $0.074 \times 10^{+9}M^{-1}$ and $0.066 \times 10^{+9}$ M^{-1} were found. Again, these are values which appear to be significantly removed from equilibrium. The finding that K_{CK} is too small would mean, if accepted at face value, that ATP could not form creatine-phosphate which is not substantiated by known facts.

A resolution of this dilemma is suggested by a series of experiments performed by Passonneau and her collaborators studying the behavior of these metabolites during the onset and relief of ischemia in gerbil brains which can easily be rendered ischemic by occlusion of the carotid arteries (46). The kinetics of the changes in metabolite levels can thus be studied during periods of rapid flux.

Table 10 shows that in 1 minute the brain can lose 75% of its ATP content and 90% in 30 minutes while AMP can rise 30-fold in 1 minute and 50-fold in 30 minutes. By contrast, measured ADP never varies by more than a factor of 1.5. The stability of measured ADP has for years been cited as evidence for the near-equilibrium of the myokinase reaction. Similar data from others formed one of the basis for the theory for adenylate "energy charge" (47) and the theory of AMP as an amplification system of ATP changes in the regulation of phosphofructokinase (48). Data of a similar type has long been known in liver, as is seen in Table 11.

Similar to the finding in brain, rat liver ATP decreased by a factor of 3 while AMP increased by a factor of 5 during 5 minutes of anoxia. ADP remained essentially unchanged during this period of rapid change.

If however, the apparent equilibrium constant of the myokinase reaction is calculated, striking differences are seen between these two tissues which show that equilibrium in fact is not maintained in brain in the adenylate kinase system and therefore the apparent stability of measured ADP could not be due to the equilibrium at myokinase.

TABLE 7. Values Apparent Equilibrium Constants Catalyzing Near-Equilibrium Reactions In Vivo

The Σ sign indicates all ionic and $[Mg^{2+}]$ species. The constants are defined at I = 0.25, t = 38° C, pH as specified and free $[Mg^{2+}]$ of 0.15 or 1 mM. Source of constant is given in references. The ratio of $[\Sigma DHAP]/[\Sigma GAP]$ is taken as 22 at equilibrium.

	Value at 1 mM free Mg	Value at 0.15 free $[Mg^{2+}]$
$K_{G+G} = \dfrac{[\Sigma 3PG]}{[\Sigma GAP]} \cdot \dfrac{[\Sigma ATP]}{[\Sigma ADP][\Sigma Pi]} \cdot \dfrac{[NADH][H^+]}{[NAD^+]} =$	1.83×10^{-4}	0.744×10^{-4} (40)
$\dfrac{K_{G+G}}{K_{LDH}} = \dfrac{[\Sigma 3PG]}{[\Sigma DHAP]/22} \cdot \dfrac{[\Sigma ATP]}{[\Sigma ADP][\Sigma Pi]} \cdot \dfrac{[\Sigma Lactate]}{[\Sigma Pyruvate]} =$	$1.65 \times 10^{+7} M^{-1}$	$0.670 \times 10^{+7} M^{-1}$
$K_{CK} = \dfrac{[\Sigma ATP][\Sigma Creatine]}{[\Sigma ADP][\Sigma Creatine\text{-}P][H^+]} =$	$1.66 \times 10^{+9} M^{-1}$	--- (41)
K_{MYK} at pH 7.2 $= \dfrac{[\Sigma ATP][\Sigma AMP]}{[\Sigma ADP]^2} =$	1.12	0.744 (42)

TABLE 8. Measured Metabolite Contents of Tissues

Metabolite values are given as $\mu mol/g$ of intracellular water $\pm$ S.E.M. The intracellular H_2O content of red cells was taken to be 0.7 x wet weight while that of other tissues was taken to be 0.8 x wet weight. (42)

	Human Erythrocytes	Rat Brain	Rat Liver	Rat Muscle
No. of Observations	7	8	9	6
Lactate	0.921 ± 0.231	1.35 ± 0.05	1.36 ± 0.05	0.924 ± 0.082
Pyruvate	0.068 ± 0.008	0.102 ± 0.002	0.258 ± 0.018	0.095 ± 0.007
3-Phosphoglycerate	0.073 ± 0.004	0.018 ± 0.001	0.387 ± 0.011	0.038 ± 0.003
Dihydroxyacetone	0.017 ± 0.001	0.019 ± 0.001	0.043 ± 0.003	0.017 ± 0.002
Creatine	~0	6.11 ± 0.07	~0	12.8 ± 0.091
Creatine-P	~0	4.72 ± 0.07	~0	26.6 ± 0.153
ATP	2.25 ± 0.13	2.59 ± 0.03	3.38 ± 0.08	8.05 ± 0.049
ADP	0.248 ± 0.009	0.726 ± 0.018	1.32 ± 0.05	0.926 ± 0.067
AMP	0.022 ± 0.001	0.059 ± 0.002	0.294 ± 0.026	0.043 ± 0.004
Pi	1.65 ± 0.12	2.72 ± 0.06	4.76 ± 0.16	8.00 ± 0.44

TABLE 9. Values of Equilibrium Constants Calculated from Measured Whole Tissue Cell Contents

Values are calculated from measurements in Table 8. The intracellular pH was 7.2 and free $[Mg^{2+}]$ = 0.15 mM in red cell and 1 mM in other tissues. The red cells are from human subjects, the other tissues from the fed rat.

	Measured _in vivo_	Predicted _in vitro_
Red Cell (7)		
K_{MYK}	0.784 ±0.037	0.744
K_{G+G}/K_{LDH}	$0.699 \times 10^{+7}M^{-1}$ ±0.085	$0.670 \times 10^{+7}M^{-1}$
Brain (8)		
K_{MYK}	0.293 ±0.021	1.12
K_{CK}	$0.074 \times 10^{+9}M^{-1}$ ±0.002	$1.66 \times 10^{+9}M^{-1}$
K_{G+G}/K_{LDH}	$0.033 \times 10^{+7}M^{-1}$ ±0.003	$1.65 \times 10^{+7}M^{-1}$

	Measured in vivo	Predicted in vitro
Muscle (9)		
K_{MYK}	0.404 ±0.082	1.12
K_{CK}	0.066 x $10^{+9}$$M^{-1}$ ±0.009	1.66 x $10^{+9}$$M^{-1}$
K_{G+G}/K_{LDH}	0.052 x $10^{+7}$$M^{-1}$ ±0.004	1.65 x $10^{+7}$$M^{-1}$
Liver (6)		
K_{MYK}	0.560 ±0.021	1.12
K_{G+G}/K_{LDH}	0.058 x $10^{+7}$$M^{-1}$ ±0.004	1.65 x $10^{+7}$$M^{-1}$

TABLE 10. Concentration of Creatine-P and Adenine Nucleotides in Gerbil Cerebral Cortex During Onset of Ischemia

The data is taken from Kobayashi, Lust & Passonneau (1977) (46). Values are given in μmoles/g wet weight ± S.E.M. N=22 in controls and 4 to 12 in each subsequent group. The protein content of brain was assumed to be 100 mg/g wet weight.

	P-Creatine	ATP	ADP	AMP	Total Adenylates
			μmoles/g wet weight		
Control	3.72 ±0.76	2.54 ±0.08	0.337 ±0.016	0.032 ±0.001	2.91
1 min Ischemia	0.419 ±0.124	0.757 ±0.155	0.539 ±0.064	1.02 ±0.21	2.32
30 min Ischemia	0.137 ±0.054	0.269 ±0.026	0.213 ±0.026	1.52 ±0.16	2.00

TABLE 11. Changes in Adenine Nucleotides in Rat Liver During Ischemia – From Brosnan, Krebs and Williamson (1970) (49)

	Values are in μmoles/g wet weight			Total Adenylates
	ATP	ADP	AMP	
Control (5)	2.45 ±0.36	1.17 ±0.23	0.30 ±0.11	3.92
2 min Ischemia (5)	1.44 ±0.57	1.42 ±0.16	0.78 ±0.31	3.64
5 min Ischemia (5)	0.86 ±0.30	1.39 ±0.11	1.18 ±0.50	3.43

TABLE 12. The Apparent Value of K_{MYK} in Liver and Brain During Anoxia

The values of K_{MYK} are calculated from the values in Table 10 and 11. The value of K_{MYK} is 1.05 at pH 7.0. Values are from reference (46).

	Apparent Value K_{MYK} in Liver		Apparent Value of K_{MYK} in Brain
Control	0.54	Control	0.72
2 min Ischemia	0.55	1 min Ischemia	2.64
5 min Ischemia	0.54	30 min Ischemia	9.00

Table 12 shows that while myokinase appears to maintain near-equilibrium, at least within a factor of 2 in liver, the values in brain are beyond any permissable K_{MYK} which could only be in a range from about 0.2 to 1.2 (41). Given the fact that K_{MYK} in brain can return almost to a permissible value as soon as 1 minute after relief of ischemia (46), this could not be due to a lack of myokinase activity.

It seems likely therefore, that the apparent disequilibrium in K_{MYK} which occurs in brain during ischemia results from the compartmentation of AMP in an area which is devoid of myokinase activity. The only obvious compartment of this type is the mitochondrial matrix.

While precise distribution figures for myokinase activity in brain are not known, a careful review of the isozyme pattern and distribution is available (50) in rat liver where approximately 68% of activity is associated with mitochondria and localized between the inner and outer mitochondrial membrane (51). Roughly 20% is cytoplasmic with a small fraction in the nucleus. It is generally thought that the mitochondrial matrix is without myokinase activity (38). If it is accepted that the obvious disequilibirium in K_{MYK} seen in ischemic brain could result from the compartmentation of AMP within the mitochondrial matrix, one must ask whether some significant portion of the measured AMP might not be in the mitochondrial matrix under more normal conditions. There is some evidence to support this view. In rat liver, which appears to maintain a lower than predicted, but at least a possible K_{MYK} during anoxia, there is an almost 3-fold elevation of K_{MYK} associated with a marked increase in the measured AMP following ethanol administration (52). One might expect excess AMP production in mitochondrial matrix during acetate activation which accompanies ethanol metabolism since acetate thiokinase is known to be located in part within the matrix (53).

Since the expression for K_{MYK} is:

$$(7) \quad K_{MYK} = \frac{[\Sigma ATP][\Sigma AMP]}{[\Sigma ADP]^2}$$

the question must arise as to why, if a significant enough proportion of AMP is in the mitochondrial matrix to affect measurements of the whole tissue contents of that metabolite, is the value of K_{MYK} in tissues containing mitochondria consistently below the value of 1.12 predicted at a free $[Mg^{2+}] = 1$ mM. One possibility is that the estimated free $[Mg^{2+}]$ is more than an order of magnitude too high. While this may be possible, there is no evidence to support this view. A more likely explanation would seem to be found in the behavior of the measured ADP as illustrated in Tables 10 and 11. It is obvious in comparing the measurements of the three adenine nucleotides that the ADP stays practically constant while the other adenine nucleotides change greatly. ATP is free to fall to 1/3 its value in liver and to 10% in brain, suggesting strongly that the major portion of ATP is not bound or segregated to an extent which precludes its use as an estimate of intracellular [ΣATP] activity.

The contrasting behavior of a rapidly changeable ATP with a more or less invariant ADP, when taken with the apparent disequilibirum in vivo of K_{G+G} and K_{CK} calculated for brain and muscle and with the fact that the measured K_{MYK} in tissues containing mitochondria are all below expected values (Table 9), strongly suggest that the measured ADP is much higher than the activity of cytoplasmic [ΣADP]. The two most logical explanations for this would be that ADP as measured in the cell represents a large component of either bound ADP or ADP that is in a non-cytoplasmic compartment. Both these possibilities are probably true. There is an extensive literature to indicate that ADP is bound with a high affinity to actin (54). Actin is estimated to make up about 20% of the myofibrillar protein content of muscle (55) and to be present in brain (56) and liver (57) and possibly red cell (58) although undoubtedly to a much lesser extent than in muscle in these latter tissues. There is, in addition, the binding of all the adenine nucleotides to the enzymes for which they are substrates, but this is likely not to be so important in the case of kinases as compared to the dehydrogenases because of the lower concentration of the former (59). An exception to this may of course be the situation with regard to the probability of extensive ATP binding in the mitochondrial matrix to carbamyl phosphate synthase (60). However, on the basis of theoretical considerations (61) and from measurements made in isolated mitochondria (62) it has for some time been thought that the free [ΣATP]/ [ΣADP] X [ΣPi] ratio would be very much lower in mitochondrial matrix than in cytoplasm. The finding of equilibrium in the K_{G+G}/K_{LDH} in red cell and the apparent lack of equilibrium in the tissues containing mitochondria is consistent with the hypothesis that ADP is significantly compartmented within the mitochondria.

If one accepts that ADP could be extensively bound or segregated and that creatine kinase is very likely to be in near-equilibrium in muscle, then one may calculate a free cytoplasmic ADP for brain and muscle in the following manner:

(8)   free cytoplasmic [ΣADP] $= \dfrac{[\Sigma\text{ATP}][\Sigma\text{Creatine}]}{K_{CK}\ [\Sigma\text{-Creatine-P}][\text{H}^+]}$

where K_{CK} = 1.66 x 10^{+9} at I = 0.25, 38°C and free $[Mg^{2+}]$ = 1.0 mM.

The result of such calculations are presented in Table 13.

TABLE 13. Measured ADP Content, Calculated Free Cytoplasmic [ΣADP] and K_{G+G}/K_{LDH}

Free cytoplasmic [ΣADP] is calculated from equation 8 and the metabolite values given in Table 8. $[H^+]$ ion concentration was taken to be 6.8 x 10^{-3}M which is equivalent to pH 7.2.

	Brain	Muscle
Measured ADP (μM)	0.726 ±0.018	0.926 ±0.067
Calculated free cytoplasmic [ΣADP] (μM)	0.032 ±0.001	0.037 ±0.001
K_{G+G}/K_{LDH} calculated from free [ΣADP](M^{-1})	0.83 x 10^{+7} ±0.06	1.30 x 10^{+7} ±0.19
K_{G+G}/K_{LDH} expected (M^{-1}) at equilibrium	1.65 x 10^{+7}	1.65 x 10^{+7}

The agreement between K_{G+G}/K_{LDH} calculated from a free cytoplasmic [ΣADP] calculated from the measured components of the creatine kinase reaction is sufficiently good to make the following conclusions.

1. The total measured cell content of ADP does not reflect the free cytoplasmic [ΣADP] in these tissues.

2. Both the creatine kinase reaction and the glyceralde-hyde-3-phosphate dehydrogenase 3-phosphoglycerate kinase system are in near-equilibirum and share a common pool of ATP and ADP.

3. The free cytoplasmic [ΣADP] is likely to be in the 30 - 40 μM region; not the 1 mM range as measured.

Since no enzymes such as creatine kinase exist in liver from which one may derive an estimate of free cytoplasmic [ΣADP], it is impossible at this time to decide definitely whether equilibrium exists in the glyceraldehyde-3-phosphate dehydrogenase

3-phosphoglycerate kinase system in liver. The fact that the liver must switch quickly from glycolysis to gluconeogenesis suggests, however, that this is likely to be the case unless new reactions are to be postulated for the gluconeogenic pathway. There have been for sometime extensive reports of the separation of glycolysis and gluconeogenesis in muscle (63) and liver (64) based on apparent isotopic disequilibrium. There are no anomeric forms of glyceraldehyde 3-phosphate and simple binding of the metabolite would be sufficient to accound for the apparent disequilibrium found so routinely in the [DHAP]/[GAP] ratio (65). The findings here with K_{G+G}/K_{LDH} in muscle do not support the view that the glycolytic and gluconeogenic pathway are compartmented within cytoplasm.

Admitting that there is no proof to say near-equilibrium exists at K_{G+G} in liver based on measured numbers, one can make the case that the apparent disequilibrium is due to the same factors as are operative in other mitochondrial containing tissues. If one simply assumes near-equilibrium at K_{G+G}/K_{LDH} in liver, a free [ΣADP] may be calculated. Using these assumptions, the free cytoplasmic [ΣADP] would be 0.046 ± 0.003 for the liver data presented in Table 8. With the figure, a cytoplasmic phosphorylation state may be calculated for the four tissues. (See Table 14).

It is obvious that if the argument that measured cell contents of ADP does not represent free cytoplasmic free [ΣADP] there will be a marked increase in the cytoplasmic phosphorylation state in the three mitochondrial containing tissues but no change in red cell. It is my opinion that this is in fact so in brain and muscle, and probably so in liver (although liver is more difficult to prove for reasons already discussed). It is worth just noting that the [ΣATP]/[ΣADP][Pi] in red cell is 5700 and 16,300 in liver, but due to the differences in free [Mg^{2+}] between the two tissues the ΔG of ATP hydrolysis is the same in both tissues although lower than the -14 Kcal/mole in the excitable tissues, muscle and brain.

Without discussing the far-reaching implications for regulation of this data, I would next simply like to point out that the cytoplasm has other potential phosphorylation states than simply the [ΣATP]/[ΣADP][ΣPi] discussed above (66). A number of reactions involve the transformation of ATP to AMP and PPi-- not ADP and Pi. The ΔG of the transformation ATP $\rightarrow$ ADP + Pi is -7.6 Kcals/mole at 38°, $I = 0.25$ and free [Mg^{2+}] = 1 mM conditions while the ΔG^0 of ATP $\rightarrow$ AMP + PPi under the same conditions is -10.0. Under cellular conditions, this discrepency in the potential energies of the two systems is even larger, being -14 Kcal/mole for an ATP $\rightarrow$ ADP + Pi and a -20

TABLE 14. Cytoplasmic Phosphorylation State in Red Cell, Brain, Muscle and Liver

The measured $[\Sigma ATP]/[\Sigma ADP][\Sigma Pi]$ is calculated for the samples given in Table 8. The calculated $[\Sigma ATP]/[\Sigma ADP][\Sigma Pi]$ is given using the calculated free cytoplasmic $[\Sigma ADP]$ and the remaining values in Table 8. The ΔG of ATP hydrolysis at pH 7.2, 38° and free $[Mg^{2+}]$ of 0.15 mM in red cell and 1.0 mM in the other tissue is taken from (42).

	Red Cell (7)	Brain (8)	Muscle (6)	Liver (9)
Measured $[\Sigma ATP]/[\Sigma ADP][\Sigma Pi]$ in (M^{-1})	5700 ±540	1320 ±40	1090 ±165	557 ±46
Calculated $[\Sigma ATP]/[\Sigma ADP][\Sigma Pi]$ in (M^{-1})	5700 ±540	30,000 ±700	27,200 ±1240	16,300 ±1620
ΔG of Hydrolysis of Free $[\Sigma ATP] \rightarrow [\Sigma ADP][\Sigma Pi]$ in the cell (kcal/mol)	-13.65 ±0.07	-14.08 ±0.01	-14.03 ±0.08	-13.69 ±0.06

to -24 Kcal/mole depending on what estimate is taken for the
cytoplasmic AMP. The situation is therefore exactly analogous
to the situation with the redox states of the two pyridine
nucleotide systems, where the low potential, high energy
[NADP$^+$]/[NADPH] system co-exists along side the higher potential, lower energy [NAD$^+$]/[NADH] system within the cytoplasm
due to the specificity confirred by the enzymes.

It is however to the low potential $\frac{[PPi]}{[Pi]^2}$ system that I wish
to address myself here, not only because it is more controversial and thus appropriate for a symposium such as this,
but also because it is an example of how different investigators draw different conclusions both in the name of thermodynamics or near-equilibirum reactions. The production of
inorganic pyrophosphate is common in many active metabolic
pathways such as in the conversion of acetate to acetyl CoA
via acetyl CoA synthetase, the synthesis of urea via argininosuccinate synthetase, the synthesis of glycogen through
UDPG pyrophosphorylase and the formation of ammoacyl-tRNA.
Rat liver contains an activity of about 50 μmoles/min/g of
UDPG pyrophosphorylase, 4 of arginino-succinate synthetase and
0.5 - 1.0 of acetyl CoA synthetase (67) although the later
enzyme is located about 80% in cytoplasm and 20% in mitochondrial matrix (53).

Measurement of enzyme activities *in vitro* can, however,
often be misleading in predicting the situation *in vivo*.
Most mammalian tissues are reported to contain very high
"pyrophosphatase" activity *in vitro* (68). The liver is known
to contain a number of pyrophosphatases including alkaline
phosphatase and glucose-6-phosphatase to name but two. It
was widely held, particularly by the molecular biologists,
that the PPi produced during the activation of aminoacids to
form aminoacyl-tRNA or through the action of DNA polymerase
is immediately hydrolysed to 2 Pi providing an even greater
ΔG for these reactions (69).

Not being a molecular biologist myself, but rather being
engaged in the archeological part of biochemistry known as
metabolism, I was concerned with the fate of glucose
1-phosphate if all the PPi were instantly hydrolysed. The
equilibrium constant of the reaction was:

(9) $K_{UDPG-PP'ase} = \frac{[\Sigma UTP][\Sigma Glucose\ 1-P]}{[\Sigma UDP-glucose][\Sigma PPi]} = 4.55 \pm 0.10$ (67)

Hexokinase activity is relatively low compared to that of UDPG
pyrophosphorylase and since that enzyme was not obviously
"controlled" it seemed possible that all the glucose-6
phosphate formed might equilibrate with glucose-1-phosphate

and then pile up in immense quantities of UDP glucose before
it could negotiate the terrible allosteric hurdles awaiting it
at phosphofructokinase.

It is now known that PPi is not hydrolysed immediately but
plays an important role in metabolism as the work of Wood and
his collaborators have shown in Propionionibacterum shermanii
(70) and Reeves (71) in E. histolytica. A new and simple
enzymatic assay has been developed using the PPi-phosphofructokinase (72) isolated from bacteria by O'Brian, Bowien &
Wood (73) which allows total PPi to be measured easily in
tissue. The finding of a PPi-phosphofructokinase in bacteria
naturally raises speculation as to what role such enzymes
might play in mammals. Even though no such enzymes with
appropriate Km's have been found, thermodynamic considerations
lead one to postulate their existence or a set of reactions
which sum to the same overall stoichiometry in mammalian cells
(66).

As an example of one possible role PPi may play in tissue
the following data was obtained in normal and insulin deficient rats 15 minutes after administration of 40 units of
regular insulin I.P. (74).

TABLE 15. Measured Metabolite Contents in Fed and Insulin-
Deficient Rats

Fed rats were given 40 units of regular insulin I.P. and
livers freeze-clamped 15 minutes later. Values are µmoles/g
wet weight ± S.E.M. with N=5 (74).

	Fed Control	Fed +Insulin	Streptozotocin Control	Streptozotocin + Insulin
Glucose	6.53 ±0.17	4.29 ±0.25	24.23 ±2.01	15.00 ±6.78
G-6-P	0.135 ±0.013	0.330 ±0.038	0.223 ±0.154	0.196 ±0.204
G-1-P	0.0104 ±0.0010	0.0221 ±0.0020	0.0183 ±0.0109	0.0166 ±0.0154
UTP	0.320 ±0.002	0.286 ±0.024	0.173 ±0.042	0.238 ±0.068
UDPG	0.503 ±0.025	0.531 ±0.013	0.474 ±0.054	0.401 ±0.070
Pi	3.94 ±0.09	4.46 ±0.14	4.80 ±0.57	4.97 ±0.99
Total PPi	0.0118 ±0.0007	0.0182 ±0.0006	0.0170 ±0.0024	0.0229 ±0.0075

The free cytoplasmic PPi was calculated from equation 9. The results of those calculations are given in Table 16 as well as the apparent equilibrium constant of a glucose-PPi transphosphorylase reaction, the nature of which is at present unknown. The equilibrium constant of this reaction may be written:

(10) $\dfrac{[\Sigma \text{Glucose-6-P}][\Sigma \text{Pi}]}{[\text{Glucose}][\text{Free } \Sigma \text{PPi}]} = 45.5$ at 38°, $I = 0.75$ and free $Mg^{+2} = 1mM$ (66)

TABLE 16. Effects of Insulin on the Calculated Free Cytoplasm [ΣPPi] in Rat Liver and the Value of K_{G6Pase} *In Vivo*

	Fed		Streptozotocin	
	Control	+ Insulin	Control	+ Insulin
Calculated Free [ΣPPi]	0.0014 ±0.0001	0.0026 ±0.0001	0.0014 ±0.0003	0.0019 ±0.0004
$\dfrac{[\Sigma \text{G-6-P}][\Sigma \text{Pi}]}{[\Sigma \text{Glucose}][\Sigma \text{ Free PPi}]}$	57 ± 6	113 ± 6	30 ± 9	25 ±16

It is noteworthy that both the total measured liver PPi and the calculated free [ΣPPi] increase within 15 minutes of giving insulin to a normal or to an insulin deficient animal. The mechanism whereby insulin exerts its blood glucose lowering effects is at present unknown, but it seems extremely unlikely to be due simply to an increased permeability of peripheral tissue to glucose (75). Liver is always permeable to glucose and the closeness of the K_{eq} of the reaction glucose + PPi → glucose 6-P + Pi to the expected value of 45 certainly calls for a re-evaluation of the mechanism of the control of the initial steps of glycolysis. Whatever ultimately proves to be the case as to the pathway of glucose phosphorylation, the effect of insulin on PPi looks significant and will have far reaching consequences on many metabolic pathways including, one would predict, protein synthesis.

The points to be made in this context, however, are that the existence of pyrophosphate was predicted on the basis of near-equilibrium studies of the type we have been discussing. Pyrophosphates offer the cell an option to phosphorylate intermediates with a much lower loss in free energy than occurs with either ATP → ADP or ATP → AMP. In terms of efficiency this lower energy phosphorylation state has many advantages for the economy of the cell.

IV. THE ACETYL CoA/CoA RATIO

In a survey of near-equilibrium reactions involving common
cofactors, the last group that needs to be mentioned following
the dehydrogenases and the kinases are those reactions
involving acetyl CoA. It is expected that the free [Acetyl
CoA]/[CoA] ratio would not be the same in the cytoplasmic and
mitochondrial compartments since acetyl CoA is not able to
penetrate the inner mitochondrial membrane (76). In cytoplasm
of rat liver, the most active acetyl CoA producing enzyme (77)
is citrate cleavage enzyme(78) which has an activity from 1.6
to 12 μmoles/min/g wet weight of liver at 38°C. This is far
higher than the rate of fatty acid synthesis which ranges from
0.02 to 1.31 μmoles of C_2 units/min/g wet weight. The activity
of citrate cleavage enzyme therefore exceeds by an order of
magnitude the capacity of the major consumer of cytoplasmic
acetyl CoA which is the process of fatty acid synthesis.
Another enzyme with a much lesser capacity but which also
favors the production of acetyl CoA in cytoplasm is the acetyl
CoA synthase reaction which has approximately half its activity
in cytoplasm in rat liver (53) although the major portion of
its activity in rat brain appears to be in mitochondria (79).

In contrast, the mitochondrial enzymes which could, at
least potentially be influenced by the [Acetyl CoA]/ [CoA]
ratio are citrate synthase in the mitochondrial matrix and
acetyl carnitine transferase which is located on the mitochondrial inner membrane. The distribution of acetyl carnitine
and carnitine is thought to be limited by the inner mitochondrial membrane by some investigators (80). However, other
investigators using different ionic media in vitro find acetyl
carnitine to be permeable throughout the entire mitochondrial
water (81). The situation in vivo has yet to be resolved. It
is however interesting in this context to review what the
thermodynamic position of the cytoplasmic versus mitochondrial
reactions would be if near-equilibrium did pertain.

Written in ionic form, the reaction for citrate cleavage
enzyme in cytoplasm would be:

(11) $oxaloacetate^{2-} + AcCoA + H_2O + ADP^{3-} + Pi^{2-} + H^+ \rightarrow$
      $citrate^{3-} + CoA + H^+ + ATP^{4-} + H_2O$

The ionic form of the citrate synthase reaction would be:

(12) $oxaloacetate^{2-} + AcCoA + H_2O \rightarrow citrate^{3-} + CoA + H^+$

The metabolites in the two reactions are the same, citrate and
oxalacetate. ATP-citrate lyase, however, balances the free

energy of the hydrolysis of ATP -7.60 Kcal/mole by the formation of acetyl CoA 8.54 Kcal/mole (32). Since the free
energies of hydrolysis of acetyl CoA and ATP are similar it
follows that the equilibrium constant of citrate synthase will
have a value which is very far from 1 while, ATP-citrate lyase
will have an equilibrium constant of about 1. Finally the
stoichiometry shows that citrate synthase will be sensitive to
pH while ATP-citrate lyase will not.

In the following table of equilibrium constants, it can be
seen that the cellular location of these enzymes is very different. ATP citrate lyase is entirely cytoplasmic, while citrate
synthase is entirely within the mitochondrial matrix. Acetyl
CoA synthase exists in both mitochondrial matrix and cytoplasm
while acetyl carnitine transferase operates in that never-never
land of the inner mitochondrial membrane. While acetyl CoA and
CoA are not permeable to the inner mitochondrial membrane,
acetyl carnitine may or may not be depending on the conditions
used in vitro. (See Table 17).

This table shows that the equilibrium constant of matrix
citrate synthase is very much different than the equilibrium
constant of the cytoplasmic enzyme ATP-citrate lyase. It is
also obvious that the equilibrium constant of citrate synthase
vastly favors the formation of CoA and citrate and the utilization of acetyl CoA. In mitochondrial matrix, therefore, to the
extent that citrate synthase tends toward equilibrium, it will
decrease the mitochondrial [acetyl CoA]/[CoA] ratio. It should
be emphasized that no one has postulated this enzyme is at
equilibrium, but none the less these calculations may be pertinent in view of attempts to understand the flux of the Krebs
cycle in vivo (59).

Cytoplasmic ATP citrate lyase, on the other hand, has an
equilibrium constant of 10, but because of the very high cytoplasmic [ΣATP]/[ΣADP][ΣPi] a very high cytoplasmic [ΣAcCoA]/
[ΣCoA] would be predicted. The same result would naturally
pertain to the extent that the cytoplasmic acetyl CoA synthetase operates where [ΣATP]/[ΣAMP][ΣPPi] is related to [ΣATP]/
[ΣADP][ΣPi] through a common cytoplasmic [AcCoA]/[CoA] ratio.
Attempts to calculate this ratio have been made (77) and values
in the range of 1000-10000 would be predicted for the free
cytoplasmic [AcCoA]/[CoA] depending upon what is taken for the
cytoplasmic concentrations of ADP and AMP.

Finally, it should be pointed out that the total tissue
contents of the components of the acetyl carnitine transferase
reaction have been measured in rat liver in a number of different states (84). The expected value at equilibrium is 1.7.
The values found were: fed 1.18; glucose fed 0.96; starved
2.77 and ethanol fed 0.65.

TABLE 17. Value of Apparent Equilibrium Constants of Reactions Using Acetyl CoA and CoA

Values are for I = 0.25, t = 38 and free $[Mg^{2+}]$ = 1 mM, except for acetyl carnitine transferase which was done at 30°C and low ionic strength and free $[Mg^{2+}]$. The activity of water was taken to be 1 by convention.

Mitochondrial Matrix – Citrate Synthase at pH 7.0

$$\frac{K_{C.S.}}{[H^+]} = \frac{[\Sigma citrate][\Sigma CoA]}{[\Sigma oxaloacetate][\Sigma acetyl\ CoA][H_2O]} = 2.24 \pm 0.11 \times 10^6 \qquad (20)$$

Cytoplasm – ATP citrate lyase

$$K_{CCE} = \frac{[\Sigma citrate][\Sigma CoA][\Sigma ATP]}{[\Sigma oxaloacetate][\Sigma acetyl\ CoA][\Sigma ADP][\Sigma Pi]} = 10.15\ M^{-1} \qquad (32)$$

Mitochondrial Inner Membrane – Carnitine Acetyl Transferase

$$K_{CAT} = \frac{[\Sigma acetyl\ carnitine][\Sigma CoA]}{[\Sigma carnitine][\Sigma acetyl\ CoA]} = 1.7 \qquad (82)$$

Mitochondrial Matrix and Cytoplasm

$$K_{AcCoAS} = \frac{[\Sigma acetate][\Sigma CoA][\Sigma ATP]}{[\Sigma acetyl\ CoA][\Sigma AMP][\Sigma PPi]} = 0.101 \qquad (83)$$

The agreement is quite good and on the face of it suggests
near-equilibrium in the carnitine acetyl transferase system
which seems surprising given the cellular location of the
enzyme and the segregation of the reactants. Like myokinase,
the transferase operates within the space between the inner
and outer mitochondrial membrane. The reactants of both
enzymes have restricted permiability through the inner mitochondrial membrane.

Clearly no definitive answer can be given to this problem
at this time except to say that the finding of equilibrium for
the carnitine acetyl transferase reaction is probably fortuitous. It points out the danger of using only one enzyme couple
to calculate free ratios of the type presented here.

V. DETERMINATION OF METABOLITE GRADIENTS BETWEEN CYTOPLASM AND MITOCHONDRIA

The measurement of metabolites was evolved as a method of
investigating the ratio of free pyridine nucleotides in various
tissue compartments which could not be determined directly
because of binding and unequal distribution of these nucleotides. The methods reported here, utilizing measurements of
total tissue contents of one or another substrate will obviously be erroneous if that substrate is extensively bound or compartmented. Our results suggest that ADP and probably AMP
are segregated within the mitochondrial matrix or bound to
unknown tissue constituents in muscle, brain, and liver.

In recent years three new methods have been developed
which attempt to estimate the content of metabolites in cytoplasm and mitochondria. One of these methods depends on
separation in non-aqueous media of mitochondria from freeze-
dried perfused liver (85). The other two utilize isolated
hepatocytes which have been disrupted either by digitonin (86)
or by turbulence (87) prior to separation. From a technical
point of view, such separations are extremely difficult, and
it seems worthwhile to view the results obtained in the light
of the information available about enzyme localization and
total metabolite contents.

The first and essential requirement is speed. Electron
microscopic studies suggest that mitochondria have dimensions
which are approximately 1 x 0.5 μm (88,89). It may be calculated (90) that the time it takes for a molecule of ATP to
diffuse from one end of the mitochondria to the other along
the long axis would be 0.03 seconds, assuming the matrix has
the viscosity of water. If the viscosity of the matrix is
ten times greater than water the diffusion time would be

0.3 seconds. Although the viscosity is not known, mitochondrial matrix is usually thought to contain about 1 μl of free
H_2O/mg total mitochondrial protein (Pfaff *et al*. Eur. J. Biochem.
5, 222-232, 1968). The time taken to either expose cells to
digitonin and then centrifuge them (86) or to transfer sheer-
disrupted cells from an inhibitor mixture and effect separation
(87) is of the order of 30 seconds. One has to be troubled
about what is diffusing into and out of damaged or non-respiring
mitochondria during this period of time.

In the methods employing freeze-clamped liver, the thickness is such that the central portion of tissue is only 1 mm
from either freezing surface (85), and it is known that the
tissue would be entirely frozen in 2.36 seconds (91). Although
this is long in comparison to the diffusion time, it is none
the less probably adequate since the cytoplasmic space and the
metabolism of the mitochondria are not disturbed until cooling.
On the other hand, drying for only 72 hours at $-70^{\circ}C$ is entirely inadequate to remove the tissue water since the vapor pressure of water is extremely low at this temperature and drying
speed is mainly a function of temperature. Storage of the
tissue subsequently at $-20^{\circ}C$ is undoubtedly when a large portion of the drying occurred. Examination of the electron
micrographs of the material used in this separation (85) show
large holes which I interpret to indicate movement of tissue
water and, presumably, small substrates. Since we have produced similar artifacts in our own laboratory, I am acutely
aware of the technical difficulties of drying tissue so as to
prevent substrate movement. A recent review of NMR data on
water in biological material suggests that a moderate amount
of H_2O remains unfrozen even at $-70^{\circ}C$ (92). These authors go
on to caution that this unfrozen water has quite high mobility
and permits considerable diffusion of water and other low
molecular weight compounds.

It is my opinion, therefore, that the methods which attempt
to separate mitochondria and, more particularly, mitochondrial
matrix from cytoplasm have not yet reached the state where the
conclusions about substrate distribution can be accepted with
confidence,but rather, these results must be viewed in the
context of other known data. Hopefully better and more rapid
methods will be devised.

As an illustration of these concerns, I will compare infer-
ences drawn from data from freeze-clamping with results obtained
by separation methods. In the first example, the inference from
the two types of methods agree; in the second they do not.

It is generally agreed that the measured ATP/ADP ratio in
mitochondria is lower than the ATP/ADP ratio of the cytoplasmic
fractions (85,86,87). This is also the implication of the data
presented in this paper. However, in the method using digitonin
and atractyloside (86) and in all but 1 of the samples (No. 41)
reported in the solvent fractionation method (85) the ratio of
[ATP][AMP]/[ADP]^2 is what one might expect in whole liver. The
values for AMP are not presented in the third method (87). In
view of the fact that adenylate kinase does not exist in mitochondrial matrix and AMP can not exit from matrix by the normal
translocation processes (93) the finding of the same K_{MYK} in
"mitochondria" as "cytosol" suggests that the particulate fraction called "mitochondria" has more cytosol than matrix space.
Thus, both because the value of K_{MYK} would indicate the bulk
of the adenine nucleotides measured are located outside the
inner membrane and also because of possible binding of mitochondrial ATP to carbamyl phosphate synthetase (60) and other
sites, the mitochondrial ATP/ADP ratios obtained by present
fractionation methods must, at best, be taken as indicating a
trend.

A second area of rough agreement between the three methods
of mitochondrial separation concerns the segregation of carboxylic acids within the mitochondria-rich fractions. The
gradients reported range from a high of 80 for citrate and 140
for isocitrate, through 5 to 20 for α-ketoglutarate using the
digitonin procedure (94); in the solvent-fractionated perfused
liver there was essentially no gradient for malate while a
citrate gradient of 3 to 8.6 was reported (95). In these
preparations, a major proportion of the cellular di- and tricarboxylic acids was found to be present in the particulate
fractions, giving a total mitochondrial concentration of these
acids of 80 - 100 mM (94).

An explanation for these observations has recently been
proposed (87) which says that citrate, isocitrate, α-ketoglutarate, malate, glutamate and puruvate are distributed in
conformity with a pH difference between mitochondrial matrix
and cytoplasm with the matrix being 0.41 units more alkaline
than cytoplasm (87). Such gradients in pH have been found
previously in isolated mitochondria (96,97) and the evidence
presented to date (87) suggests that mitochondria obtained by
the cell fractionation procedures discussed here have the same
pH gradients as mitochondria isolated by classical methods.

The evidence presented in this paper indicates that
gradients of this magnitude do not occur <u>in vivo</u>. If citrate
were 20-to 60-fold higher in mitochondria which comprise 10
to 20% of the total cellular volume, this would be expected

to lead to a disagreement of 4-to 8-fold in the free cytoplasmic $[NADP^+]/[NADPH]$ ratio calculated from reactants of isocitrate dehydrogeanse and 6-phosphogluconate dehydrogeanse. We do not find such discrepancies in vivo.

Secondly, if a pH gradient of 0.41 units existed between cytoplasm and mitochondria in vivo, one would expect a number of consequences in regard to the distribution of NH_4^+ and HCO_3^- since both these substrates have gaseous forms, NH_3 and CO_2, which diffuse rapidly through biological membranes. The liver cell pH in vivo, calculated by $[CO_2]/[HCO_3^-]$ ratios is 7.22 (43) and 7.23 by 5,5-dimethyl-2, 4-oxazolidinedione (44). We have recently redetermined the $[CO_2]/[HCO_3^-]$ ratio in liver and can confirm a pH of 7.2 with a liver $[HCO_3^-]$ of 22.8 ± 0.6 (n = 9) (42). The postulated pH gradient would require a mitochondrial matrix $[HCO_3^-]$ of about 60 mM since CO_2 would diffuse freely across mitochondrial membrane. Such concentration of HCO_3^- in mitochondria, have not been reported in mitochondria to date.

While the speed of the diffusion of NH_3 across cell membranes may not be sufficient to achieve equilibrium according to pH gradients in all cases (98), particularly where blood flow is rapid and the Na-K ATP'ase is also likely to be active in pumping NH_4^+ (99), it seems unlikely that NH_3 would be distributed unevenly between mitochondria and cytoplasm. There a steady state of NH_4^+ level of 0.5 mM exists and it would be expected that NH_3 would be equal inside and outside mitochondria. If a pH gradient of 0.41 occurred in vivo, it follows that NH_4^+ concentration would be 2.5 times less in mitochondrial matrix than in cytoplasm which should lead, at least theoretically, to a lower $[NAD_m^+]/[NADH_m]$ calculated from the

$$\frac{[NH_4^+][\alpha\text{-ketoglutarate}]}{[glutamate]}$$

than that calculated from the [acetoacetate]/[β-hydroxybutyrate] (7). While in practice this degree of error would be difficult to determine it is a point worth considering.

Finally, in vivo the ratio of measured citrate/measured isocitrate suggests that the free $[Mg^{2+}]$ is approximately 1 mM (31) regardless of where the citrate and isocitrate are located. From the stability constant of Mg-citrate ($10^{3.3}$) and a free $[Mg^{2+}]$ of 1 mM, one would expect that in vivo citrate exists 67% in the univalent $[Mg\text{-citrate}^{1-}]$ form rather than as the $[citrate^{3-}]$ form as required by the proposed theory (87). Thus, while a citrate distribution according to the pH gradient presented is very likely in isolated mitochondria, the evidence from freeze-clamped material presented here suggests that gradients of this type are unlikely to occur in vivo.

It has long been recognized that isolated mitochondria accumulate metabolites, particularly citrate (100) and that some accumulations do not require respiration (101) and can even occur at $0^{\circ}C$ (102). Endogenous citrate in mitochondria isolated in the usual fashion is about 3.8 mM (100,102). Assuming that matrix space is 10% of cell volume, this would indicate that all the citrate measured in freeze-clamped liver is within the mitochondria. If, instead, mitochondria occupy 17-20% of liver space, there would be more citrate in isolated mitochondria than is found by analysis of freeze-clamped liver.

Thus while in some respects, the data from freeze-clamped data agree with those obtained by the newer cell fractionation procedures, this is not true in all cases. There is an apparent agreement in regard to the distribution of some of the adenine nucleotides and an apparent disagreement in regard to the distribution of di- and tri- carboxylic acids. Clearly more rapid methods of cell fractionation would be desirable. However, as with the pyridine nucleotides, an equilibrium form of analysis will have to be applied in order to differentiate "bound" and "free" substrates.

REFERENCES

1. Bayliss, W.M., in "Principles of General Physiology", 1915. Preface to first edition.
2. Holtzer, H., Schultz, G., and Lynen, F., Biochem. Z. 328: 252 (1956).
3. Borst, P., in "Funktionelle und Morphologische Organisation der Zelle" (P. Karlson, ed.), p. 137. Springer Verlag, Berlin.
4. Hohorst, H.J., Kreutz, F.H., and Bücher, Th., Biochem. Z. 332:18 (1959).
5. Lehninger, A.L., in "The Mitochondrion", p. 32. W.A. Benjamin, New York.
6. Wollenberger, A., Ristau, O., and Schoffa, G., Pfluegers Arch. Gesamte Physiol. Menschen Tiere 270:399 (1960).
7. Williamson, D.H., Lund, P., and Krebs, H.A., Biochem. J. 103:514 (1967).
8. Brosnan, J.T., Krebs, H.A., and Williamson, D.H., Biochem. J. 117:91 (1970).
9. Hems, D.A., and Brosnan, J.T., Biochem. J. 120:105 (1970).
10. Miller, A.L., Hawkins, R.A., and Veech, R.L., J. Neurochemistry 20:1393 (1973).
11. Eggleston, L.V. (unpublished observations).
12. Rall, T.W., and Lehninger, A.W., J. Biol. Chem. 194:119 (1952).
13. Schneider, W.C., and Hogeboom, G.H., J. Nat'l Cancer Inst. 10:969 (1950).
14. Veech, R.L. Dissertation, Oxford, 1969.
15. Veech, R.L., Eggleston, L.V., and Krebs, H.A., Biochem. J. 115:609 (1969).
16. Kraupp, O., Adler-Kastner, L., Niessner, H., and Plank, B., Eur. J. Biochem. 2:197 (1967).
17. Goldberg, N.D., Passonneau, J.V., and Lowry, O.H., J. Biol. Chem. 241:3997 (1966).
18. Kauffman, F.C., Brown, J.G., Passonneau, J.V., and Lowry, O.H., J. Biol. Chem. 244:3647 (1969).
19. Veech, R.L., Neilsen, R., and Harris, R.L., in "Frontiers of Pineal Physiology" (M.D. Altschule, ed.), p. 177. MIT Press, Cambridge, 1975.
20. Guynn, R.W., Gelberg, H.J., and Veech, R.L., J. Biol. Chem. 248:6957 (1973).
21. Russman, W.. Dissertation, Munchen, 1967.
22. Londesbourgh, J., and Dalziel, K., Biochem. J. 110:217 (1968).
23. Villet, R., and Dalziel, K., Biochem. J. 115:633 (1969).
24. Engel, P.C., and Dalziel, K., Biochem. J. 105:691 (1967).

25. Krebs, H.A., and Veech, R.L., in "The Energy Level and
    Metabolic Control in Mitochondria" (S. Papa, J.M. Tager,
    E. Quagliariello, and E.C. Slater, eds.), p. 329.
    Adriatica Editrice, Bari, 1969.
26. Miller, A.L., Hawkins, R.A., and Veech, R.L., J. Neuro-
    chem. 25:553 (1975).
27. Robinson, B.H., Oei, J., Cheema-Dhadli, S., Halperin,
    M.L., J. Biol. Chem. 252:5661 (1977).
28. Brand, M.D., Reynafarje, B., and Lehninger, A., Proc.
    Nat'l Acad. Sci. U.S.A. 73:437 (1976).
29. Veech, R.L., Raijman, L., and Krebs, H.A., Biochem. J.
    117:499 (1970).
30. Rose, I.A., Proc. Nat'l Acad. Sci. U.S.A. 61:1079 (1968).
31. Veloso, D., Guynn, R.W., Oskarsson, M., and Veech, R.L.,
    J. Biol. Chem. 248:4811 (1973).
32. Guynn, R.W., and Veech, R.L., J. Biol. Chem. 248:6966
    (1973).
33. Burton, K., in "Energy Transformations in Living Matter"
    (H.A. Krebs and H.L. Kornberg, eds.), p. 275, 1957.
34. Collins, R.C., Posner, J.B., and Plum, F., Am. J.
    Physiol. 218:943 (1970).
35. Lowry, O.H., Passonneau, J.V., Hasselburger, F.X., and
    Schultz, D.W., J. Biol. Chem. 239:18 (1964).
36. Newsholme, E.A., and Start, C., in "Regulation of Metab-
    olism", p. 111. John Wiley, London, 1973.
37. Kielley, W.W., and Kielley, R.K., J. Biol. Chem. 191:485
    (1951).
38. Sottocasa, G.L., Kuylenstierna, B., Ernster, L., and
    Bergstrand, A., in "Methods in Enzymology" (R.W.
    Estabrook and M.E. Pullman, eds.), Vol. X, p. 448.
    Academic Press, New York, 1967.
39. Chappell, J.B., and Crofts, A.R., Biochem. J. 95:707
    (1965).
40. Cornell, N., Leadbetter, M., and Veech, R.L. (Submitted
    for publication, 1978.)
41. Lawson, J.W.R., and Veech, R.L. (Submitted for publica-
    tion, 1978.)
42. Veech, R.L., Lawson, J.W.R., and Krebs, H.A. (Submitted
    for publication, 1978.)
43. Krebs, H.A., Adv. Enz. Reg. 5:409 (1967).
44. Masoro, E.J., and Siegel, M.E., in "Acid-Base Regulation:
    Its Physiology and Pathophysiology", p. 35. W.B.
    Saunders, Philadelphia, 1971.
45. Minikami, S., and Yoshikawa, H., J. Biochem. (Toyko) 59:
    139 (1966).
46. Kobayashi, M., Lust, W.D., and Passonneau, J.V., J.
    Neurochem. 29:53 (1977).
47. Atkinson, D.E., Biochemistry 7:4030 (1968).

48. Newsholme, E.A., in "Essays in Cell Metabolism (W. Bartley, H.L. Kornberg, and J.R. Quayle, eds.), p. 189. Wiley-Interscience, London, 1970.

49. Brosnan, J.T., Krebs, H.A., and Williamson, D.H., Biochem. J. 117:91 (1970).

50. Noda, L., in "The Enzymes", 3rd Edition (P.B. Boyer, ed), Vol. 8, p. 279, 1973.

51. Criss, W.E., J. Biol. Chem. 245:6352 (1970).

52. Veech, R.L., Guynn, R., and Veloso, D., Biochem. J. 127: 387 (1972).

53. Aas, M., and Bremer, J., Biochim. Biophys. Acta 164:157 (1968).

54. Perry, S.V., Biochem. J. 57:495 (1952).

55. Hasselbach, W., and Schneider, G., Biochem. Z. 321:462 (1951).

56. Weihing, R.R., in "Cell Biology" (P.L. Altman and D.D. Katz, eds.), p. 341. FASEB, Bethesda, 1976.

57. Brandon, D.L., Eur. J. Biochem. 65:139 (1976).

58. Guidotti, G., Ann. Rev. Biochem. 41:731 (1972).

59. Srere, P.A., in "Energy Metabolism and the Regulation of Metabolic Processes in Mitochondria" (M.A. Mehlman and R.W. Hanson, eds.), p. 79. Academic Press, New York, 1972.

60. Raijman, L., in "The Urea Cycle" (S. Grisolia, R. Baguena, and F. Mayor, eds.), p. 243. John Wiley, New York, 1976.

61. Krebs, H.A., and Veech, R.L., in "Pyridine Nucleotide-Dependent Dehydrogenases (H. Sund, ed.), p. 413. Springer-Verlag, Berlin, 1970.

62. Klingenberg, M., Heldt, H.W., and Pfaff, E., in "The Energy Level and Metabolic Control in Mitochondria" (S. Papa, J.M. Tager, E. Quagliariello, and E.C. Slater, eds.), p. 237. Adriatica Editrice, Bari, 1969.

63. Kalant, N., and Beitner, R., J. Biol. Chem. 246:504 (1971).

64. Threlfall, C.J., and Heath, D.F., Biochem. J. 110:303 (1968).

65. Veech, R.L., Raijman, L., Dalziel, K., and Krebs, H.A., Biochem. J. 115:837 (1969).

66. Lawson, J.W.R., Guynn, R.W., Cornell, N., and Veech, R.L., in "Gluconeogenesis" (R.W. Hanson and M.A. Mehlman, eds.), p. 481, 1976.

67. Guynn, R.W., Veloso, D., Lawson, J.W.R., and Veech, R.L., Biochem. J. 140:369 (1974).

68. Bergmeyer, H.U., Holtz, G., Klotzch, H., and Lang, G., Biochem. Z. 338:114 (1963).

69. Stadtman, E.R., in "The Enzymes", 3rd Edition (P.D. Boyer, ed.), Vol. 8, p. 1, 1973.

70. Wood, H., O'Brian, W.E., and Michaels, G., in "Adv. in Enzymology" (A. Meister, ed.), Vol. 45, p. 85, 1977.
71. Reeves, R.E., South, D.J., Blytt, H.J., and Warren, L.G., J. Biol. Chem. 249:7737 (1974).
72. Cook, G.E. (Unpublished data, 1978.)
73. O'Brian, W.E., Bowien, S., and Wood, H.G., J. Biol. Chem. 250:8690 (1975).
74. Cook, G.A., and Veech, R.L. (Unpublished data, 1978.)
75. Felig, P., in "Diabetes: Its Physiological and Biochemical Basis" (J. Vallance-Owen, ed.), p. 93, 1975.
76. Fritz, I.B., Physiol. Rev. 41:52 (1961).
77. Veech, R.L., and Guynn, R.W., in "Regulation of Hepatic Metabolism" (F. Lundquist and N. Tygstrup, eds.), p. 337. Academic Press, New York, 1974.
78. Srere, P.A., and Lipmann, F., J. Am. Chem. Soc. 75:4874 (1953).
79. Neidle, A., van den Berg, C.J., and Grynbaum, A., J. Neurochem. 16:225 (1969).
80. Haddoch, B.A., Yates, D.W., and Garland, P.B., Biochem. J. 119:565 (1970).
81. Brosnan, J.T., and Fritz, I.B., Biochem. J. 125:94 (1971).
82. Fritz, I.B., Schultz, S.K., and Srere, P.A., J. Biol. Chem. 238:2509 (1963).
83. Guynn, R.W., Webster, L.T., and Veech, R.L., J. Biol. Chem. 249:3248 (1974).
84. Kondrup, J., and Grunnet, N., Biochem. J. 132:373 (1973).
85. Elbers, R., Heldt, H.W., Schmucker, P., Soboll, S., and Wiese, H., Hoppe-Seyler's Z. Physiol. Chem. 355:378 (1974).
86. Zuurendonk, P.F., and Tager, J.M., Biochim. Biophys. Acta 333:393 (1974).
87. Tischler, M.E., Hecht, P., and Williamson, J.R., Arch. Biochem. and Biophys. 181:278 (1977).
88. Loud, A.V., J. Cell Biol. 37:27 (1968).
89. Weibel, E.R., Stäubli, H.R., Gnägi, H.R., and Hess, F.A., J. Cell Biol. 42:68 (1969).
90. Cornell, N. (Unpublished observations, 1978.)
91. Veech, R.L., and Hawkins, R.A., in "Research Methods in Neurochemistry" (N. Marks and R. Rodnight, eds.), Vol. 2, p. 171. Plenum Press, New York, 1974.
92. Kuntz, I.D., and Zipp, A., N. Eng. J. Med. 297:262 (1977).
93. Heldt, H.W., and Schwalbach, K., Eur. J. Biochem. 1:199 (1967).
94. Zuurendouk, P.F., Akerboom, T.P.M., and Tager, J.M., in "Use of Isolated Liver Cells and Kidney Tubules in Metabolic Studies" (J.M. Tager, H.D. Söling, and J.R. Williamson, eds.), p. 17. North-Holland, Amsterdam, 1976.

95. Soboll, S., Scholz, R., Freisel, M., Elbers, R., and
     Heldt, H.W., in "Use of Isolated Liver Cells and Kidney
     Tubules in Metabolic Studies" (J.M. Tager, H.D. Söling,
     and J.R. Williamson, eds.), p. 29. North-Holland,
     Amsterdam, 1976.
96. Stucki, J.W., Hoppe-Seyler's Z. Physiol. Chem. 354:221
     (1973).
97. Williamson, J.R., in "Use of Isolated Liver Cells and
     Kidney Tubules in Metabolic Studies" (J.M. Tager, H.D.
     Söling, and J.R. Williamson, eds.), p. 79. North-Holland,
     Amsterdam, 1976.
98. Brosnan, J.T., in "The Urea Cycle" (S. Grisolia, R.
     Báquena, and F. Mayor, eds.), p. 443. John Wiley,
     New York, 1976.
99. Hawkins, R.A., Miller, A.L., Neilsen, R.C., and Veech,
     R.L., Biochem. J. 131:1001 (1973).
100. Schneider, W.C., Streibich, M.J., and Hogeboom, G.H.,
     J. Biol. Chem. 222:969 (1956).
101. Gamble, J.L., J. Biol. Chem. 240:2668 (1965).
102. Amoore, J.E., Biochem. J. 70:718 (1958).

DISCUSSION

F. LIPMANN: I would like to comment on Dr. Veech's talk. I
was very pleased to see that he mentioned pyrophosphate as a
frequent reaction product of ATP. But, I wonder why he
didn't say anything about pyrophosphatase which very often is
mentioned as being an ubiquitous enzyme. On the other hand,
you alluded to the Pi/PPi ratio which implies that you think
there is a transfer of phosphate from PPi to an acceptor. Is
that what you meant to say? Do you know anything about such
a possible reaction in animal tissues?

R. VEECH: We think the PPi measurements are accurate and the
changes in the concentration seen after insulin treatment are
real. The measured equilibrium constants for a glucose-PPi
transphosphorylase are as you saw them if you measure the
glucose, glucose-6-phosphate and Pi in liver. I didn't have
time to discuss the possibility of a fructokinase working
with PPi too. Our problem is that the thermodynamics of the
system forces us to postulate reactions in vivo for which
we have no equivalent enzymatic pathway in mammals. In
regard to your first comment, the paper by Bergmeyer et al.
(Biochem. Z., 338, 114, 1963) argues that the pyrophosphatase
is ubiquitous and very active in mammals. This is the paper

which is usually quoted. I think this is the danger of
taking in vitro enzyme measurements and applying them to the
in vivo situation, because we can confirm Bergmeyer's measured pyrophosphatase activity in vitro. I would, however,
suggest that this activity doesn't express itself in a cell.
I think your comments earlier that we didn't mention it in
regard to the adenyl cyclase system and the effect of PPi on
cyclic AMP should also be considered. I think you made those
comments earlier - a couple of years ago at least. Not
everyone ignores PPi.

F. LIPMANN: I just want to continue this line a little bit
more. There is the question of what becomes of the AMP
because a lot of it is formed in protein synthesis as well
as by the acetyl-CoA ATP reaction etc.

H. KREBS: I think I can answer the question of what happens
to AMP arising in the mitochondrial matrix. Klingenberg
(Essays in Biochemistry, $\underline{6}$, 119-159, 1970) has shown that
AMP cannot leave the matrix as such because there is no
transport mechanism. But the matrix possesses a specific
phosphotransferase which catalyses the reaction GTP + AMP
$\rightleftharpoons$ GDP + ADP. The required GTP is generated either by the
oxoglutarate dehydrogenase system or by nucleotide diphos-
phokinase.

C. deDUVE: I have a question for both Dr. Krebs and Dr.
Veech. In some of their equations the number of terms above
and below the fraction line is unequal. This introduces the
actual volume of the microcompartment involved as a significant variable. How is this taken into account? Could apparent departures from equilibrium reflect the lack of an
appropriate volume correction?

R. VEECH: The ratios that we calculated were based on whole
tissue measurements. It is therefore implied that if large
gradients of the measured metabolites occur, near equilibrium measurements of the type given will be meaningless.
The importance of the Williamson, Lund and Kreb's paper
(Biochem. J. $\underline{103}$, 514, 1967) is that measurements of NH_4^+,
α-ketoglutarate and glutamate in whole tissue apparently
gives the redox state of the mitochondrial free $[NAD^+]/[NADH]$
ratio. No correction for mitochondrial volume would be
needed unless concentration gradients were proven for these
intermediates. In the case of the myokinase equilibrium,
the number of reactants are equal and therefore volume considerations will not pertain.

J. LOWENSTEIN: I would like to make a few comments about
Dr. Veech's presentation. I get the impression from what
he says that there is no need to postulate special pools,
for example for adenine nucleotides, because a comparison of
mass action ratios with equilibrium constants seems to make
them unnecessary. Now, when one does metabolite measurements, for example of skeletal muscle, one gets concentrations of ATP, ADP, and AMP which appear to be in the equilibrium which one would expect from the myokinase reaction.
If one examines this more closely one finds that most of
the ADP measured is not in fact free at all; it is bound to
actin (1.5 μmol per gram dry weight, which can be converted
to about 0.6 mM if it is assumed that it is evenly distributed throughout the intracellular water). I don't know why
Dr. Veech said he is uncertain about this - it is a fact
accepted by everyone in the muscle field. In order to poly-
merize actin one needs 1 mol of ATP per monomer of actin.
The ADP that is formed is trapped in such a way that it
cannot be released without depolymerizing the actin. The
amount of actin in muscle is also about 0.6 mM. This is
the basis for saying that most of the ADP in muscle is
tightly bound and is not metabolically available. Now, once
you agree to this, you are in trouble because now the myokinase reaction is apparently no longer in equilibrium. If
it is assumed that it is in equilibrium, and also that the
creatine kinase reaction is in equilibrium, one can calculate
the content of free ADP and AMP. One then discovers that the
calculated amount of AMP is somewhere between 50 and 500 times
smaller than the measured amount. Thus simply to measure
metabolites such as AMP, ADP, and ATP, and to say "all is
well in the garden" because they appear to be in equilibrium,
does not prove that they actually are in equilibrium (Goodman
and Lowenstein, J. Biol. Chem. 252, 5054-5060, 1977). We
don't know yet where to put this AMP in skeletal muscle.
We have done other experiments in the perfused rat heart using
a totally different approach. The adenine nucleotide pool
was labeled in two different ways. When labeled adenosine is
used then ATP, ADP, and AMP quickly acquire the same specific
activities. When labeled AMP is used then ADP and ATP are
are found to have the same specific activity, but there is a
separate pool of AMP which has a much higher specific activity
than that of ADP and ATP. This difference persists. One is
led to the conclusion that there is a separate pool of AMP
(Frick and Lowenstein, J. Biol. Chem. 253, 1240-1244, 1978).
Again we don't know yet where to put this pool, but one can
calculate its size.

H. KREBS: Muscle presents a very special situation because
most other tissues contain extremely little actin.

J. LOWENSTEIN: Even brain contains actin.

H. KREBS: Some, but not of the same order of magnitude.

R. VEECH: I know the figure that you are quoting, 0.6 mM.
The question comes to the actin content in red blood cells.
According to a review by Guidotti (Ann. Rev. Biochem. 41, 731,
1972) there is actin in red blood cells - we don't have good
figures on how much actin there is in red cells and there is
no need to invoke this from the figures I have presented;
nor do I know how much actin there is quantitatively in liver
as opposed to muscle. In liver we have the same degree of
discrepancy that we have in muscle. Therefore, I felt that
to explain the results on the basis of the binding of ADP
to actin would not be possible for liver. I think for that
reason the mitochondrial matrix is also a candidate for an
AMP pool. I agree essentially with what you are saying.

INFLUENCE OF METABOLIC COMPARTMENTATION
ON THE QUANTITATIVE ANALYSIS
OF INTERMEDIARY METABOLISM

J. J. Blum[1]

Department of Physiology
Duke University
Durham, North Carolina

About 5 years ago we became interested in developing a
procedure for quantitating the flow of metabolites along some
of the major pathways of intermediary metabolism. For a
number of reasons, not least of which was the ease with which
they can be grown, we chose to work with the ciliate Tetrahymena pyriformis. In order to be able to obtain quantitative
information on metabolite flux patterns in vivo, one has to
either have available or to develop enough information to
construct a realistic diagram of the structure of intermediary
metabolism in that cell. This necessarily includes not only
the various enzymes that are present and - equally important -
absent, but also their location in the cell. At the time we
began this work it was already known that isocitrate lyase
and malate synthase, the key enzymes of the glyoxylate bypass,
were localized in the peroxisomes of Tetrahymena (1), and it
had been shown that there were at least two pools of acetyl
CoA in this cell (2). One of these, derived most directly
from acetate, was associated with lipid synthesis, whereas
the other, derived from pyruvate, was associated with CO_2
production and presumably mitochondrial. Connett and Blum (2)
then developed a model for the structure of intermediary
metabolism in Tetrahymena which assumed that one of the pools
of acetyl CoA was localized in the peroxisomes, a choice that
was dictated both by the requirement for acetyl CoA in the
formation of malate by malate synthase and by the finding (4)

---

[1]Supported by NIH grant 5 RO1 HD01269

Copyright © 1978 by Academic Press, Inc.
All right of reproduction in any form reserved.
ISBN 0-12-660550-5

that acetyl CoA synthetase was localized in the peroxisomes of this organism. The latter finding, coupled with the discovery that the peroxisomes of castor bean seedlings contained a complete system for the β-oxidation of fatty acids (5,6) led us to ascertain whether the peroxisomes of Tetrahymena also contained enzymes of the β-oxidation sequence. Data obtained from zonal centrifugation runs (7) of homogenates of Tetrahymena showed that several enzymes of the β-oxidation sequence were present as were short, medium, and long chain fatty acid activating enzymes (Table I). Similar studies showed that LDH[2], PFK, and hexokinase were localized on the mitochondria of Tetrahymena, suggesting that at least part of the glycolytic sequence in this cell was mitochondrial. Table II presents a summary of our present knowledge concerning the compartmentation of some key enzymes of intermediary metabolism in Tetrahymena.

STRUCTURAL ORGANIZATION OF INTERMEDIARY METABOLISM IN TETRAHYMENA

In our initial studies of intermediary metabolism in Tetrahymena we assumed that there were two pools of acetyl CoA (3). This yielded a reasonable fit to the relatively limited data we had at that time, but the two-pool model required that there be two pathways for lipid synthesis, with the mitochondrial pool contributing heavily to lipogenesis. Since several authors had suggested that there were two pools of acetyl CoA in mitochondria (17,18) we set up experiments to test for the possible presence of three pools of acetyl CoA (19). Cells were exposed to a mixture of octanoate, acetate, and pyruvate, but with only one substrate at a time labeled with ^{14}C in such a position that any acetyl CoA formed would be labeled in the carboxyl carbon. The results from experiments on cells at the end of the logarithmic phase of growth (referred to as transition phase) (Table III) show that the ratios of label incorporated from [1-^{14}C] acetate to that from [2-^{14}C]pyruvate[3] into CO_2, lipids, and

---

[2]Abbreviations used are: LDH, lactic dehydrogenase; PFK, phosphofructokinase; FDPase, fructose diphosphatase; PEP carboxykinase, P-enolpyruvate carboxykinase; PEP carboxylase, P-enolpyruvate carboxylase.

[3]Pyruvate enters the pathways of intermediary metabolism only via pyruvate dehydrogenase (2). [2-^{14}C]pyruvate therefore becomes [1-^{14}C]acetyl CoA.

TABLE I. Localization of Some Enzymes of Fatty Acid
Catabolism in Tetrahymena

Enzyme	Activity in peroxisomal fraction / Activity in mitochondrial fraction
Glutamic dehydrogenase	0.082
Lactic dehydrogenase	0.088
Isocitrate lyase	20.0
Catalase	65.0
Acetyl CoA synthetase	2.2
Octanoyl CoA synthetase	1.3
Palmitoyl CoA synthetase	2.2
3-β-hydroxyacylCoA dehydrogenase	5.0
Thiolase	1.8

Tetrahymena were grown to transition phase and homogenized
in a Potter-Elvejhem grinder in a buffer consisting of 0.25 M
sucrose, 0.05 M $MgCl_2$, 0.5 mM dithiothreitol, and 0.01 M
glycyglycine, pH 8.0. Zonal centrifugation was performed in
a Type TiXIV rotor for ∿ 15 min at 5000 rpm using a 10-50%
sucrose gradient in the above buffer. The numbers presented
in the table are the ratios of activities in the fraction
containing the highest activities of the peroxisomal marker
enzymes (catalase and isocitrate lyase) to the activities in
the fraction containing the highest activities of the mitochondrial marker enzymes (glutamic dehydrogenase and lactic
dehydrogenase). For further details, see (7).

glycogen were 7.3, 68, and 3.0, respectively. These ratios
clearly differ from one another, proving that there are 3
pools of acetyl CoA. The ratios of label incorporated from
[1-^{14}C]acetate to those from [1-^{14}C]octanoate were 86, 4.7,
and 40 into CO_2, lipids, and glycogen, respectively. The
value of 4.7 into lipids, however, is too low, since a large
part of the octanoate appeared in lipid by a direct pathway
(see Fig. 1). When correction is made for the amount of
label from octanoate that entered via β-oxidation, the value
of 4.7 increases to about 14, but the conclusion remains the
same. Thus both the acetate/pyruvate ratios and the acetate/
octanoate ratios require at least 3 pools of acetyl CoA in
these cells. It should also be noted that the data for label
appearing in glutamate (which is released in small amounts
into the medium by these cells) suggested that glutamate was
being labeled from the same pool of acetyl CoA that yielded
CO_2.

TABLE II.   Compartmentation of Some Enzymes of
Intermediary Metabolism in Tetrahymena

Enzyme	Location	Reference
Present		
PEP carboxykinase	M	8,9
PEP carboxylase	M	8
	M and C	9
Lactic dehydrogenase	M	10,11,12
Glutamic dehydrogenase	M	12
Glyceraldehyde-3-P-dehydrogenase	M?	13
Alanine transaminase	M	12
Aspartic transaminase	M(and P?)	1,12
Hexokinase	M	11
Phosphofructokinase	M	14
Transaldolase	C	15
Transketolase	C	15
Acetyl, octanoyl, and palmitoyl CoA synthetases	M and P	7
β-oxidation sequence	M and P	7
Absent		
Malic enzyme		16
Pyruvate carboxylase		16
Citrate cleavage enzyme		16
Glucose-6-phosphate dehydrogenase		15
6-Phosphogluconate dehydrogenase		15

Given that there are three (or more) pools of acetyl CoA
in this cell, a second problem to be resolved is how are
these pools connected and what reactions contribute to each,
i.e. the structural organization of intermediary metabolism.
To approach this, we set up steady state rate equations which
would describe the flow of label from any of the labeled substrates used into all of the products measured, and programmed
the resulting equations for convenient interactive work with
the computer.   Figure 1 shows the general structure of
intermediary metabolism which was required to obtain the fits
shown in Table IV to data obtained on transition phase cells
incubated in a mixture of acetate, pyruvate, and octanoate
with only one substrate labeled in any given flask.   The
first point to notice in Table IV is that it is possible to
pick up a set of fluxes, which give a virtually perfect fit

TABLE III. Appearance of Label in CO_2, Lipids,
Glycogen, and Glutamate from Cells
Incubated in a Mixture of Acetate,
Pyruvate and Octanoate

| Labeled Substrate | Amount of Label Appearing in | | | |
| | CO_2 | Lipids | Glycogen | Glutamate |
	nmoles/10^6 cells·hr			
[1-^{14}C]acetate	496±25	142±9	16.1±3.2	7.6±2.0
[2-^{14}C]pyruvate	67.8±4.0	2.1±0.5	5.3±1.5	<1.0
[1-^{14}C]octanoate	5.8±1.8	30.4±3.0	0.40±0.13	<0.1
Ratios:				
$\frac{[1-^{14}C]acetate}{[1-^{14}C]pyruvate}$	7.3	68	3.0	<7.6
$\frac{[1-^{14}C]acetate}{[1-^{14}C]octanoate}$	86	4.7	40	<76

Cells were grown to transition phase and incubated for 1 hour with a mixture of 6.2 mM sodium acetate, 6.2 mM sodium pyruvate, and 1.5 mM octanoate, with one of these substrates labeled with ^{14}C, i.e. [1-^{14}C]acetate or [2-^{14}C]pyruvate or [1-^{14}C]octanoate. At the end of the hour incubation at 25° flasks were analyzed for label incorporated into the products shown. Values are means ± standard deviation for 8 experiments. For further details, see (19).

to the data. This comes about in part because there are only 12 measurements with which to specify 12 independent parameters. The lack of excess measurements is not, however, the sole reason for the ability to achieve such a fit, for it was shown that any other arrangement of the three-pool structure would not yield an acceptable fit to the data (19). This emphasizes the importance of understanding the organization of fluxes into and out of compartments if one is to undertake large scale network analysis of intermediary metabolism. We shall see below how this structural scheme was expanded to form a more realistic model of intermediary metabolism, but we first consider some of the metabolic implications of the flux pattern shown in Fig. 1.

TABLE IV. Comparison of Experimental with Calculated
Values of Label Incorporation into Products

Labeled Substrate	CO_2	Amount of Label Appearing LIPIDS	GLYCOGEN	GLUTAMATE
		nmoles/10^6 cells·hr		
[1-^{14}C]Acetate				
Observed	501	130	13.7	8.4
Calculated	501	130	13.7	8.3
[2-^{14}C]Pyruvate				
Observed	69.8	2.0	4.8	<1
Calculated	69.6	2.0	4.8	1.2
[1-^{14}C]Octanoate				
Observed	4.1	28.6	0.26	0.15
Calculated	4.1	28.7	0.26	0.07

Cells were grown and incubated with a mixture of acetate,
pyruvate, and octanoate as described in the legend to Table
III. The calculated results tabulated here for a single
experiment were obtained with flux values close to the
average values shown in Fig. 1.

Under the conditions of these experiments almost equal
amounts of octanoate were β-oxidized in the mitochondrial and
peroxisomal compartments. In order to fit the data, however,
it was required that over twice as much octanoate as was β-
oxidized be utilized via a hypothetical direct pathway for
lipid synthesis. When pentanoate was used instead of
octanoate, about 108 nmoles/10^6 cells·hr were β-oxidized
(about 12% of this occurring in the peroxisomes as compared
to 42% for octanoate) and 25 nmoles/10^6 cells·hr appeared in
lipid by the presumed direct pathway. The subsequent
demonstration of a direct pathway for fatty acid chain
elongation in Tetrahymena (20) strengthened our confidence in
the validity of the structural scheme shown in Fig. 1. It has
recently been reported (21) that acyl CoA-dihydroxyacetone-
phosphate:acyl transferase (and possibly several other enzymes
involved in glycerolipid synthesis) is present in liver
peroxisomes. If this enzyme were present in Tetrahymena
peroxisomes, it could provide for peroxisomal utilization of
the elongated fatty acid.
It should also be noted that about 75% of the total flux
of acetyl groups being utilized for glyconeogenesis is

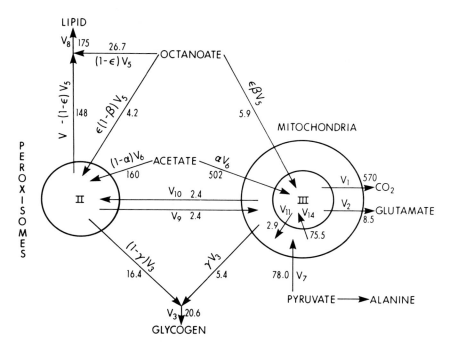

FIGURE 1. Structural organization of intermediary metabolism in Tetrahymena according to an abbreviated model with three pools of acetyl CoA. Cells were grown to transition phase and incubated with a mixture of acetate, pyruvate, and octanoate as described in the legend to Table III. The flux values shown (in units of nmoles/10^6 cells·hr) were obtained by fitting the average values for 8 experiments, one of which is presented in detail in Table IV. For further details, see (19).

represented as coming from the peroxisomal compartment in Fig. 1, even though only 10% of the acetate entering into the peroxisomes was used for glyconeogenesis. Thus although the peroxisomes were clearly important for glyconeogenesis, as expected from the presence of the glyoxylate bypass enzymes, these experiments were the first to reveal the quantitatively important role that the peroxisomes played in both β-oxidation and lipogenesis in Tetrahymena.

Further confidence in the structural organization shown in Fig. 1 came from the ability to achieve excellent fits in studies with cells grown in the presence of tolbutamide (22), AMP (23), with 4-pentenoic acid (24), and under partial anaerobiosis (25), treatments that both increased and

decreased the flux values computed in the glyconeogenic and
other pathways. We then proceeded to the development of a
more realistic model that would retain the structural organization shown in Fig. 1 but account for most of the metabolic
details which were absent from Fig. 1.

DEVELOPMENT OF A REALISTIC MODEL
OF INTERMEDIARY METABOLISM

Figure 2 is essentially an expanded version of the
structural organization of intermediary metabolism in Tetrahymena deduced from the experiments described in Table III
and Fig. 1.   In expanding the purely formal diagram of Fig.
1 to the more realistic scheme of Fig. 2, most of the
available information of the enzymology of intermediary
metabolicm in this cell was used (cf. Table I).   Thus malic
enzyme (NADP; decarboxylating), pyruvate carboxylase, and
citrate lyase are not present, and alanine transaminase is
entirely in the mitochondria. A direct pathway for fatty
acid elongation (V_{29}) is included, and the glycerol required
for lipid synthesis is shown as derived from a single pool of
P-enolpyruvate.   Since P-enolpyruvate carboxykinase (and,
probably, P-enolpyruvate carboxylase) is present in both the
mitochondria and cytosol, it is likely that there are two
pools of P-enolpyruvate.   Since we were able to obtain an
acceptable fit to the data (26; see below), it was unnecessary
to include more than one pool of this metabolite. If there
are, indeed, two pools of P-enolpyruvate present, then our
ability to fit the data by using just one pool may result
from the highly oversimplified representation of the glycolytic and pentose phosphate pathways used in the scheme in
Fig. 2.   The three pools of acetyl CoA are shown as being
localized in the peroxisomes and in the inner and outer
mitochondrial compartments. Either the peroxisomal or the
outer mitochondrial pool, but not both, may be identical
with the cytosolic pool of acetyl CoA or a separate cytosolic
pool of acetyl CoA may exist and may have to be taken into
account in future studies. It is, however, required that
the initial step of pyruvate metabolism occur in a separate
compartment from the initial step of mitochondrial acetate
metabolism (2).

The scheme shown in Fig. 2 has 33 flux parameters of
which 10 are determined by conservation equations. If the
ability to achieve a satisfactory fit to experimental data
is to constitute a stringest test of the model the number of
measurements made must be in considerable excess of the
number of independent parameters (23 in this case).   Data

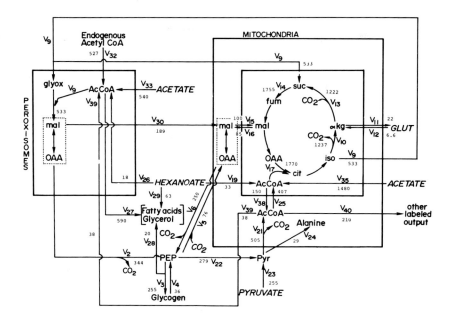

FIGURE 2. Carbon flow scheme for intermediary metabolism in <u>Tetrahymena</u>. V_i refers to the flux of reactant through the indicated pathway. The associated smaller numbers are the steady state <u>in vivo</u> flux rates (in nmol/10^6 cells·hr) for cells incubated in a salt solution containing 3.1 mM acetate, 1.6 mM pyruvate, 0.31 mM glutamate, 0.62 mM hexanoate, and 0.31 mM bicarbonate. Reactions enclosed by dotted lines are assumed to be in equilibrium. Abbreviations used are: AcCoA, acetyl coenzyme A; cit, citrate; iso, iso-citrate; αkg, α-ketoglutarate; GLUT, glutamate; suc, succinate; fum, fumarate; mal, malate, OAA, oxaloacetate; glyox, glyoxylate; PEP, phosphoenolpyruvate; Pyr, pyruvate. For further details, see (26).

were obtained by incubating cells grown under carefully con-trolled conditions with a mixture of acetate, pyruvate, bicarbonate, hexanoate, and glutamate, with only one substrate in any given flask labeled with ^{14}C in a known position. Twenty-seven measurements were made of label incorporation into various metabolites - CO_2, glycogen, lipids, and glutamate were chosen for this study (26). These, plus 4 measurements of label distribution into fatty acid and

glycerol moieties of lipids and one measurement each of
glycogen breakdown and of Q_{O2} yielded a total of 33 independent measurements. In addition, there were many measurements
which yielded values too small for reliable quantitation.
The exact contribution of these "limit" measurements to
determining the fit to the model cannot be quantitated, but
they obviously place significant constraints on the fit since
if the computed values for any of these measurements were
large enough so that they should have been measurable, the
fit or the model would have to be revised.

DERIVATION OF STEADY STATE EQUATIONS

In the isotopic steady state the following equation holds:

$$\sum_i V_{ik} \, S_i(m) = S_k(n) \sum_o V_{ok},$$

where $S_i(m)$ is the specific activity of the carbon m of the
ith metabolite and V_{ik} and V_{ok} are the input and output
fluxes, respectively, to the kth metabolite. This equation
simply says that in the steady state the rate of label flow
into a particular carbon atom from all reactions leading to
that atom equals the rate of label outflow from this carbon
atom to all products derived from it. By repeated algebraic
manipulations of these equations (one equation for each
carbon atom of each metabolite), it is possible to express
the specific activity of every carbon atom in the kinetic
scheme in terms of the independent flux parameters and the
known specific activities of the exogenous substrates.
Expressions can then be written for the rate of appearance
of label into any product that one wishes to measure as well
as for the rate of oxygen consumption. These equations are
then programmed on a digital computer in such a form as to
provide for convenient interactive trial and error fitting.
The investigator chooses a trial set of independent flux
parameters and the computer then prints out the expected
values of label incorporation into each of the products
measured and the expected value of the Q_{O2}. The investigator
then compares these with the experimental values and chooses
a new set of flux values, until a satisfactory agreement is
reached. Questions of uniqueness of fit and goodness of fit
are discussed elsewhere (26).
The flux pattern shown in Fig. 2 yielded a good fit to
the data, and thus must be considered as a quantitative
representation of carbon flow in this cell for the particular
set of growth and incubation conditions chosen. Several
points of interest emerge from this flow chart. Net malate

transport for example, is from peroxisomes to mitochondria. This is required to maintain continued operation of the Krebs cycle in the face of the glyconeogenic drain by the glyoxylate bypass. About one-third of the citrate formed in the Krebs cycle (V_{17}) enters the glyoxylate bypass in the peroxisomal compartment (V_9) and two-thirds of the malate formed in the peroxisomes is decarboxylated to P-enolpyruvate where much of it enters the glyconeogenic pathway. A considerable flux of P-enolpyruvate through the pyruvate kinase reaction (V_{22}) was necessary to fit the data. Since pyruvate was present in the substrate mix, a non-zero value for V_{22} implies a "futile" cycle at this metabolic crossroads. Recent theoretical studies of futile cycling at the P-enolpyruvate-pyruvate-oxaloacetate junction (similar to but not identical with the cycle present in Tetrahymena) suggest that the futile cycle at this junction may function as a complex switching system that directs metabolic flux towards gluconeogenesis of glycolysis in response to the inputs of these three metabolites as well as to the combined action of allosteric modulators of the individual enzymes of this substrate cycle[4]. Factors affecting the rate of substrate cycling at this metabolic crossroads in Tetrahymena have not yet been investigated.

An appreciable exchange of acetyl CoA between the inner and outer mitochondrial compartments is implied by V_{25} and V_{38}. The functional significance of this apparently futile exchange is unknown.

It was mentioned above that studies with the abbreviated three-compartment model (Fig. 1) required the inclusion of a direct pathway for lipid synthesis from pentanoate and octanoate. Figure 2 shows that hexanoate is also subject to chain elongation (V_{29}) and that more hexanoate flows along this pathway than is β-oxidized. It is also seen that about twice as much hexanoate is β-oxidized in the mitochondria than in the peroxisomes (cf. V_{19} and V_{26}). Studies with the abbreviated 3-pool model showed that about 7 times as much pentanoate was β-oxidized in the mitochondria as in the peroxisomes (24), while octanoate was β-oxidized at almost equal rates in the two β-oxidation compartments (19). It appears, therefore, that in Tetrahymena short chain fatty acids are β-oxidized preferentially in the mitochondria, and that the locale shifts towards the peroxisomes with increasing chain length. This could account for the puzzling finding

---

[4]Stein, R.B., and Blum, J.J. On the analysis of futile cycles in metabolism. Submitted for publication.

that endogeneously produced acetyl CoA (V_{32}) appeared to be
utilized entirely in the peroxisomal compartment (Fig. 2).
The absence of carnitine in Tetrahymena (27) may also require
that long chain fatty acids be β-oxidized only in the
peroxisomal compartment.

       During the course of finding the flux pattern that would
best fit the data it was found that V_5, V_6, V_2 and V_{30}
constitute a linked set of parameters. Measurement of [^{14}C]
bicarbonate fixation into glycogen specified the relation
between V_5 and V_6 but did not uniquely define either. The
values of V_5 and V_6 actually used had, therefore, to be
determined by a criterion outside the ^{14}C-incorporation
data. (The criterion used was to adjust the ratio of V_2:V_6
to match the relative activities of the cytosolic and particulate forms of P-enolpyruvate carboxykinase in cells grown
under identical conditions.) This shows that a considerable
excess of data to undetermined parameters does not necessarily
enable one to determine all the parameters in a complex
metabolic network. Indeed, we were unable to suggest any
experimental measurements (using the original substrates)
which would resolve the ambiguity. Since then we have
discovered (28) that there are at least 2 pools of CO_2 in
Tetrahymena, as demonstrated in Table V. Since the first
steps in the metabolism of [1-^{14}C]pyruvate and of [1-^{14}C]
leucine in Tetrahymena are to produce $^{14}CO_2$, the finding of
different ratios of incorporation of label into lipids and
into CO_2 requires that there be at least two pools of CO_2 in
this cell. The data further indicate that CO_2 arising from
leucine decarboxylation is preferentially used for lipid
synthesis (via fixation onto β-methylcrotonyl CoA and subsequent formation of acetyl CoA) as compared to CO_2 arising
from pyruvate decarboxylation. This information does not
seem to provide any better way to determine V_5 and V_6
unambigously, but it is clear that the scheme used in Fig. 2
should be modified to include the compartmentation of CO_2,
though this may not be feasible until further information is
obtained about the structural organization of the CO_2 pools.

                  MODELS FOR THE GLYCOLYTIC AND PENTOSE
                          PHOSPHATE PATHWAYS

       It was pointed out above that in the scheme used in Fig.
2 all the reactions of the glycolytic and pentose phosphate
pathways were symbolized by a single pair of fluxes, V_3 and
V_4. A more realistic scheme for this portion of intermediary
metabolism is shown in Fig. 3 (29). It will be noted that
these reactions are all depicted as occurring in a single

TABLE V. Compartmentation of CO_2 in Tetrahymena

Labeled Substrate	Lipid nmol incorporated/10^6 cells·hr	CO_2
[1-^{14}C]Pyruvate	7.44±1.54	1018±65
[1-^{14}C]Leucine	5.45±1.13	169±9
$\dfrac{[1\text{-}^{14}C]\text{Pyruvate}}{[1\text{-}^{14}C]\text{Leucine}}$	1.4(1.0-1.7)	6.0(5.6-6.4)

Cells were grown for 17 hours at 26° with shaking, from an initial cell density of ∿ 1.5·10^5 cells/ml and incubated with a mixture of 3 mM pyruvate and 3 mM leucine with either [1-^{14}C]pyruvate or [1-^{14}C]leucine. Incorporation of label into CO_2 and into lipid was measured in 3 experiments, and results are expressed as the mean ± S.E. The numbers in parentheses represent the range of ratios obtained in three paired experiments. For further details, see (28).

compartment, despite the evidence (Table I) that PFK, LDH, hexokinase, and a portion of glyceraldehyde-3-phosphate dehydrogenase are localized on the mitochondria. A comprehensive discussion of the compartmentation of the glycolytic and pentose phosphate pathways in other species has recently been published (30) and will not be summarized here. We wish only to emphasize that if the various glycolytic enzymes found on the mitochondria were bound on the outer surface of the outer mitochondrial membrane, the entire glycolytic and pentose phosphate pathways could effectively occur in a single (cytosolic) compartment regardless of whether the enzymes were associated in a loose glycolytic complex and/or attached to mitochondria. In the absence of any compelling evidence that there were two pools of glycolytic intermediates in Tetrahymena, we chose to attempt to fit the data collected for analysis of this portion of intermediary metabolism with the one-compartment model shown in Fig. 3. That we were able to achieve a good fit to the data does not, of course, rule out the possibility that the system has mutiple pools of some intermediates. The scheme shown in Fig. 3 has 18 independent flux rate parameters. Cells were incubated with a mixture of glucose, fructose, ribose, and glycerol, with only one substrate labeled in a specified position, and a total of 29 measurements of label incorporation into selected products were made at each time point. While this provides a comfortable excess of measurements over parameters

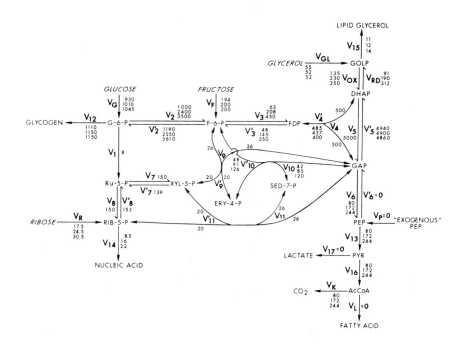

FIGURE 3. Metabolic scheme for glycolysis and the pentose phosphate pathway in Tetrahymena. Cells were incubated in a mixture of glucose (6 mM), fructose (6 mM), ribose (3 mM), and glycerol (3 mM), with only one substrate labeled in a specified position. The small numbers represent the values for the indicated fluxes, in units of nmol/10^6 cells·hr, which gave the best fit to experimental data on incorporation of label into CO_2, glycogen, RNA, and lipids. For reactions with a constant flux throughout the hour of incubation, a single number is given. For those reactions which have changing rates, these are listed vertically. The top, middle, and bottom are those in the 0 to 20-min, 20 to 40-min, and 40 to 60-min intervals, respectively. Abbreviations used are: FDP, fructose 1,6-diphosphate; DHAP, dihydroxyacetone-P; GAP, glyceraldehyde-3-P; PYR, pyruvate; PEP, phosphoenolpyruvate; RU-5-P, ribulose-5-P; XYL-5-P; xylulose-5-P; RIB-5-P, ribose-5-P; ERY-4-P, erythrose-4-P; SED-7-P, sedoheptulose-7-P; GOLP, Sn-glycerol-3-P; AcCoA, acetyl coenzyme A; G-6-P, glucose-6-phosphate; F-6-P, fructose-6-phosphate. For further details, see (29).

to be determined, it is of course possible that had more
measurements been made the fit would have become unacceptable
and either the reactions assumed to be occurring could have
to be modified or experiments would have had to be devised to
clarify the pool structure. Since a good fit to the data
was obtained at each of the three times (29), one is
justified for the present in continuing to treat this portion
of intermediary metabolism in Tetrahymena as occurring in a
single compartment.

The flux values presented in Fig. 3 show that metabolism
changes with time following the addition of a mixture of
glucose, fructose, ribose, and glycerol to cells that had
been growing in a proteose-peptone medium. By arguments that
will not be repeated here it was shown that this adaptation
to the addition of carbohydrates to the growth medium occurred
slowly enough so that the system could be considered as being
in a quasi-steady state for each of the 3 time intervals
during the 1-hour incubation. Several points of metabolic
interest become evident on studying the flux rates in Fig. 3.
Glycogen synthesis (V_{12}), for example, started almost
immediately (i.e. within the first 20-min interval) at its
maximal rate. If glycogen synthetase had been present in a
"dependent" form, it must have been converted to the active
form within a very few minutes. Fructose utilization (V_F),
which appears to occur via hexokinase in Tetrahymena (11),
occurred at about one-fifth the rate of glucose utilization
(V_G) throughout the hour incubation, while glycerol utilization (V_{GL}) was one-quarter of that of fructose. Ribose
utilization (V_R), while very small, almost doubled between
the first 20-min interval and the third 20-min interval,
most of it, apparently, being used for RNA synthesis (V_{14}).

It will also be noted that flux through glucose-6-P
dehydrogenase is almost nil. This accords well with the
apparent absence of this enzyme from Tetrahymena (Table I).
Although the NADPH-generating function of the pentose
phosphate pathway is absent (and is probably performed by
NADP-linked isocitrate dehydrogenase) the non-oxidative
steps of this pathway [catalyzed by transaldolase (V_{10}, V_{10}')
and transketolase (V_9, V_9', V_{11}, V_{11}') are clearly operating.
The net flux through these steps is very small, but exchange
through transaldolase increased over 2-fold during the hour
incubation, and contributes an appreciable amount of label
to the pool of glyceraldehyde-3-phosphate. Although this
marks the first analysis of flux through the non-oxidative
steps of the pentose phosphate pathway, the metabolic
significance of this pathway in Tetrahymena will not be fully
apparent until experiments are done with cells grown under
different conditions and incubated with different substrate
mixtures.

Of particular interest is the flux pattern through phosphofructokinase (V_3 in Fig. 3) and fructose diphosphatase
(V_3' in Fig. 3). Flux through PFK increases over 7-fold
during the course of the hour incubation, consistent with
the widely held view that PFK is one of the main regulatory
steps of the glycolytic pathway. The increase in flux
through FDPase, however, was also over 7-fold, so that
although net flux increased almost 7-fold, a futile cycle of
considerable magnitude was present throughout the incubation.
This is consistent with computer simulation studies[4] which
suggest that the F-6-P/F1,6diP cycle acts to gate bidirec-
tional flux but does not appreciably enhance the regulation
of unidirectional flux. It can be shown (29) that even in
the 40 to 60-min interval, when flux through PFK and FDPase
was large, ATP consumption was increased by less than 10% of
the amount that would have been consumed by the reactions
shown in Fig. 3 if there had been no futile cycling. It
seems likely that this futile cycle has no function in
Tetrahymena, i.e. that it was not "worthwhile" to develop
highly effective controls on these two enzymes. Perhaps in
nature Tetrahymena rarely finds itself in an environment
rich in carbohydrates, and a costly control mechanism never
evolved. Other points of metabolic significance, such as
the magnitude of the exchange rates at hexosephosphate
isomerase (V_2, V_2'), triosephosphate isomerase (V_5, V_5'), and
glycerol phosphate dehydrogenase (V_{OX}, V_{RD}) are discussed in
the original paper (29).

In Fig. 2, the glycolytic and pentose phosphate pathways
were symbolized by V_3 and V_4. In Fig. 3, the reactions of
the Krebs cycle, and the glyoxylate bypass, etc., are
symbolized by V_K, with $V_L=0$. The question arises as to
whether, when a single kinetic scheme is formulated embodying
all the reactions shown in Figs. 2 and 3, it will be possible
to obtain fits to a large body of data without being forced
to modify the structural arrangement (3 pools of acetyl CoA
in Fig. 2, 1 pool of intermediates in Fig. 3) of metabolism
used so far. If so, this would argue that the ability to
achieve a fit to the limited data in each of the previous
studies was not dependent on the presence, in each case, of
a portion of the system that was represented in essentially
symbolic form, and this would support the view that the
schemes used are adequate representations of the metabolic
configurations of this cell. Such experiments are currently
in progress.

REFERENCES

1. Muller, M., Hogg, J.F., and DeDuve, C., J. Biol. Chem. 243:5385 (1968).
2. Connett, R.J., Wittels, B., and Blum, J.J., J. Biol. Chem. 247:2657 (1972).
3. Connett, R.J., and Blum, J.J., J. Biol. Chem. 247:5199 (1972).
4. Levy, M.R., Biochem. Biophys. Res. Commun. 39:1 (1970).
5. Cooper, T.G., and Beevers, H., J. Biol. Chem. 244:3514 (1969).
6. Hutton, D., and Stumpf, P.K., Plant Physiol. 44:508 (1969).
7. Blum, J.J., J. Protozool. 20:688 (1973).
8. Diesterhaft, M., Hsieh, H.-C., Elson, C., Sallach, H.J., and Shrago, E., J. Biol. Chem. 247:2755 (1972).
9. Liang, T., Raugi, G.J., and Blum, J.J., J. Protozool. 23:473 (1976).
10. Eichel, H.J., Goldenberg, E.K., and Rem, L.T., Biochim. Biophys. Acta 81:172 (1964).
11. Risse, H.J., and Blum, J.J., Arch. Biochem. Biophys. 149:329 (1972).
12. Porter, P., Blum, J.J., and Elrod, H., J. Protozool. 19:375 (1972).
13. Conger, N.E., Fields, R.D., and Feldman, C.J., Fed. Proc. 30:1158 (1971).
14. Eldan, M., and Blum, J.J., J. Biol. Chem. 248:7445 (1973).
15. Eldan, M., and Blum, J.J., J. Protozool. 22:145 (1975).
16. Shrago, E., Brech, W., and Templeton, K., J. Biol. Chem. 242:4060 (1967).
17. Fritz, I.B., Perspect. Biol. Med. 10:643 (1967).
18. Chase, J.F.A., and Tubbs, P.K., Biochem. J. 129:55 (1972).
19. Raugi, G.J., Liang, T., and Blum, J.J., J. Biol. Chem. 248:8064 (1973).
20. Conner, R.L., Koo, K.-E., and Landrey, J.R., Lipids 9:554 (1972).
21. Jones, C.L., and Hajra, A.K., Biochem. Biophys. Res. Commun. 76:1138 (1977).
22. Liang, T., Raugi, G.J., and Blum, J.J., J. Biol. Chem. 248:8073 (1973).
23. Raugi, G.J., Liang, T., and Blum, J.J., J. Biol. Chem. 248:8079 (1973).
24. Raugi, G.J., Liang, T., and Blum, J.J., J. Biol. Chem. 250:4067 (1975).
25. Raugi, G.J., Liang, T., and Blum, J.J., J. Biol. Chem. 250:445 (1975).

26. Raugi, G.J., Liang, T., and Blum, J.J., J. Biol. Chem. 250:5866 (1975).
27. Wittels, B., and Blum, J.J., Biochim. Biophys. Acta 152:220 (1968).
28. Borowitz, M., Raugi, G.J., Liang, T., and Blum, J.J., J. Biol. Chem. 252:3402 (1977).
29. Borowitz, M.J., Stein, R.B., and Blum, J.J., J. Biol. Chem. 252:1589 (1977).
30. Ottaway, J.H., and Mowbray, J., in "Current Topics in Cell Regulation" (B.L. Horecker and E.R. Stadtman, eds.), Academic Press, N.Y., 12:107 (1977).

DISCUSSION

F. GAERTNER: I would like to ask Joe Blum about possible transient times. Were you able to get an estimate of these?

J. BLUM: Most of the rates of incorporation were linear within a few moments after the addition of the mixture of acetate, pyruvate, bicarbonate, hexanoate, and glutamate to the cells. In a few cases there was an appreciable lag before incorporation began, and this was accounted for in determining the steady-state rates used in our data. In the experiments in which the cells were exposed to a mixture of glucose, fructose, ribose, and glycerol, the increase in pool size of glucose-6-P and of fructose-6-P was largely accomplished within the final 5 minutes of incubation, and the subsequent slow changes in rate of incorporation of label into product were merely due to a slow change in enzyme activity, so that the system was in a quasi-steady state. We did not make any measurements of isotopic transit times.

F. GAERTNER: Is there anything in your data that would indicate compartmentation, that is, is the flux so rapid to the end product that the label has to go directly to the end to equilibrate with the intermediates along the way? I think I saw one example of that.

J. BLUM: I can not quite answer that question. The model cannot tell you anything about compartmentation directly. A good fit to the data implies that the compartmental structure you have assumed in formulating the model is a reasonable approximation to the *in vivo* situation. If you fail to obtain a fit to the data you will presumably be driven to deduce a more realistic model of the structure of metabolism in the cell under study. Once a sufficiently realistic model is formulated and the equations describing isotopic flow in that model are derived, you should then be able to obtain a good fit to the data. If the data are of good quality and you have a sufficient excess of data to independent flux parameters, the ability to obtain a good fit will constitute a strong argument in favor of that particular compartmental structure.

S. BESSMAN: I would like to ask questions both of Dr. Veech and Dr. Blum, and to present data concerning pyrophosphate. We can detect pyrophosphate by the technology to be described in my paper (This volume, pgs 111-126). When you label ATP with ^{32}P you never see a peak of ^{32}P labeling nor a net change in pyrophosphate on incubating the ATP with metabolizing tissue. There is only one instance where this occurs, and Dr. Ben-Or in our laboratory did this using the retina of the fetal chicken where you can detect a considerable net increase in the content of radioactive pyrophosphate. The only trouble is that this occurs only when you incubate the tissue under extremely traumatic conditions.

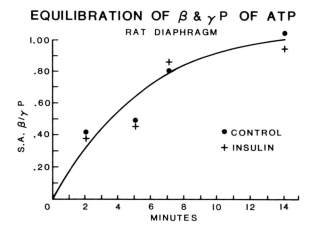

Figure 1. The equilibration of labeled ATP with rat diaphragm (S. Bessman).

Now, to turn to myokinase, I can show a slide on this subject. This slide (Figure 1) shows you the equilibration
of the beta and gamma phosphate of ATP in an intact rat
diaphragm respiring in a medium containing inorganic ^{33}P.
You can see that it is about 14 minutes before equilibration
occurs in this system; so the myokinase activity, in general,
is not very great. This is similar to mitochondria. These
are data on the measurement of the gamma and beta phosphates
of ATP and does not involve measuring ADP as well as ATP.
Dr. Blum claims that there is no compartmentation in glycolysis at equilibrium. The time course in which this was
measured is critical because we have had the same problem
with the creatine kinase system using mitochondria. The
equilibrium between some compartments probably takes place
within a minute. If you measure before a minute you will
discover that there is compartmentation. I question the
time course you use when you measure these compounds.

J. BLUM: In these experiments, we first write what we
think is a correct structural scheme for the metabolic pathways under investigation. We then make a large number of
measurements of label incorporation into selected products.
If we can obtain a set of flux parameters which give a good
fit to the large number of measurements, we must assume that
the structural scheme we used was an adequate description
of the system. In the experiments that we did to study metabolite flux along the glycolytic and pentose-phosphate pathways we were able to fit the data using a single well mixed
compartment. This does not prove that this system is not
compartmented. We merely assume that within the limits of
our experimental data it behaves as if it were not compartmented.

S. BESSMAN: The important point here is that we can deny the
presence of compartmentation simply because the rates of
equilibration are faster than the frequency of our analytical system. We can look at a whole liver and say the whole
liver behaves as if it were in equilibrium or a steady
state, but that doesn't mean that things are not happening
individually in liver compartments. So, it is very nice
to say that we can make a balance sheet for the whole cell,
but it does not mean that these reactions do not occur in
discrete places.

J. BLUM: That is true. But neither does the evidence indicate that they do exist. We do not deny the possibility
that compartmentation may exist in these pathways in

<u>Tetrahymena</u>.   Since we need not invoke it to interpret our
data, we must continue to consider these two pathways as
occurring in a single compartment until compelling evidence
to the contrary is obtained.

THE LIPOPROTEIN RECEPTOR SYSTEM AND THE CELLULAR REGULATION OF CHOLESTEROL METABOLISM[1]

Michael S. Brown
Joseph L. Goldstein

Departments of Molecular Genetics and Internal Medicine
University of Texas Health Science Center
Dallas, Texas

I. INTRODUCTION

Cholesterol is required for the normal function of the plasma membrane of all mammalian cells. Studies over the past 20 years have demonstrated that most of the cholesterol found in the membrane of nonhepatic cells is not synthesized locally, but rather it is derived from cholesterol that is synthesized in the liver or absorbed from the intestine (1,2). The liver distributes endogenously-synthesized or intestinally-derived cholesterol to extrahepatic tissues by means of lipoproteins that are secreted into the plasma. The main cholesterol-carrying lipoprotein in human plasma is low density lipoprotein (LDL). LDL consists of a core of neutral lipid that is composed predominantly of cholesteryl esters. Surrounding this neutral lipid core is a polar coat composed of phospholipid, free cholesterol, and a protein called apoprotein B. Body cells require free cholesterol for their membranes and not cholesteryl esters. So the cells require a mechanism by which they can extract the cholesteryl esters from LDL and hydrolyze those esters so as to generate free cholesterol for metabolic use.

II. THE LDL PATHWAY

A. Biochemical Aspects

The pathway by which cells are able to utilize the cholesteryl esters of LDL was elucidated through studies of human fibroblasts in tissue culture (2-4). Figure 1 summarizes this pathway as it emerged from studies conducted in Dallas over the past several years. When cultured human fibroblasts are in need of cholesterol, they synthesize a receptor molecule that becomes localized to the plasma membrane. This receptor speci-

[1]Supported by NIH grant P01-HL-20948

Copyright © 1978 by Academic Press, Inc.
All right of reproduction in any form reserved.
ISBN 0-12-660550-5

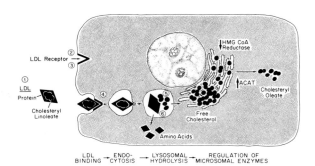

<u>Figure 1</u>.   Sequential steps in the LDL pathway in cultured
human fibroblasts.   The numbers indicate the sites at which
mutations have been identified: 1. abetalipoproteinemia; 2.
familial hypercholesterolemia, receptor-negative; 3. familial
hypercholesterolemia, receptor-defective; 4. familial hypercholesterolemia, internalization defect; 5. Wolman syndrome;
and 6. cholesteryl ester storage disease. HMG-CoA reductase
denotes 3-hydroxy-3-methylglutaryl coenzyme-A reductase, and
ACAT denotes acyl-coenzyme A: cholesterol acyltransferase.

fically binds the protein component of the lipoprotein.   Once
LDL binds to the receptor on the surface of these cells, the
lipoprotein is internalized by adsorptive endocytosis and
delivered to cellular lysosomes.   Within the lysosomes the
protein component of LDL is hydrolyzed to amino acids and the
cholesteryl esters of LDL are exposed to an acid lipase that
hydrolyzes the cholesteryl esters so as to generate free
cholesterol.   The free cholesterol is able to cross the lysosomal membrane to enter the cellular compartment where it is
used by the cell for membrane synthesis.
      Within the cell the cholesterol derived from the catabolism
of LDL regulates three metabolic events.   First, it suppresses
the activity of 3-hydroxy-3-methylglutaryl coenzyme A reductase
which is the rate-controlling enzyme in cholesterol biosynthesis (5).   Second, the cholesterol activates an acyl CoA:cho-
lesterol acyltransferase which re-esterifies the incoming
cholesterol. The newly formed cholesteryl esters are stored
within the cell as cytoplasmic lipid droplets (6). Third, the
incoming cholesterol turns off the synthesis of the LDL receptor itself.   This feedback regulation of LDL receptor synthesis stops the uptake of LDL and prevents cells from becoming
overloaded with cholesterol when exposed to LDL (7).

B. Morphological Aspects

The LDL pathway was elucidated through biochemical studies
in which the metabolism of various types of radio-labeled LDL
was studied in human fibroblasts. To study this pathway at the
morphological level, we have recently worked in collaboration
with Dr. Richard Anderson to attach LDL covalently to an electron dense probe, ferritin. When this ferritin-labeled LDL was
incubated with fibroblasts, we observed that the lipoprotein
bound to specialized regions of the plasma membrane where the
membrane is indented and where it appears to be coated on both
of its sides by a fuzzy material (8,9). These so-called coated
pits have been observed in many other cell types but their
precise function has not been known.

Even though the coated pits only account for about 2% of
the surface of the human fibroblast, they contain 50–80% of the
LDL receptors. The importance of the binding of LDL to the
coated pits lies in the observation that these regions are
specialized for the rapid endocytosis of receptor bound molecules. For example, if one binds LDL-ferritin to the cell at
4° and then warms up the cell for only 1 min, the majority of
the ferritin-labeled coated pits have invaginated into the
cell. Within 2 min, they pinch off to form coated endocytic
vesicles that carry the bound LDL-ferritin into the cell.
Within 5 min, the LDL-ferritin particles that were bound to the
coated pits have reached cellular lysosomes (9).

C. Genetic Aspects

All of the studies discussed above were performed on
normal human fibroblasts. The inference that this pathway is
important in vivo was based upon studies of human mutants who
have specific biochemical blocks in the degradation of LDL.
These mutant cells are cultured from humans with genetic disorders of lipoprotein metabolism. The most informative of
these has been the mutation that occurs in the disease called
Familial Hypercholesterolemia (FH) (2,10).

FH exists in the population in two forms (11). Patients
have either the heterozygous form or the homozygous form of the
disease. Heterozygotes number 1 in 500 among the general
population in the United States. These heterozygotes have a two
to three-fold elevation in the plasma level of LDL which ultimately gets them into trouble because the lipoprotein deposits
in their arteries and they develop myocardial infarctions,
typically between the ages of 35 and 45. Rarely, two heterozygotes marry and produce a homozygote. About one in a million

children in the population is affected with the homozygous form
of FH. These children exhibit six-fold elevations in the
plasma LDL level with massive deposition of cholesterol in
tissues. Myocardial infarctions generally occur before the age
of 15. These homozygotes held the key to solving FH. Every
homozygote whose fibroblasts have been studied has exhibited a
genetic defect in the LDL receptor. This defect leads to a
reduction in the ability of body cells to take up LDL. As a
result, the lipoprotein accumulates to massive levels in plasma
and myocardial infarctions result (12).

 By studying fibroblasts from 43 of these homozygous children, we have been able to identify three different mutant
alleles at the LDL receptor locus. The first of these is
termed $\underline{R^{b^\circ}}$ which indicates an allele that specifies a receptor
that is not able to bind LDL. The second is termed $\underline{R^{b-}}$, which
indicates an allele that specifies a receptor that is able to
bind LDL, but in amounts that are only 1-10% of normal. The
third allele, designated $\underline{R^{b+,i^\circ}}$ specifies a receptor that is
able to bind LDL normally but is not able to carry the LDL into
the cell. Among the 43 homozygotes that we have studied, 24
are homozygous for the $\underline{R^{b^\circ}}$ allele and have no ability to bind
LDL. Eighteen subjects have detectable but markedly reduced
binding ability. These latter subjects have one $\underline{R^{b-}}$ allele and
either one $\underline{R^{b^\circ}}$ allele or a second $\underline{R^{b-}}$ allele. And finally, we
have studied a unique patient with the internalization defect.
This child turns out to be a genetic compound who has one $\underline{R^{b^\circ}}$
allele and one $\underline{R^{b+,i^\circ}}$ allele at the LDL receptor locus. We
have also studied fibroblasts from 31 FH heterozygotes. The
cells from each of these patients have shown evidence of one
normal allele and one of the mutant alleles as expected from
the genetics of the disease.

 Recent studies of LDL metabolism in fibroblasts from the
patient with the internalization defect have taught us a great
deal about the way in which the LDL receptor finds its way into
the coated pits (13-15). These studies have demonstrated that
the $\underline{R^{b+,i^\circ}}$ allele specifies a receptor that can bind LDL
normally but has lost the ability to become localized to the
coated pits. As a result when LDL binds to these receptors, it
is not internalized by the cell. The patient with the internalization defect inherited one copy of this allele and one
copy of the $\underline{R^{b^\circ}}$ allele, whose product does not bind LDL.
Hence, all of the ^{125}I-LDL that binds to this patient's cells
binds to the product of the $\underline{R^{b+,i^\circ}}$ allele, and consequently
none of the bound lipoprotein enters the cell. The father of
this patient is a heterozygote for the $\underline{R^{b+,i^\circ}}$ allele (geno-
type, $+/R^{b+,i^\circ}$). Approximately half of his LDL receptors
(i.e., those specified by the normal + allele) are able to

carry their bound LDL into the cell. The other half, specified
by the $\underline{R^{b+,i^\circ}}$ allele, are unable to reach the coated pits and
so they do not carry their bound LDL into the cells. These
observations have been made biochemically using ^{125}I-LDL
(13,14) and confirmed at the ultrastructural level using ferritin-labeled LDL (15).

III. MODEL FOR INCORPORATION OF LDL RECEPTORS
INTO COATED PITS

From the properties of the $\underline{R^{b+,i^\circ}}$ allele, we have formulated a working model for the way in which LDL receptors are
incorporated into coated pits on the cell surface. This model
is based on our genetic studies of the LDL receptor (15) as
well as on studies by others of the assembly of lipid envelope
viruses in mammalian cells (16,17). As shown in Figure 2, we
envision that the LDL receptor is a transmembrane protein that

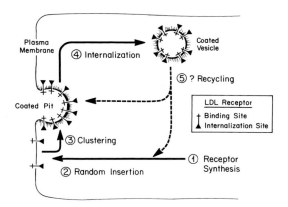

Figure 2. Schematic illustration of the proposed pathway by
which LDL receptors become localized to coated pits on the
plasma membrane of human fibroblasts. The sequential steps in
this process are as follows: 1) synthesis of LDL receptors on
polyribosomes, 2) insertion of LDL receptors at random sites
along non-coated segments of plasma membrane, 3) clustering
together of LDL receptors in coated pits, 4) internalization of
LDL receptors as coated pits invaginate to form coated endocytic vesicles, and 5) recycling of internalized LDL receptors
back to the plasma membrane.

is made within the cell where it presumably is glycosolated and inserted into the plasma membrane. The receptor is postulated to have two active sites. One of these, on the external surface of the membrane, is the binding site for LDL. A second site, on the cytoplasmic side of the membrane, contains an amino acid sequence that is necessary for the receptor to become incorporated into coated pits. We call this site the internalization site. The receptor is initially inserted into the plasma membrane at random. However, if the LDL receptor has an active internalization site, it is clustered together with other receptors to form a coated pit. This clustering possibly occurs under the influence of a cytoplasmic protein that is not yet identified. Once the LDL receptors are clustered together and the coated pit becomes full, it invaginates, pinches off, and forms a coated vesicle. The vesicles then fuse with lysosomes and the LDL is degraded. A great deal of indirect kinetic evidence suggests that the receptors are recycled back to the cell surface after they discharge their LDL within the lysosomes.

When the receptor carries a mutation in the internalization site, as in the patient with the internalization defect, the receptor is inserted into the membrane but it is unable to become incorporated into coated pits. As a result, the receptor accumulates at a site just proximal to the metabolic block, i.e., at random locations on the plasma membrane.

IV. IMPLICATIONS OF THE MODEL

The mechanism for internalization of receptor-bound LDL may be a general one for receptor-bound macromolecules (15). Thus, the studies of Carpenter and Cohen demonstrate that ^{125}I-labeled epidermal growth factor binds to receptors on fibroblasts and is rapidly internalized and degraded (18). The kinetics of the uptake process for this polypeptide hormone are similar to those of the LDL uptake process. Similar kinetics have been demonstrated for the cellular uptake of transcobalamin II, the transport protein for vitamin B_{12} in plasma (19). It may be that many receptor molecules whose function is to carry bound ligands into the cell are localized over coated pits so that the internalization process can be enhanced. It is attractive to speculate that these other receptors, like those for LDL, may have internalization sites that allow this incorporation to take place. Further studies of the coated pit mechanism should provide much information into the manner in which membrane compartmentation helps to control a variety of metabolic processes in eukaryotic cells.

REFERENCES

1. Dietschy, J. M., and Wilson, J. D. (1970). New Engl. J. Med. 282:1128, 1179, 1241.
2. Brown, M. S., and Goldstein, J. L. (1976). Science 191:150.
3. Goldstein, J. L., and Brown, M. S. (1976). Curr. Topics Cell. Reg. 11:147.
4. Goldstein, J. L., and Brown, M. S. (1977). Ann. Rev. Biochem. 46:897.
5. Brown, M. S., Dana, S. E., and Goldstein, J. L. (1974). J. Biol. Chem. 249:789.
6. Goldstein, J. L., Dana, S. E., and Brown, M. S. (1974). Proc. Nat. Acad. Sci. USA. 71:4288.
7. Brown, M. S., and Goldstein, J. L. (1975). Cell 6:307.
8. Anderson, R. G. W., Goldstein, J. L., and Brown, M. S. (1976). Proc. Nat. Acad. Sci. USA. 73:2434.
9. Anderson, R. G. W., Brown, M. S., and Goldstein, J. L. (1977). Cell 10:351.
10. Brown, M. S., and Goldstein, J. L. (1976). N. Engl. J. Med. 294:1386.
11. Fredrickson, D. S., Goldstein, J. L., and Brown, M. S. (1978). In "The Metabolic Basis of Inherited Disease" (J.B. Stanbury, J.B. Wyngaarden, and D.S. Fredrickson, eds.), p. 604, 4th edition. McGraw Hill Book Co., New York.
12. Goldstein, J. L., and Brown, M. S. (1977). Metabolism 26:1257.
13. Brown, M. S., and Goldstein, J. L. (1976). Cell 9:663.
14. Goldstein, J. L., and Brown, M. S. (1977). Cell 12:629.
15. Anderson, R. G. W., Goldstein, J. L., and Brown, M. S. (1977). Nature 270:695.
16. Lenard, J., and Compans, R. W. (1974). Biochim. Biophys. Acta 344:51.
17. Knipe, D. M., Baltimore, D., and Lodish, H. F. (1977). J. Virol. 21:1128.
18. Carpenter, G., and Cohen, S. (1976). J. Cell Biol. 71:159.
19. Youngdahl-Turner, P., Rosenberg, L. E., and Allen, R. H. (1978). J. Clin. Invest. 61:133.

DISCUSSION

C. deDUVE: If nobody is making any comment, I would at least
like to congratulate the authors on this beautiful work. In
our laboratory we have for several years now been investigating
the mechanism of lipid deposition in the arterial smooth muscle cells of rabbits fed on a cholesterol-rich diet. Much of
this lipid is intralysosomal and was believed first to consist
of undigested cholesterol esters. But present indications
are that it is made up largely of free cholesterol. I would
like to ask Drs. Brown and Goldstein whether they have encountered a similar situation where lysosome overloading seems
to occur as a result not of deficient digestion, but of inadequate clearance of a digestion product.

M. BROWN: Thank you very much, Dr. deDuve. No we have not
seen that in the fibroblast. In the fibroblast, once you start
saturating the system with cholesterol esters the synthesis of
the receptor is turned off so you can't really overload the
cell using native LDL. Now, we have recently made an analog
of LDL which has a positive charge so that it sticks non-
specifically to the membrane and goes into the lysosomes. In
that case we can overload the cell, but even so, we see mostly
the accumulation of cholesterol ester.

F. LIPMANN: The cholesterol content in the blood of the homozygotes you mentioned is very high. If you have a high blood
level of cholesterol you have to be very careful and eat very
little cholesterol and if you don't have high blood cholesterol
you don't need to. Now please answer this.

M. BROWN: I wish I could. The situation is that there are
many different genetic diseases and environmental diseases
responsible for high cholesterol. In these particular indi-
viduals who have the high cholesterol due to the FH mutation,
a low cholesterol diet doesn't seem to do much good. In fact
the body tries to restore the high level of blood cholesterol
no matter what you do. That is, in the absence of the receptors the cells sense a deficiency of cholesterol and the cells
actually overproduce cholesterol despite the high level in the
plasma. Thus, these patients are not affected by diet. But
the FH patients only account for 1 in 500 in the population.
Of all the others in the population who have high blood cholesterol, a fraction of them seem to be sensitive to the diet
and another fraction is not. What we are trying to do with
all of these studies is to dissect out the different forms of
hypercholesteroleria so we can begin to rationally say to
someone, "you should not eat cholesterol" or "you should".

L. RAIJMAN: You said at the beginning of your talk that most of the cholesterol that is found in the membrane of different cells is of hepatic origin. Am I right to assume that the increased levels of cholesterol that you find in peripheral cells in some people are due to the fact that they don't have the proper receptors to incorporate hepatic cholesterol and inhibit peripheral cell synthesis of cholesterol? Can you speculate at all why cells have retained this double system for control of cholesterol metabolism?

M. BROWN: This is the question that Dr. Srere always asks us. This dual system is clearly a fact. Now in terms of teleology, we don't know why such a dual system should have been chosen by evolution. One thing we do know is that cholesterol is absolutely required by cells. If you take away lipoproteins and block the synthesis of cholesterol by tissue culture cells they die very quickly, so it may be that the synthetic system is a backup that is retained in case lipoproteins can't supply cholesterol. There may be some conditions of cell growth in which endogenous synthesis is important, perhaps in rapidly dividing cells. It is known that if you take lymphocytes from the blood stream that are not dividing, they have low rates of cholesterol synthesis and they derive all of their cholesterol from lipoprotein. If you incubate them in the absence of LDL, they increase their synthesis of cholesterol. It may be that under certain specific conditions cells may need to produce their own cholesterol.

J. PATERNITI: When we speak of cholesterol as a feedback inhibitor of HMG-CoA reductase and decreasing the synthesis of the low density lipoprotein receptor are we speaking of the cholesterol molecule itself or is it the 7-keto derivative or the 25-hydroxy derivative; in other words, a metabolite of cholesterol? What is your feeling about that, and are the derivatives doing both of these things?

M. BROWN: If one adds to the exterior of the cell certain polar derivatives of cholesterol, such as 25-hydroxy and 7-keto cholesterol, they are more effective than free cholesterol in regulating the enzyme that you mentioned. We think that this may be a problem of cellular compartmentation. These derivatives are more polar than cholesterol and cross membranes more easily when added in an ethanol solution. However, if you add the cholesterol in the form of low density lipoprotein so that it can utilize the specific uptake mechanism, then it clearly can achieve regulation. If you block the hydrolysis of the cholesterol ester of the lipoprotein within the cell you don't get any regulatory effects.

Therefore, the effective component of LDL has to be the free
cholesterol that is generated from the lysosomal hydrolysis
of cholesteryl esters. We don't find any hydroxylated
steroids in the lipoprotein or in the cells incubated with
lipoproteins.

EFFECT OF COMPARTMENTATION OF HEART PHENYLALANINE ON
MEASUREMENTS OF PROTEIN SYNTHESIS AND AMINO
ACID TRANSPORT

Howard E. Morgan, Edward E. McKee, and
Joseph Y. Cheung

Department of Physiology
The Milton S. Hershey Medical Center
The Pennsylvania State University
Hershey, Pennsylvania

An apparent acceleration of protein synthesis by a hormonal or nonhormonal factor, as measured by incorporation of radioactive amino acids, may be due either to a genuine increase in the synthetic rate or to an increase in the specific radioactivity of the pool of amino acids serving as the immediate precursor. Identification of the precursor pool is complicated by compartmentation of amino acids within interstitial, intracellular, mitochondrial, lysosomal and perhaps other membrane-limited spaces. An approach to measuring the specific activity of the precursor pool of amino acids is to determine the specific activities of amino acids acylated to tRNA, the immediate precursor for protein synthesis (1-3).

Similarly, an apparent stimulation of substrate transport by an agent depends not only on its effect on transmembrane flux, but also on the nature of compartmentation of the substrate within the cell and on changes in the subsequent metabolism of the substrate. For example, insulin accelerates glucose transport in a wide variety of tissues, including heart muscle (for review, 4). However, insulin also shifts the rate-limiting step in glucose metabolism from transport to glucose phosphorylation. The resultant accumulation of intracellular glucose makes evaluation of the effect of insulin on transport kinetics extremely difficult and, at best, imprecise (5). Studies of amino acid transport is made even more complex by the involvement of multiple transport systems, each serving a subgroup of amino acids. Insulin has been reported to accelerate transport of

Copyright © 1978 by Academic Press, Inc.
All right of reproduction in any form reserved.
ISBN 0-12-660550-5

α-aminoisobutyric acid, a nonmetabolized analog transported
by the A system, in rat myocardium (6). The significance of
the finding in relation to an effect of insulin on protein
synthesis is uncertain because the natural amino acids,
instead of remaining in a static pool, are dynamically
involved in protein synthesis and degradation, pathways
which are affected by insulin (3,7).

   The purpose of this paper is to summarize evidence
indicating that phenylalanine and other amino acids are
compartmented within heart and to define conditions that
allow for accurate estimates of the rate of protein synthesis. The difficulties in interpreting initial rates of
amino acid entry and the possible effect of insulin are
considered in relation to models of amino acid compartmentation.

II. EVIDENCE FOR AMINO ACID COMPARTMENTATION AND ITS EFFECT ON MEASUREMENTS OF PROTEIN SYNTHESIS

   In studies from this laboratory, [^{14}C]phenylalanine has
been used to measure rates of protein synthesis in the
perfused rat heart (3,8). This amino acid was chosen because it is not synthesized nor degraded in the perfused rat
heart. Rates of protein synthesis were calculated from the
incorporation of radioactivity into heart protein and the
specific activities of perfusate, intracellular, and tRNA-
bound phenylalanine (Fig. 1). When the specific activity of
[^{14}C]phenylalanyl-tRNA was used, the same rate of protein
synthesis was obtained at phenylalanine concentrations in
the perfusate varying from 0.01 to 0.4 mM. On the other
hand, use of the specific activity of phenylalanine in the
perfusate gave a lower rate of synthesis at low phenylalanine concentrations, while use of the intracellular
specific activity gave a higher rate. A constant rate of
synthesis, based upon phenylalanyl-tRNA specific activity,
coupled with a constant rate of histidine incorporation
(Fig. 1) indicated that protein synthesis was not affected
in these time periods by this range of concentration of
phenylalanine in the perfusate. These findings also indicated that neither a well-mixed interstitial or intracellular pool of phenylalanine could serve as the sole
source of phenylalanine used for amino acid activation.

   Addition of insulin accelerated the rate of protein
synthesis (Table I). As in control hearts, use of the
specific activity of phenylalanyl-tRNA gave the same rate of
synthesis at phenylalanine concentrations of 0.01 and 0.4
mM, while the specific activity of phenylalanine in the

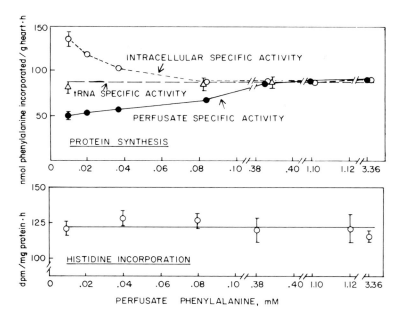

Figure 1. Effect of perfusate phenylalanine concentration on rates of protein synthesis and histidine incorporation. A preliminary perfusion of 10 min with buffer containing phenylalanine at the concentrations indicated, 15 mM glucose, and normal plasma levels of other amino acids (3) was followed by recirculation of the same buffer containing [14C]phenylalanine for either 90 (phenylalanyl-tRNA specific activity) or 180 minutes (specific activity of perfusate and intracellular phenylalanine and histidine incorporation). The volume of perfusate that was recirculated in the 180 min experiments was varied from 25 to 170 ml to minimize the fall in phenylalanine specific activity in the perfusate. Because of the large amount of radioactivity needed to measure [14C]phenylalanyl-tRNA specific activity, the volumes of perfusate in these experiments was kept at 25 ml. Intracellular specific activity was calculated as described previously (3) as was determination of the specific activity of phenylalanyl-tRNA. Each value represents the mean ± S.E. In the phenylalanyl-tRNA experiments, 6 hearts were pooled for each determination.

TABLE I. Effect of phenylalanine concentration in the perfusate on rates of protein synthesis and histidine incorporation in insulin-treated hearts.

Parameter	Phenylalanine concentration, mM	
	0.01	0.4
Protein synthesis, nmol/ g heart · h, calculated from specific activity of phenylalanine in the:		
perfusate	108 ± 4	162 ± 8
intracellular compartment	286 ± 12	162 ± 8
tRNA	160 ± 6	160 ± 8
Histidine incorporation, dpm/ mg protein · h	301 ± 15	337 ± 12

Hearts were perfused as in Fig. 1 for 90 min with buffer containing insulin (25 mU/ml). Values represent the mean ± S.E. of 5-6 determinations.

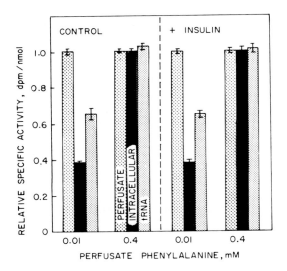

Figure 2. Relationship of the specific activities of phenylalanine in the perfusate, intracellular compartment, and tRNA. Hearts were perfused for 90 min as described in Fig. 1. Insulin (25 mU/ml) was added as indicated. Relative specific activities of [^{14}C]phenylalanine in the intracellular compartment and tRNA were calculated by dividing these values by the specific activity in the perfusate. Values represent the mean ± S.E. of 5-6 determinations.

perfusate underestimated and that of the intracellular compartment overestimated the rate when the concentration in the perfusate was 0.01 mM. Histidine incorporation was unchanged when phenylalanine concentration was increased from 0.01 to 0.4 mM.

Measurement of the specific activities of phenylalanine in the perfusate, intracellular compartment, and tRNA revealed that the specific activity of phenylalanyl-tRNA was intermediate between the two other values in either control or insulin-treated hearts perfused with buffer containing 0.01 mM phenylalanine (Fig. 2). When the concentration in the perfusate was increased to 0.4 mM, the intracellular concentration of phenylalanine increased proportionally (3), and the differences in specific activities disappeared. These observations indicated that heart phenylalanine was compartmented because neither a well-mixed interstitial or intracellular pool could serve as the sole precursor. Two models of compartmentation that are consistent with these findings were the two-site activation model (3,9-11) and the compartmented intracellular pool model (1,3,12) (Figures 3 and 4). In both models, the concentration and specific activity of phenylalanine in the perfusate, heart phenylalanine content and specific activity, rates of protein synthesis and degradation, and the rate constant of sorbitol flux across the capillary were known. In the two-site activation model, a unique solution for the rate constants into and out of the intracellular pool and into phenylalanyl-tRNA could be obtained (3). In the compartmented

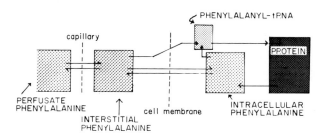

Figure 3. Model of amino acid compartmentation involving acylation of phenylalanine from two sites. The solution of this model by compartmental analysis and the derived rate constants and equations have been presented elsewhere (3).

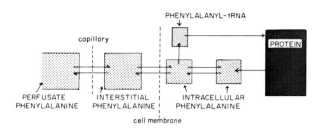

<u>Figure 4.</u> Model of amino acid compartmentation involving two intracellular pools. The solution of this model by compartmental analysis and the derived rate constants and equations have been presented elsewhere (3).

intracellular pool model, a unique solution for the trans-membrane fluxes of phenylalanine was possible, but a range of sizes of the two intracellular pools of phenylalanine fitted equally well. In this model, the intracellular pool of phenylalanine serving as the precursor for aminoacylation of tRNA could range from a value approaching zero to a maximum of about 15% of intracellular phenylalanine. From the point of view of measurements of protein synthesis, these models were operationally the same since both provided for a specific activity of phenylalanyl-tRNA intermediate between the interstitial and intracellular values. The implications of these models of compartmentation for measurement of transmembrane fluxes of phenylalanine will be described in the remaining section of this paper.

III.   EFFECT OF COMPARTMENTATION ON MEASUREMENTS OF AMINO ACID TRANSPORT

Effects of hormones on entry of amino acids into the cell often are evaluated by comparing the initial rates of amino acid equilibration (13-15). Insulin increased the rate of phenylalanine equilibration from 2.7 to 4.7 nmol/g · min (Fig. 5). In deriving these values the assumptions were made that rapid equilibration of about 45% of heart water with phenylalanine was due to fill-up of the extracellular volume and that the second, slower phase of equilibration represented fill-up of a well-mixed intracellular pool (Fig. 6). Superficially, these data could be interpreted to indicate that insulin accelerated phenylalanine transport. This conclusion, however, ignores other important factors in

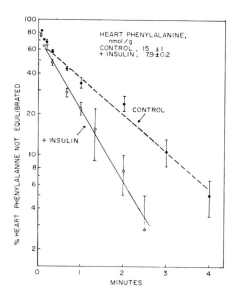

Figure 5. Rates of equilibration of heart phenylalanine. Hearts were perfused for 30 min with buffer containing 15 mM glucose, 0.01 mM phenylalanine, and normal plasma levels of other amino acids. Insulin (25 mU/ml) was added as indicated. After this period, perfusion was continued for the time indicated with the same buffer containing [^{14}C]phenylalanine. Results are plotted as the percent of [^{14}C]phenylalanine of the heart not at equilibrium. Values represent the mean ± S.E. of 6-8 determinations. Lines were drawn by linear regression using data collected between 40 and 150 sec. Rates of phenylalanine entry were calculated by the following equation:

$$\frac{\text{phenylalanine influx,}}{\text{nmol/g} \cdot \text{heart} \cdot \text{min}} = \frac{0.693 \cdot W_i \cdot [\text{Phe}]_o}{t \; 1/2}$$

where W_i equals the volume of intracellular water (ml/g); [Phe_o], the perfusate concentration of phenylalanine (nmol/ml); and t 1/2, the half-time of equilibration (min).

evaluating equilibration of radioactivity in heart phenylalanine. These factors include 1) the concentration of
intracellular phenylalanine, 2) rates of protein synthesis
and degradation, and 3) compartmentation of phenylalanine.
The concentration of phenylalanine could influence the rate
constant in two ways. As the intracellular concentration
increased, a longer time interval would be required for
equilibration; on the other hand, at higher intracellular
concentrations, the entry of [^{14}C] phenylalanine was more
rapid, presumably due to exchange diffusion (16). As noted
in Fig. 5, insulin reduced the intracellular concentration
of phenylalanine by approximately 50%. The effect of this
change in concentration on phenylalanine influx as compared
to an effect of insulin directly on influx cannot be deduced
intuitively from these measurements. The effect of intracellular phenylalanine concentration, as well as rates of
protein synthesis and degradation, could be taken into
account in the formulation of a well-mixed intracellular
pool model (Fig. 6). In these calculations, rates of protein synthesis were based on the specific activity of phenylalanyl-tRNA, while rates of degradation were measured by
release of phenylalanine from hearts perfused with buffer
containing cycloheximide (7). When intracellular phenylalanine concentration and rates of synthesis and degradation
were considered, influx of phenylalanine was reduced by the
addition of insulin rather than accelerated (Fig. 7). In

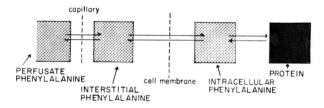

Figure 6. Model of amino acid compartmentation in the heart
involving a well-mixed intracellular pool. Values for
influx and efflux of phenylalanine were obtained by compartmental analysis as previously described (3). The values are
given in Fig. 7.

most experiments involving evaluation of transport rates, estimates of influx were more uncertain than these because the intracellular concentrations of the amino acids were not measured, and reliable rates of synthesis and degradation were not available.

Evaluation of transmembrane flux of phenylalanine becomes more complicated when compartmentation of amino acids is introduced (3). In the two-site activation model (Fig. 3), only a portion of phenylalanine influx enters the intracellular pool and is measured by determining the rate of equilibration of heart phenylalanine. Influx into the intracellular pool accounted for 83% of total influx in control hearts but decreased to 63% in the presence of insulin. It is apparent that the role of amino acid transport in restricting protein synthesis cannot be evaluated by measurement of influx into the intracellular pool if this model of compartmentation applies.

In the compartmented intracellular pool model (Fig. 4) the compartment of intracellular phenylalanine that receives amino acid from the interstitial space does not amount to more than 15% of intracellular phenylalanine (3). As a result, a plot of phenylalanine equilibration, such as in

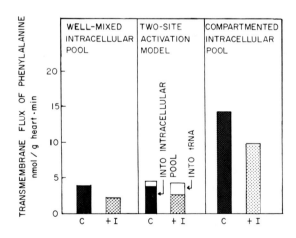

Figure 7. Transmembrane influx of phenylalanine in three models of amino acid compartmentation. Rate constants for the well-mixed intracellular pool were obtained as described in Fig. 6; the remaining values have been published earlier (3). Values for control hearts are denoted by bars labeled "C," while those of insulin-treated hearts are denoted as "+I."

Fig. 5, cannot resolve the rate of equilibration of this compartment. Instead, data derived from the second exponential reflect movement of phenylalanine from one intracellular compartment to another rather than transmembrane flux. When influx across the membrane was calculated for this model, the rate was 3-4 times faster than in the two-site activation model, but as in the other models, the rate of influx was reduced in insulin-treated hearts.

Meaningful evaluation of the effect of insulin on entry of phenylalanine would require definition of the model of compartmentation and evaluation of the effects of extracellular and intracellular concentrations of phenylalanine (as well as other amino acids sharing the L system) on phenylalanine entry in control and insulin-treated hearts.

IV. SUMMARY

Calculation of rates of protein synthesis, based upon incorporation of [^{14}C]phenylalanine into protein, depended upon use of the specific activity of phenylalanyl-tRNA. At 0.01 mM phenylalanine in the perfusate, specific activity of phenylalanyl-tRNA was intermediate between that of phenylalanine in the perfusate and intracellular compartments in both control and insulin-treated hearts. This evidence indicated that neither a well-mixed interstitial nor intracellular pool of phenylalanine could serve as the sole precursor for protein synthesis. Two models of amino acid compartmentation involving 1) aminoacylation of tRNA from both the extracellular and intracellular compartments or 2) aminoacylation of tRNA from a compartmented intracellular pool were consistent with these data. Difficulties in measuring rates of amino acid transport are discussed in relation to amino acid compartmentation and changes in the size of amino acid pools.

ACKNOWLEDGMENT
    This research was supported by grants from the National Heart, Lung and Blood Institute (HL-20388, HL-18258, and HL-07223).

REFERENCES

  1. Khairallah, E. A., and Mortimore, G. E., J. Biol. Chem. 251:1375 (1976).

2. Martin, A. F., Rabinowitz, M., Blough, R., Prior, G., and Zak, R., J. Biol. Chem. 252:3422 (1977).
3. McKee, E. E., Cheung, J. Y., Rannels, D. E., and Morgan, H. E., J. Biol. Chem., in press.
4. Morgan, H. E., and Whitfield, C. F., in "Current Topics in Membranes and Transport" (F. Bronner and A. Klein-zeller, eds.), Vol. 4, p. 255. Academic Press, New York, 1973.
5. Cheung, J. Y., Conover, C., Regen, D. M., Whitfield, C. F., and Morgan, H. E., Amer. J. Physiol., in press.
6. Manchester, K. L., and Wool, I. G., Biochem. J. 89: 202 (1963).
7. Rannels, D. E., Kao, R., and Morgan, H. E., J. Biol. Chem. 250:1694 (1975).
8. Morgan, H. E., Earl, D.C.N., Broadus, A., Wolpert, E. B., Giger, K. E., and Jefferson, L. S., J. Biol. Chem. 246:2152 (1971).
9. Airhart, J., Vidrich, A., and Khairallah, E. A., Biochem. J. 140:539 (1974).
10. Hod, Y., and Hershko, A., J. Biol. Chem. 251:4458 (1976).
11. Vidrich, A., Airhart, J., Bruno, M. K. and Khairallah, E. A., Biochem. J. 162: 257 (1977).
12. Mortimore, G.E., Woodside, K. H., and Henry, J. E., J. Biol. Chem. 247:2776 (1972).
13. Guidotti, G. G., Borghetti, A. F., Gazzola, G. C., Tramacere, M., and Dall'asta, V., Biochem. J. 160: 281 (1976).
14. Manchester, K. L., Guidotti, G. G., Borghetti, A. F., and Luneburg, B., Biochim. Biophys. Acta 241:226 (1971).
15. Narahara, H. T., and Holloszy, J. O., J. Biol. Chem., 249:5435 (1974).
16. Oxender, D. L., and Christensen, H. N., J. Biol. Chem. 238:3686 (1963).

DISCUSSION

R. WEISS: I would like to make a suggestion to Dr. Morgan. I believe that the model of two charging sites or charging at mammalian plasma membranes originated in 1962 by Hendler (Nature, 193, 821–823, 1962) and is still with us. It really has never been tested by very simple experimental techniques that we have used in Neurospora. Since you can determine the rate of protein synthesis, the easiest way to check for preferential charging at the plasma membrane is to generate your amino acids inside the cell by using a precursor to the ultimate amino acids. If preferential utilization is an effect of having distinct pools within the cell, then, amino acids generated intracellularly should also be preferentially incorporated into protein and you should be able to calculate the pool sizes. This would be independent of any preferential charging at the plasma membrane.

H. MORGAN: Yes, those sorts of experiments were tried in muscle by Manchester and Krahl (J. Biol. Chem. 234, 2938, 1959). The problem is that amino acids generated in the intracellular compartment rapidly exchange with those in the interstitial compartment. The major point is that there is no evidence, at the moment, upon which to decide which model is better. Resolution of the problem will depend upon a more complete understanding of the localization of the enzymes that are involved.

S. BESSMAN: May I comment on Dr. Morgan's paper. I think this is really a beautiful piece of work. We published many years ago (American J. Medicine, 40, 740, 1966) an article on the theory of insulin action. Muscle, pretreated with radioactive amino acids at 4° and then washed and incubated in the presence of non-radioactive carrier, will concentrate the amino acid and will use preferentially the internal amino acid on insulin stimulation. That could not be due to pushing it out and pulling it back in. Udenfriend and I, in studying phenylketonuria gave radioactive phenylalanine to human beings. We isolated albumin with labeled phenylalanine and tyrosine. We found that the half-life of tyrosine in the purified albumin was much longer than the half-life of phenylalanine. It looks like there is a special compartment adjacent to the resynthesis of protein where phenylalanine is converted to tyrosine.

H. MORGAN: When one considers the overall effect of insulin on protein synthesis in the heart, the physiologically important site of action is on peptide chain initiation and not on amino acid transport. In fact, one of the results of studies of compartmentation is an appreciation of how difficult it is to accurately measure transport rates in a system where compartmentation is present. If one determines the half-time of equilibration of specific activity of heart phenylalanine, equilibration is faster in the presence of insulin than in the control. On the other hand, transmembrane fluxes calculated from either one of these models are lower in the presence of insulin. In the two-site activation model, only the portion of transmembrane flux going into the intracellular pool is measured by following accumulation of heart phenylalanine. In the compartmented intracellular pool model, accumulation of heart phenylalanine reflects movement between the intracellular compartments and not transmembrane flux. Much more care must be taken in making transport measurements if reliable values are to be obtained.

MITOCHONDRIAL CREATINE KINASE AND HEXOKINASE
TWO EXAMPLES OF COMPARTMENTATION PREDICTED
BY THE HEXOKINASE MITOCHONDRIAL BINDING
THEORY OF INSULIN ACTION

Samuel P. Bessman
Borgar Borrebaek[1]
Paul J. Geiger
Sarah Ben-Or[2]

Department of Pharmacology and Nutrition
University of Southern California
Los Angeles, California

All of the observed effects of insulin on tissues could be
the result of facilitated delivery of energy to anabolic processes. The hexokinase-mitochondrial theory of the mechanism
of insulin action (1,2,3) proposes that insulin causes the
binding of hexokinase to mitochondria to produce an increase
of efficiency of respiratory control, thereby facilitating
delivery of energy to all of the anabolic processes known to
be accelerated by insulin (Fig. 1, Fig. 2). It is proposed
that hexokinase is bound at a site of generation of ATP so
that the delivery of ATP would be immediately followed by the
return of ADP with its resultant respiratory control. This
process would be facilitated by the proximity of the active
site of hexokinase to the phosphorylation site. The juxtaposition of these two active sites would form a "compartment"

---

[1]Present address: Institute for Medical Biochemistry,
University of Oslo, Norway
[2]Present address: Department of Physiology, The Hebrew
University, Jerusalem, Israel

Copyright © 1978 by Academic Press, Inc.
All right of reproduction in any form reserved.
ISBN 0-12-660550-5

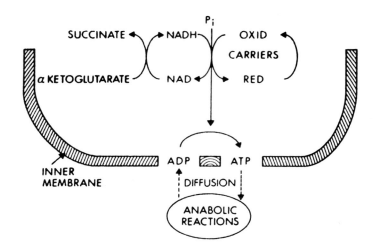

FIGURE 1. The rate of oxidative phosphorylation depends upon the supply of ADP and the removal of ATP. Where there is no kinase close by control of the mitochondrial rate occurs by diffusion of ATP from the mitochondrion to the site where it is converted to ADP which must then diffuse back to the appropriate mitochondrial sites. In this case energy generation is diffusion limited.

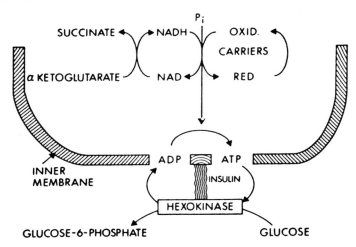

FIGURE 2. The attachment of hexokinase or a similar kinase such as creatine kinase to the mitochondrion provides an efficient mechanism for utilization of ATP and immediate resupply of ADP. It is proposed that the role of insulin in stimulating metabolism is to connect hexokinase to the appropriate sites on the mitochondrion.

such as described by Srere (4). This hormone generated compartmentation would explain a number of observed physiological
phenomena and experimental findings not interpretable in the
light of any other theory of insulin action.

1. Although the brain derives a preponderance of its
energy from glucose, insulin has no significant effect on
glucose metabolism by brain. It has been shown by Crane and
Sols (5) and confirmed by many others, that most of the hexokinase of brain is bound to the mitochondria. Any action of
insulin in binding hexokinase to brain mitochondria must therefore be superfluous.

2. The effect of insulin on tissues is inversely related
to the percentage of hexokinase bound to the mitochondria
(6a, 6b).

3. Antibodies to insulin cause hexokinase to be released
from mitochondria of lactating mammary gland (7).

4. Incubation of fat pads with insulin causes increased
binding of hexokinase to the mitochondria (8).

5. The control of respiration in ascites cells seems to
be related to the binding of hexokinase to the mitochondria
(9).

6. The insulin stimulation of protein synthesis in diaphragm muscle does not occur if the hexokinase pathway is
interrupted (10).

7. Gots has shown the close relation of the active site
of mitochondrial bound hexokinase to the ATP generation site
by demonstrating the preferential use of intra-mitochondrial
ATP to form glucose-6-phosphate. Fig. 3 shows that the initial glucose-6-phosphate formed by mitochondrial bound hexokinase has the same specific activity as the inorganic phosphate of the medium rather than of the free ATP of the medium
(11).

These observations on the insulin-hexokinase relation suggest the formation of a compartment as the mechanism of insulin action. The well-known effects of exercise in stimulating
metabolism in muscle equivalent to the effect of insulin, suggests another compartment which obviates the need for insulin
in exercising skeletal muscle and heart. The creatine-
creatine phosphate pathway provides an acceptor system for the
rate of generation of creatine increases with exercise. If
the sarcosome responded to creatine as it does to ADP, exercise could cause an acceleration of energy delivery (Fig. 4).
This would presume a compartment including creatine phosphokinase in juxtaposition to the ATP generating site of the sarcosome analagous to the hexokinase compartment. This unit
would be effective only in exercise - generation of creatine -
and the muscle would require insulin only at rest. This compartment was established by the work of Klingenberg, who
showed that an isozyme of creatine phosphokinase was bound to

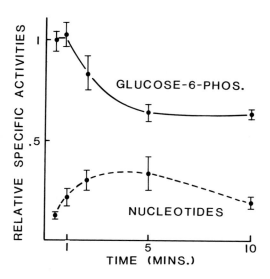

FIGURE 3. Relative specific activities of G-6-P and labile nucleotide phosphates as a function of time. Unlabeled ADP, ATP and $^{32}P_i$ (1 mM each) were supplied to the respiring mitochondria with attached hexokinase. Three of four separate experiments were performed for each point. They are represented as relative specific activities (initial $^{32}P_i = 1$) ± SD. Experimental details are discussed in the text and in Table I.

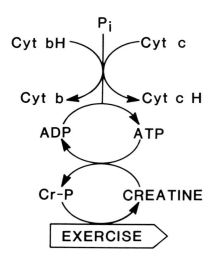

FIGURE 4. The acceptor role of exercise.

sarcosomes, and Fonyo and Bessman, who showed that creatine could produce respiratory control in sarcosomes (12). These observations have been confirmed and extended by Jacobus and Lehninger (13). The picture of a shuttle system of creatine-creatine phosphate for energy translocation from mitochondria to muscle fiber has been completed by the discovery by Turner (14) of an isozyme of creatine phosphokinase attached to the M line of muscle. Saks has provided confirmation of this shuttle in an elegant kinetic analysis (15).

As a result of the hexokinase-mitochondrial binding theory, the mitochondrion was visualized as a "cafeteria" for selective delivery of energy to coenzymes bound at appropriate sites (3). Bachur (Fig. 5) demonstrated that the addition of hexokinase and glucose to a mitochondrial ATP generating system would increase the delivery of ATP to a system with a very high Km and low V-max for ATP (16). The system he chose was the Chou-Lipmann acetyl activating-transfer system of pigeon liver. This crude mixture of enzymes with added CoA activated acetate and transferred it to 4-aminoazobenzene-4'-sulfonic acid (17). He incubated rat liver mitochondria with ketoglutarate and glucose substrate and added increasing amounts of yeast hexokinase. Figure 5 shows that the more hexokinase added, the more acetylation of dye occurred. This result is not to be expected if the added enzymes have equally free access to mitochondrial generated ATP. It provided support for the proposal that both hexokinase and the acyl-activating system have sites at which they preferentially receive ATP.

It was also proposed that the acyl-activating system could not have the same acceptor (respiratory control) effect as hexokinase because the hexokinase reaction utilizes ATP and returns ADP, an effective respiratory control substrate, whereas the acyl-activating enzyme utilized ATP and forms pyrophosphate and AMP, neither of which is effective in respiratory control. The control role of hexokinase (and creatine kinase) is established in preference to all other ATP utilizing anabolic systems which do not deliver ADP but pyrophosphate.

In order further to investigate the properties of the two compartments postulated by the hexokinase-mitochondrial binding theory it was necessary to develop technology to study pool size and turnover of a number of individual glycolytic and nucleotide intermediates. An apparatus was constructed which automatically separates and measures most of the glycolytic and nucleotide intermediates (18-20). A typical chromatogram of an extract of 20 mg of rat diaphragm muscle shows the degree of separation achieved. Fig. 6 is a chromatogram of one milligram of embryo chick retina incubated for 1 minute with

inorganic ^{32}P showing how specific activity, as well as pool
size, can be obtained for minute quantities of glycolytic and
nucleotide intermediates.

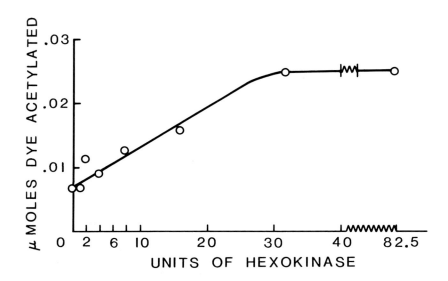

FIGURE 5. The effect of varying yeast hexokinase on 4-
aminoazobenzene-4'-sulfonic acid acetylation in the arylamine
acetylation-mitochondrial system.

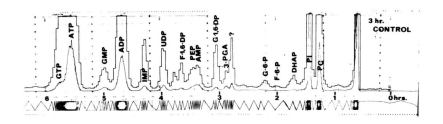

FIGURE 6. Radioactivity of collected fractions shown
superimposed on peaks of chromatogram.

In view of the need for information on the specific activity of both beta and gamma phosphate groups of ATP the following procedure was developed. A chromatogram is run with measurement of specific activity of all intermediates. An aliquot of the initial filtrate is incubated with hexokinase and glucose, causing the formation of glucose-6-phosphate with the same specific activity as the gamma phosphate of the ATP and the transfer of the ATP peak to the ADP area. This provides a direct count of both the beta and gamma phosphate. Fig. 7 and 8 are chromatograms of 50 micrograms of sarcosomes incubated with creatine and ATP for ten seconds. Note the clear separation of creatine phosphate, in this case about 14 nanomoles. The tiny peak in Fig. 8, proximal to glucose-6-phosphate, contains the fructose-6-phosphate formed by a small amount of phosphohexose isomerase contaminating the preparation of hexokinase used. We have found this peak always to have the same specific activity as the glucose-6-phosphate.

Two types of experiments were done to explore the metabolic effect of changes in the hexokinase mitochondrial compartment brought about by the action of insulin in vivo and in vitro. In the first set of experiments, quarter diaphragms of groups of 4 rats, 8 quarters to a flask, were incubated for varying lengths of time in the presence of glucose and inorganic ^{32}P, with and without insulin, 10 milliunits per milliliter. At the end of the incubation period, at varying intervals, the diaphragm pieces were frozen in liquid nitrogen, powdered, and filtrates prepared by a modification of the method of Lowry (21). Aliquots of the filtrates, equivalent to approximately 20 mg wet weight of tissue were subjected to column

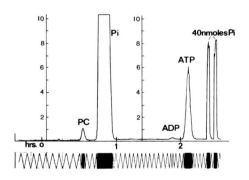

FIGURE 7. Typical chromatogram illustrating separation of the compounds of interest: PC, P_i, ADP, ATP. The 40-nmole P_i standards used for quantitation of the individual peaks were measured in duplicate in order to improve precision. The integrator tracing is also shown at the bottom of the figure.

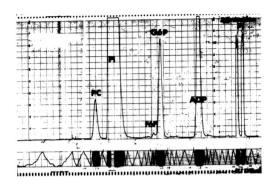

FIGURE 8. Sample similar to that shown in Fig. 7 but
sample treated with hexokinase in order to determine the
specific activity of the gamma and beta phosphate of ATP.

chromatography and counting of each peak both before and after
charcoal treatment to remove nucleotides, and hexokinase treatment to permit the measurement of specific activity of the beta
and gamma phosphate of ATP.

Figure 9 shows the net change in glucose-6-phosphate in
comparison to the non-insulin treated specimens over 14 minutes
of incubation as percent of the parallel control values.   The
data are reported this way because each time period represents
a different group of rats and there were differences between
groups of rats in the net amounts of intermediates.   The relative changes with insulin were always the same, however.

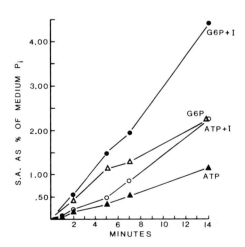

FIGURE 9.   Effect of insulin on the specific activities
of ATP (γ-^{32}P) and G6P in rat diaphragm.

Table I

The effect of insulin on the specific radioactivities of various phosphate compounds of the isolated rat diaphragm incubated in the presence of ^{33}P-labelled inorganic phosphate and glucose.

The data are presented as percent of the specific radioactivity of the inorganic phosphate of the incubation medium. The numbers in brackets indicate percent stimulation by insulin.

Incubation time (min)	Insulin	CP	Intracellular P_i	F6P	G6P	PGA	PEP	FDP	UDPG	βADP	UTP	γATP	βATP	GTP
1	−	0.042	0.708									0.052	0.011	
	+	0.032	0.898									0.063	0.012	
		(−24)	(27)									(22)		
2	−	0.164	1.35	0.282	0.420	0.661	0.296	0.251	0.146	0.084		0.154	0.038	
	+	0.168	2.12	0.414	0.588	0.772	0.368	0.283	0.178	0.113		0.203	0.048	
		(2)	(57)	(46)	(40)	(17)	(24)	(13)	(22)	(35)		(32)	(26)	
5	−	0.391	3.01		1.13	1.75	0.502	0.399	0.346	0.182	0.559	0.351	0.122	0.586
	+	0.433	3.90		1.49	2.15	0.611	0.495	0.457	0.235	0.667	0.490	0.159	0.721
		(11)	(30)		(32)	(23)	(22)	(24)	(32)	(29)	(21)	(40)	(30)	(23)
7	−	0.460	3.94	0.500	1.31	2.21		0.522		0.361		0.508	0.341	
	+	0.649	6.92	0.741	1.96	2.56		0.790		0.596		0.874	0.582	
		(41)	(75)	(48)	(50)	(16)		(51)		(65)		(72)	(71)	
14	−	1.22	7.24	1.40	2.29	3.83	1.12	0.950	0.842	0.990	2.07	1.18	0.88	1.81
	+	1.88	13.4	2.35	4.43	4.29	1.68	1.44	1.20	1.73	3.77	2.28	1.48	3.11
		(54)	(85)	(68)	(94)	(12)	(50)	(52)	(42)	(75)	(82)	(93)	(68)	(72)

Table I shows the specific activity of several phosphate compounds of interest with time, as percent of specific activity of intracellular inorganic phosphate. It is clear that glucose-6-phosphate has a much higher specific activity than the gamma phosphate of ATP or any other phosphate compound. We interpret this to mean that the phosphorylation of glucose is taking place primarily through the mitochondrial bound hexokinase.

In these experiments it can be calculated that approximately 75% of the glucose phosphorylated was phosphorylated on the mitochondrion even though less than 20% of the total hexokinase activity of muscle cell is attached to the sarcosomes (22). This experiment also is consistent with the data of Insel et al (23) who showed by mathematical analysis that there are two "compartments" for the utilization of glucose - the one increased by insulin and the other one apparently diminished in proportion to the increase of the first one. This is consistent with our proposal that insulin increases the functional attachment of hexokinase to the mitochondrion creating a special compartment. It would appear metabolically as an inverse relation between two compartments.

The second group of experiments was done as follows: Rats were anesthetized and a tourniquet was placed as high as possible up one hind leg. The leg was then amputated, the muscle excised, defatted, and put into ice-cold mannitol EDTA-Tris phosphate buffer, pH 7.2, 10 volumes. Immediately after the tourniquet was placed, 10 units of insulin were injected intraperitoneally. Five minutes after the injection of insulin a tourniquet was placed on the other leg and the muscles stripped and placed in 10 volumes of cold buffer solution in the same way as the first leg. Homogenates were then prepared from both tissues, centrifuged at 500 g to remove large cellular debris and incubated with added inorganic ^{33}P (20 µCi).

Figure 10 shows the specific activities of glucose-6-phosphate and the gamma phosphate of ATP during the course of incubation. There are several noteworthy effects. In the first place, in the insulin treated leg muscle homogenate practically all of the glucose-6-phosphate is formed in the first two minutes. This probably represents exhaustion of the endogenous glucose of the medium. The maintenance of the glucose-6-phosphate specific activity is in fact caused by the fact that there is not much turnover of the glucose-6-phosphate that has been formed. In the non-insulin treated homogenate the glucose-6-phosphate increases in specific activity during the course of the incubation but does not attain, in 10 minutes, the specific activity of the glucose-6-phosphate of the insulin-treated

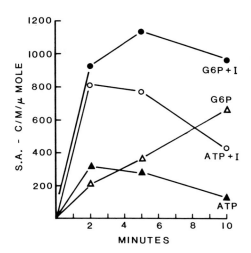

FIGURE 10.   Specific activities of glucose-6-phosphate and
ATP from homogenates of rat leg muscle before and after insulin treatment <u>in vivo</u>.

muscle homogenate. On the other hand, in both the insulin-
treated and the control homogenates the ATP reaches a maximum
in two minutes and then falls off.   This suggests, again, that
insulin makes a more efficient connection of hexokinase with
mitochondria and stimulates the turnover of mitochondrial ATP.
    The second form of compartmentation proposed by the insu-
lin-hexokinase theory is the creatine phosphate shuttle.
Quantitative experiments to test the degree of connection of
creatine kinase to the mitochondrion or the specificity of the
mitochondrial bound creatine kinase for mitochondrial generated ATP have not shown the same type of compartmentation as
were revealed for hexokinase by the experiments of Gots (11).
    Experiments similar to those in which Gots showed direct
incorporation of labelled P_i into glucose-6-phosphate independent of the presence of large amounts of unlabelled ATP in
the medium failed to show the same direct connection between
creatine kinase and the mitochondrion.   In all cases the
specific activity of creatine phosphate was lower than the
gamma phosphate of ATP and the activity of the gamma phosphate
of ATP could not account for the lower specific activity of
the creatine phosphate.

   Experiments were then undertaken using gamma ^{32}P labelled
ATP. The experiments again showed that the creatine phosphate
formed during incubation for 5 to 15 seconds could not all have
come from the gamma phosphate of ATP; the creatine phosphate
was always approximately 1/3 as active as the gamma phosphate
of ATP. The question then arose as to where the phosphate for
creatine phosphate formation actually came from. It could not
come from the inorganic phosphate of the medium the way glu-
cose-6-phosphate came, nor could it come from the gamma phosphate of ATP primarily. Experiments were then undertaken using inhibitors of oxidative phosphorylation or of nucleotide
transport and the data in Table II were obtained.
   Here we see that in the control experiment a certain
amount of creatine phosphate is formed when it is incubated
with gamma labelled ATP and this has 1/3 the specific activity
of ATP. Incubation with either an inhibitor of oxidative
phosphorylation CCCH* or with atractyloside, an inhibitor of
nucleotide transport, permits the formation of approximately
1/3 of the control amount of creatine phosphate, but this
creatine phosphate now has exactly the same specific activity
as the gamma phosphate of ATP. We conclude that the creatine
phosphate formed by the sarcosome is made 1/3 from exogenous,
or cytoplasmic, ATP and 2/3 from some other source. It may
be noted that the net amount of creatine phosphate formed is
equal to more than 10 times the total pre-existing organic
phosphate of the mitochondrion so that there is no question of
dilution by pre-formed high energy phosphate.
   The experiments with labelled inorganic phosphate show an
incorporation of label into creatine phosphate such that a
deficit of approximately 35-40% in the identifiable sources of
ATP for creatine phosphate formation is observed. Incubation
with beta-gamma labelled ATP results in the formation of
creatine phosphate of very high specific activity, almost
equal to the phosphate label of ATP.
   We have, therefore, tentatively concluded that there is a
special connection of creatine kinase to the mitochondrion
which involves myokinase. In order to account for the observed phenomena there must be two molecules of myokinase
bound to an oxidative phosphorylation site and to a second
molecule of myokinase to which is bound a molecule of creatine
kinase. This proposed arrangement is shown in Figure 11 as a
sequence of reactions with M-1 and M-2 indicating simply two
different molecules of myokinase.

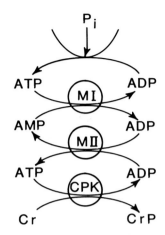

FIGURE 11. Schematic representation of the way in which myokinase connects creatine phosphokinase to oxidative phosphorylation in the mitochondrion.

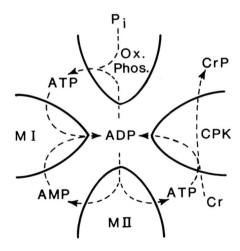

FIGURE 12. A possible architectural arrangement of enzymes comprising the "comparticle".

Figure 12 shows a tetrahedral arrangement of these four units, the oxidative phosphorylation site, the two myokinase molecules, and the creatine kinase molecule around a common

Table II

Effect of Atractyloside and CCH on mitochondrial CP formation*

	Incubation Time (sec.)	CP			ATP			ADP	Total Nucleotides
		nmol	cpm/nmol	Total Counts	nmol	cpm/nmol	Total Counts	nmol	nmol
Control	5	8.58	8644	74167	29.4	24039	706728	2.40	31.8
	10	12.20	10133	123625	28.5	19870	566294	2.86	31.4
CCH 4×10^{-6} M	5	2.26	26475	59833	26.0	30673	797494	4.98	31.0
	10	3.49	30424	106181	24.7	29187	702705	6.43	31.1
Atractyloside 5×10^{-8} M	5	2.81	24953	70119	25.9	29866	773521	4.38	30.2
	10	3.31	30890	102274	24.8	29977	743432	6.65	31.5

*One ml of incubation mixture contained α-KG, 5mM; ATP [γ-^{32}P], 0.8 mM; Mg^{++}, 1.5 mM; P_i, 5 mM; Cr, 10 mM; DTT, 0.1 mM. Incubation temperature, 30°C. CCH is Carbonylcyanide m-chlorophenyl hydrazone, DTT is Dithiothreitol. Values shown were contained in 200 µl of neutralized acid extract.

pool of ADP. This would provide two portals of entry of ATP and one of AMP and an exit portal of creatine phosphate. This hypothetical unit we would like to name "comparticle".

This hypothesis fits many requirements. In the first place, creatine kinase differs remarkably from hexokinase in its sensitivity to inhibition by product ADP. This mechanism would provide a prompt and efficient process for removal of ADP. It would also explain the efficiency of totally labelled ATP in labelling creatine phosphate and it would provide an explanation for the inability of mitochondrial generated phosphate directly to label creatine phosphate. It would also provide an explanation of the inability of gamma labelled ATP totally to label creatine phosphate. What is of further interest is that it might give us an opportunity, for the first time, to understand the role of myokinase which has been relegated at present to a scavenger role in recognition only of our lack of understanding of its actual metabolic role. Experiments are underway further to test this hypothesis which grows out of a theory for the mechanism of insulin action which has already been fruitful in explaining a number of physiologic phenomena.

REFERENCES

1. Bessman, S.P., in Fat Metabolism (V. Najjar, Ed.) p. 133. Johns Hopkins Press, Baltimore, Md. (1954)
2. Bessman, S.P., J. Pediatr. 56:191 (1960)
3. Bessman, S.P., Am. J. Med. 40:740 (1966)
4. Srere, P.A. and Mosbach, K., Ann. Rev. Microbiol. 29 (1974)
5. Crane, R.K. and Sols, A., J. Biol. Chem. 203:273 (1953)
6a. Katzen, H.M., Adv. in Enz. Reg. 5:335 (1967)
6b. Katzen, H.M., Soderman, D.D. and Wiley, C.E., J. Biol. Chem. 245:4081 (1970)
7. Walters, E. and McLean, P., Biochem. J. 109:737 (1968)
8. Borrebaek, B., Biochem. Med. 3:485 (1970)
9. Gumaa, K.A. and McLean, P., Biochem. Biophys. Res. Commun. 36:771 (1969)
10. DeSchepper, P.J., Toyoda, M. and Bessman, S.P., J. Biol. Chem. 240:4 (1965)
11. Gots, R.E. and Bessman, S.P., Arch. Biochem. Biophys. 163:7 (1974)
12. Bessman, S.P. and Fonyo, A., Biochem. Biophys. Res. Commun. 22:597 (1966)
13. Jacobus, W.E. and Lehninger, A.L., J. Biol. Chem. 21: 4803 (1973)
14. Turner, D.C., Wallimann, T. and Eppenberger, H.M., Proc. Nat. Acad. Sci. USA 70:702 (1973)

15. Saks, V.A., Chernousova, G.B., Gukovsky, D.E., Smirnov, V.N. and Chazov, E.I., Eur. J. Biochem. 57:273 (1975)
16. Bachur, N., Doctoral Thesis, University of Maryland (1961)
17. Bessman, S.P. and Lipmann, F., Arch. Biochem. 46:252 (1953)
18. Bessman, S.P., Anal. Biochem. 59:524 (1974)
19. Bessman, S.P., Geiger, P.J., Lu, T.C. and McCabe, E.R.B., Anal. Biochem. 59:533 (1974)
20. Geiger, P.J., Ahn, S. and Bessman, S.P., in Methods in Carbohydrate Chemistry (R. Whistler, ed.), in press 1977
21. Lowry, O.H. and Passonneau, J.V. in A Flexible System of Enzymatic Analysis, p. 123, Academic Press, N.Y. (1972)
22. Katzen, H.M., Soderman, D.D. and Wiley, C.E., J. Biol. Chem. 245:4081 (1970)
23. Insel, P.A., Liljenquist, J.E., Tobin, J.D., Sherwin, R.S., Watkins, P., Andres, R. and Berman, M., J. Clin. Invest. 55:1057 (1975)

DISCUSSION

R. WELCH: I have a couple of questions for Dr. Bessman. One specific question: When hexokinase binds to the mitochondrial membrane, does the inhibition effect seen with glucose-6-phosphate change? Second is a more general question concerning this "cafeteria table model" for the dispensation of nascent ATP. I find it very enticing. Would you go so far as to suggest that all kinase-type reactions, for example those involved in biosynthetic processes, might be subject to this type of dispensation? As you may know, some years ago Robert Wagner (in "Organizational Biosynthesis, ed. H. J. Vogel, J. O. Lampen, and V. Bryson, p. 267, Academic Press, New York, 1967) suggested that the mitochondria were cellular centers for the biosynthesis of amino acids. Wagner and coworkers showed that the isoleucine-leucine-valine pathway binds reversibly to the outer mitochondrial membrane, depending upon the metabolic state of the mitochondrion (Proc. Natl. Acad. Sci. (USA), 71, 4352, 1974). So, would you be willing to generalize that concept?

S. BESSMAN: Anytime - delighted. The work by a number of people, including Dr. Raijman, who is doing some work with mitochondrial synthesis of carbamyl phosphate, and others who are doing work with various kinases, all seem to indicate the cafeteria principle. We call the mitochondria a little outboard motor that goes around the cell and supplies

energy. It may be interesting to point out that when mitochondrial energy generation is stimulated by insulin, it
spews out energy wherever it happens to be. The cell in
which insulin is most effective in stimulating transport is
the fat cell. The interesting thing here is that other cells
have the mitochondria floating around in various places and
very few adjacent to the membrane, but the fat cell has the
mitochondria all plastered up against the cell membrane. Apparently their transport systems are very well endowed when
you supply insulin. The second part of your question about
inhibition by glucose-6-phosphate is interesting. Work by
I. Rose (J. Biol. Chem. <u>242</u>, 1635, 1967) and a number of
others on the glucose-6-phosphate inhibition of hexokinase
showed that it removes or splits off the bound hexokinase
from the mitochondria. So, the kinetics are very complicated and studies to determine what is really taking place
with the mitochondrial bound hexokinase is very hard work.
There is evidence from a number of laboratories that the
kinetics of the "bound enzyme" are different from what
we call a "free enzyme".

<u>R. WELCH</u>: One related question. What do you think of the
situation in cells, like certain tumor cells or brain cells,
where it is thought that hexokinase might be bound to mitochondria all the time?

<u>S. BESSMAN</u>: I am glad you asked that question. We de-
scribed this in the first paper we wrote in 1954 (Fat Metabolism, V. Najjar (Editor), Johns Hopkins Press, Baltimore,
Md., p. 133). Dr. Lipmann, incidentally was chairman of that
meeting. We pointed out that the lack of effect of insulin
on brain is caused by the fact that it already has hexokinase
attached. Two physiological phenomena, exercise, and the
autonomy of brain in relation to insulin, are both explained
by the hexokinase-mitochondrial complex. It is noteworthy
that all of the stress hormones are designed to generate glucose in order to keep the machinery going in the head-that is
a teleological explaination - but in fact that appears to be
the way the organism survives. Glucose is absolutely necessary; it is not the only substrate of brain metabolism, but
it is necessary for everything else to be oxidized efficient-
ly. A level of approximately 50 milligrams per deciliter
of glucose keeps the hexokinase system saturated.

<u>J. KATZ</u>: I have two questions. First of all I would like
you to explain - if you presume that mitochondria make
phosphorylation more efficient - how phosphorylation is
faster in anaerobic cells than in the presence of oxygen.
That seems to indicate that mitochondria have very little

to do with it.   Second, have you done a control experiment
incubating your homogenates without mitochondria?

S. BESSMAN: I could put it a different way.   We have incubated red cells without mitochondria, which have the
whole glycolytic system, and there is no effect of insulin.
Second, you can also say that mitochondria oxidize faster
when you poison them.   We could give dinitrophenol and
increase the rate of oxidation, but we know now that it
starts a new acceptor system which destroys itself.   I don't
think we can use that kind of information to discuss this
issue.

METABOLIC POOLS

MICROHETEROGENEITIES OF REDOX STATES
OF PERFUSED AND INTACT ORGANS

Britton Chance
Clyde Barlow
John Haselgrove
Yuzo Nakase
Bjørn Quistorff
Franz Matschinsky
Avraham Mayevsky

Johnson Research Foundation
University of Pennsylvania
Philadelphia, Pennsylvania

Microheterogeneity or metabolic activity is an essential
property of some tissues in the normal state and of many in
pathological states. Rapid methods for nondestructive, non-
invasive evaluation of metabolic heterogeneity due to spatio-
temporal variations of metabolic activity can most readily be
evaluated by a two-dimensional flying spot scanner that reads
out in real-time a histogram display of the distribution of
redox states as measured by the fluorescence of mitochondrial
flavoprotein or NADH. Another nondestructive technique is
that of ^{31}P NMR which, while global in its signal averaging,
discriminates the pH value of different tissue compartments.
Three dimensional resolution of metabolic microheterogeneity
can be obtained by redox scanning and sectioning of tissues in
appropriate states of heterogeneity, for example, model infarcts
of heart, metabolic states of liver, and local ischemias of
brain. Sections scanned at distances of 100 microns can be
assembled into three dimensional displays of tissue volumes in
which homogeneous redox states are obtained. Microanalytical
biochemistry using 50 ng samples gives results which control
and amplify those of redox scanning.

I. INTRODUCTION

The classical approach of analytical biochemistry and
indeed of surface fluorometry has been to average the metabolic states of all the cells in the particular tissue under

Copyright © 1978 by Academic Press, Inc.
All right of reproduction in any form reserved.
ISBN 0-12-660550-5

observation (1). Scanning micro-fluorometry of NADH fluorescence of the brain cortex (2) and more recently the development of 2- and 3-D redox scanning procedures for NADH and flavoprotein (Fp)(3), together with the deoxyglucose labelling techniques (4) clearly show the intrinsic complexity and heterogeneity of cell and tissue metabolism as suggested by other methods (5).

The apparently tried and true concept of homogenization of cells and tissues that made it possible to obtain large samples appropriate to the low sensitivities of the method apparently obscured the real distribution of metabolic states prior to homogenization. There are two types of heterogeneity that are readily demonstratable; temporal and spatial.

A.   Temporal Heterogeneity

Metabolic oscillations (Figure 1) have been studied together with Estabrook (6) and Hess (7) in yeast cell suspensions and found to occur in heart (8) and in heart extracts by Frenkel (9). Here the amplitude of the oscillations is so large that ignoring the temporal heterogeneity would lead to "nonsense" assays in biochemical recording. In optical recording the assays can be timed to occur at the peaks or nodes of the oscillatory cycle (10) and thus be extremely useful.

B.   Spatial Heterogeneity

The current discussion and the papers at this symposium emphasize inhomogeneities of distribution of enzymes in the liver lobule and the consequent differences of metabolism in different parts of the liver lobule (5,11).

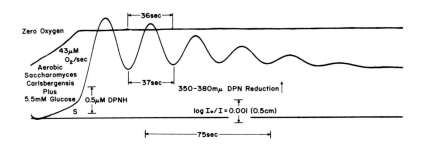

FIGURE 1.   Temporal heterogeneities of metabolic control: NADH oscillations in anaerobic yeast cells (Saccharomyces carlsbergensis).

C. Spatio-temporal Heterogeneity

Spatio-temporal heterogeneities may occur in unstirred
solutions as in Prigogine's "phase separations" (12), and in
solid tissues as for example in the propagated disturbances
such as spreading depression or epilepsy in the brian (13,14)
(Figure 2). Preliminary spectroscopic observations of cytochrome $\underline{a}$ and oxymyoglobin indicated spatio-temporal heterogeneities of O_2 delivery to perfused heart (15).

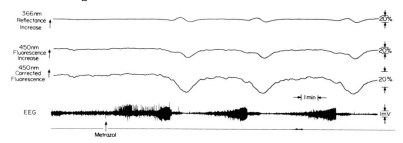

FIGURE 2. NADH oscillations due to spatio-temporal
metabolic heterogeneity represented by periodic electrical and metabolic activity introduced by an intra-
venous metrazol injection in an anesthetized rat
(Unpublished data of Mayevsky, A. and Chance, B.)

II. METHODOLOGICAL ASPECTS

A. Localized Indicators of Metabolic Activities

The identification of heterogeneities requires resolution
of the metabolic state to intracellular dimensions and for this
purpose mitochondria have proved themselves to be appropriate
indicators of the metabolic intensity in tissue, affording a
"consumer report" on metabolic activity and tissue oxygen
delivery. The responses in various metabolic states are indicated by Figure 3A which indicates the correlation between
metabolic state (16,17) and oxidation-reduction level of reduced pyridine nucleotide. Since oxygen delivery to tissue is
intrinsically discrete and heterogeneous due to the nature of
the capillary bed, changes in response to variations of the
oxygen concentration (Figure 3B) are very useful. A quantitation of this response is indicated in Figure 3D, which shows
how the pyridine nucleotide component (NADH) is a more sensitive indicator of tissue oxygen tension than is cytochrome $\underline{c}$.
The most important aspect of the PN response is that it
precisely follows the energy coupling response for mitochondria
and thus serves as an indicator of both oxygen tension and
energy coupling (18,19).

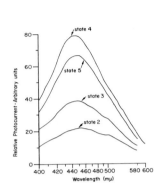

FIGURE 3A. Effect of metabolic state upon NADH redox level in rat liver mitochondria (18).

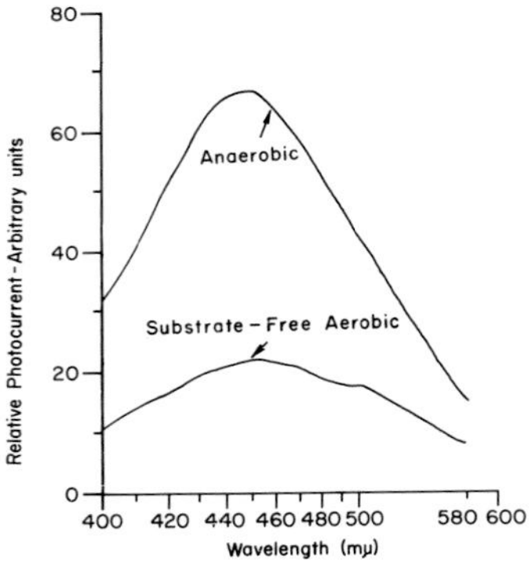

FIGURE 3B. Effect of oxygen upon NADH fluorescence in rat liver mitochondria (18).

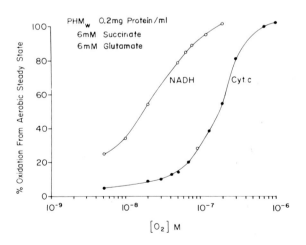

FIGURE 3C. A titration of NADH and cytochrome <u>c</u> with oxygen in isolated mitochondria (19).

B.   The Flavoprotein Component of Mitochondria

The excitation-emission spectra for NADH and flavoprotein are compared in Fig. 4 which indicates that the oxidized state of flavoprotein will be observed exclusively in oxidized mito- chondria whereas in reduced mitochondria, the pyridine nucleo- tide component is exclusively observed.   Thus the ratio of the two signals gives a redox ratio largely independent of distribution and screening errors (20). These excitation-emis- sion spectra were taken at low temperatures, although back- ground pigments interfere more at the higher temperature.

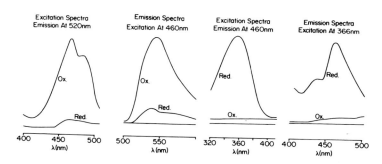

FIGURE 4.   Low temperature excitation-emission spectra for PN (366 → 460 nm) and Fp (460 → 520 nm) for cardiac mitochondria (pigeon).

The localization of the highly fluorescent flavoprotein signal is within the mitochondrial space with the α-ketoglu- tarate and pyruvate dehydrogenases.   The NADH signal at low temperature originates almost exclusively from the mitochon- drial space while at room temperature in the perfused liver NADH signals may also be observed from the cytoplasm and from the NADPH pool.

C.   Two-dimensional Ratio Recording

By time-sharing the excitation-emission wavelengths for Fp and PN it is possible to obtain signals from tissues whose ratio will represent the redox state of the material.   The calibration procedure is described elsewhere (21).   Such an instrument coupled to a lightguide of 20 to 80 microns in tip diameter can be used to scan a smoothed tissue section as indicated in the diagram of Figure 5.

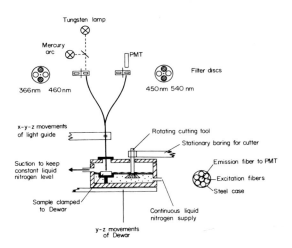

FIGURE 5. Illustrating the method of time-sharing Fp
and PN signals, 2-D lightguide scanning of tissue section, and low temperature grinding of tissue surface
for scans of consecutive sections.

The motion of the lightguide across the tissue is precisely controlled by a computer and Fp/PN fluorescence ratio
recordings are acquired from over the surface of the tissue
section. When one scan is finished the tissue may be ground
in the rotating mill (22) and sections between 20 and 50
microns may be removed. The scan is then repeated so that a
series of sections is accumulated, affording a series of 2-D
presentations which can be displayed in 3-D.

III.   RESULTS

A.   Metabolic Heterogeneity in Cardiac Ishemia

The topical question of the nature and extent of the border
zone in cardiac infarcts (23 - 25) is clarified by a series of
sections of heart tissue containing a model coronary occlusion
that are displayed in Figure 6. It seems that each one of the
successive 100 µ tissue sections has borders that are quite
sharp, as sharp as the 80 µ resolution of the scanner. In
addition, the shape of the model infarct can be followed
from the epicardium to the endocardium (see Figure 9).

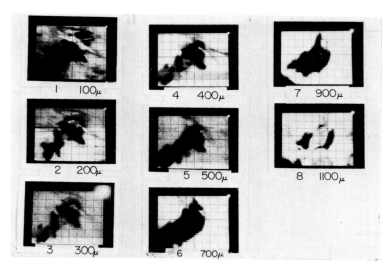

FIGURE 6. Consecutive 2-D scans of a model cardiac infarct from epi- to endocardium. The initial layer of the heart is scanned by the Fp/PN fluorometer at 80 μ resolution and the results are plotted as a 2-D redox picture with the reduced state black (low Fp/PN ratio) and the oxidized state white (high Fp/PN ratio). The initial scan represents a surface somewhat distorted by freeze-clamping, but later surfaces clearly outline the shape of the infarct proceeding from 100 μ below the epicardium to the endocardium (section 8).

B. The Steepness of the Border Zone in Model Infarcts

   (a)   Redox measurements

In order to compare three methods for evaluating the nature of the border zone, redox data are presented in Figures 7 and a combination of redox and analytical biochemical data in Figure 8. In Figure 7 a model coronary occlusion has been applied to a rabbit heart, the heart has been freeze-trapped and sectioned across the model infarct. Five identifying dots (actually drilled holes) appear as indices for the subsequent analysis. Figure 7A illustrates the use of NADH flash photography as applied to the freeze-trapped tissue; the bright areas represent reduced NAD and the dark areas oxidized NAD. The center mark of the indices is the reference point for the three subsequent displays (Figures 7B-D) illustrating the use of the lightguide scanner in evaluating the redox state of the ischemic and normoxic areas as was employed in the scan of Figure 6. Figure 7B shows the scan for NADH fluorescence. Contours of

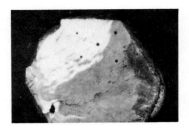

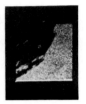

B. NADH Fluorescence Scan

A. NADH Fluorescence Photograph

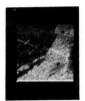

C. Flavoprotein Fluorescence Scan   D. Ratio Scan

FIGURE 7. Comparison of redox scanning methods on a
freeze-trapped section of rabbit heart with model
coronary occlusion. A, NADH flash photography.
B, Lightguide scan, NADH excitation and emission.
C, Lightguide scan, flavoprotein excitation and
emission. D, Lightguide Fp/PN ratio. Note that
the central marker of the left figure appears in
each one of the subsequent ones.

the border zones of Figures 7A and 7B are nearly identical
testifying to the equality of performance of the two methods
for 2-D NADH assay. Figure 7C is the scan of the ischemic and
the normoxic areas with excitation and emission appropriate to
flavoprotein and the figure is clearly complementary to Figure
7B. This illustrates how the ratio of these two quantities
(Figure 7D) gives a redox state diagram less dependent upon
variable distribution of mitochondria or an effect of screening
pigments as indicated by the "smoothing" of the irregular signals introduced by the index signals in the heart.
    Figure 8 displays quantitative analysis of the NADH scan
of Figure 7B (circled dots) showing the rise of NADH fluorescence as one progresses from the dark aerobic portion to the
index marker in the bright ischemic portion. The trace rises
from 20-80% in a distance of 200 μ.

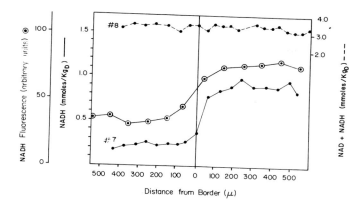

FIGURE 8. A comparison of the border zone delineated by redox scan of Figure 7B (Circle dot) and microanalytical biochemistry of NADH (solid trace) with total pyridine nucleotides (dashed trace). The microtome sections were 15 μ apart. The NADH assay (solid) was 105 μ below the surface of that represented by Figure 7. The top trace (dashes) was 120 μ below the surface.

(b) Microanalytical biochemistry

Microanalytical biochemistry can also be used to define the border between the two zones. Analyses of NADH (solid trace) is made along the same line across the border zone of the same specimen, but a section deeper below the surface; the particular section was 105 μ below the surface of Figure 7 and was 15 μ thick. The sample volume was 50 ng and and each point corresponds to a different sample. A quantitative assay in terms of millimoles per kilo dry weight (m moles/kg_D) is afforded. The two traces are very similar and both give the same contour for the border zone. In order to ensure that no pyridine nucleotides were lost from the ischemic portion of the heart under the conditions of the experiments, the top trace gives the total of NAD plus NADH which is maintained at 3 millimoles per kg dry weight.

These data clearly identify the border zone in rabbit heart to involve the transition from normal aerobic respiring tissue to ischemic anoxic tissue in a distance of 200 μ. It appears that adequate resolution is obtainable from both redox scanning and analytical biochemistry to precisely identify the position of the border zone between normoxic and anoxic ischemic areas in model cardiac infarcts.

These values may be compared to the distance of 8-15 mm obtained by Hearse, et al (24) who used a much larger sample volume in the dog heart. Presumably the use of more highly

resolved analytical techniques would give sharper border zones
in model infarcts in the dog heart.

(c)   Three dimensional redox display

The possibility of a three dimensional display of such
data has been explored recently and an assembly of the sections
of Figure 6 are displayed in Figure 9.   Here sections corresponding to the border zone of the 8 scans of Figure 6 are displayed in the three dimensional series giving the general shape
of the infarct proceeding from the endocardial side to the epi-
cardial side.   Each section in this figure is 100 μ thick, very
nearly equal to the maximum depth from which fluorescent signals
can be obtained from the frozen tissue.   For this reason, no
correction for material lying at a depth greater than 100 μ from
the surface of the frozen heart is necessary.
One of the noteworthy features of the three dimensional
display is that the ischemic area does not appear to increase
in size as one proceeds from the epicardium to the endocardium.
Thus, we have demonstrated the general principles of the redox
scanning combined with the micro-analysis and its applicability
to a variety of systems.

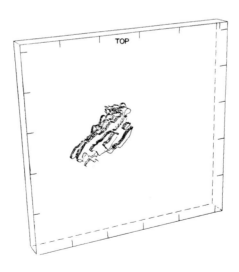

FIGURE 9.   A 3-D assembly of sections 2-D of the
infarct of Figure 6 from endo- to epicardium.

B.   Kinetics of Changes in Two-dimensional Metabolic Heterogeneity

As convenient as the 3-D method is, the data are based upon one sample of tissue trapped at a moment of time and does not permit further following the metabolic events in that particular portion of the organ.   For this reason we have considered a method that would read out in real time the metabolic hetero-geneity from the surface of the organ in order to provide a maximally "interesting" metabolic state (presumably one in which there is maximal deviation from the average) for freeze-trapping analytical biochemistry and redox scanning (3,25,26).   The principles of the scanner are indicated in Figure 10.   Here, a source illuminates two vibrating mirrors which afford a faster scan over the sample of about 1 cm^2 in area.   The fluorescent light is focused by a Fresnel lens, measured by a photomul-tiplier via a secondary filter.   The analysis circuit provides a histogram of the intensity of the signal versus the number of signals having a given intensity level for 64 levels.   20,000 points may be gathered in one second to form an extremely precise histogram.

Using laser light appropriate to the excitation of reduced pyridine nucleotide (350/363 nm) or flavoprotein (457.9 nm) it is possible to generate histograms for both of these pigments as shown in Figure 11 for a perfused liver.

In this case the histograms for the normoxic state have been matched so that they are superimposed one upon the other for the condition of normal flow through the liver (30 ml/min). If the flow is diminished to 5 ml/min the pyridine nucleotide fluorescence increases while the flavoprotein fluorescence

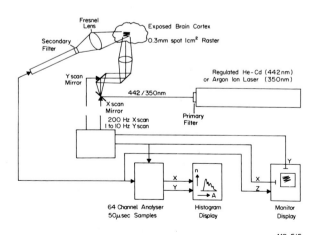

FIGURE 10.   Block diagram of 2-D flying spot fluorometer with on-line histogram display.

decreases.   The diagrams show how pyridine nucleotide
and flavoprotein change in their respective opposite directions.
Changes of heterogeneity are indicated also.   In the anoxic state,
the reduced pyridine nucleotide histogram becomes broader and the
flavoprotein histogram becomes narrower.

Flying Spot Fluorometer
Flavoprotein (457.9 → 540 nm)
NADH (350/363 → 450nm)
Perfused Rat Liver   4 x 4mm Raster

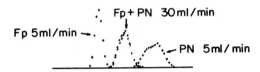

FIGURE 11.   Illustrating the opposite response of Fp
and PN histograms in a high-flow, low-flow hypoxia of
a perfused rat liver.

C. Perfused Heart

The application of this technique to the heterogeneity of
perfused heart is indicated in terms of flavin fluorescence in
Figure 12.   The normoxic histogram is distributed over most of
the register as indicated in the left-hand diagram.   This is
characteristic of the "average" perfused heart where microheterogeneities in the redox pattern are due to small ischemic
areas.   In diagram B a major ischemic is imposed upon the heart
by occlusion of a portion of the coronary artery resulting in
intracellular anoxia in a portion of the tissue under observation.
The histogram maintains its characteristics at 15, 30 and 60 sec.
Thereafter, the ligature is released and the recovery pattern 5 min
later is nearly identical to that prior to the coronary occlusion.
The difference of the two histograms is emphasized by the
superimposed diagrams of Figure 12D.   A cut-out and weighing of
the differences between the two portions indicates that 20% of the
area scanned is rendered anoxic by the model infarct.   Those portions affected mostly by the model infarct are those having the
highest fluorescence intensity and hence the most normoxic state.
These histograms are recorded once every second but can be recorded in 0.1 sec.   Thus, the mirror scan can be synchronized with
the heart beat so that the histogram can be attributed to systole
or diastole.

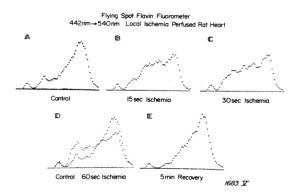

FIGURE 12.   Changes of Fp histogram of a perfused rat
heart following a model coronary occlusion.

D.   Metabolic Heterogeneities in Brain Tissue

Scans of a portion of the left brain cortex of a gerbil (Fig.
13 - experiments in collaboration with A. Mayevsky) indicate in
the top left-hand diagram the histogram in response to NADH fluorescence excitation in normoxia (left) and anoxia (30 sec).

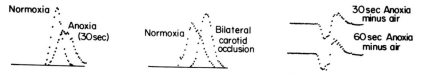

FIGURE 13.   Comparison of NADH histograms of gerbil brain
before and after bilateral carotid artery occlusion and
systemic anoxia

The normoxic histogram which extends over 65% of the scale
is replaced by the anoxic histogram which extends over 62%
of the scale.   The heterogeneity of NADH redox states in
anoxia seems significantly greater than that of normoxia as
indicated by the smaller height and greater breadth of the
anoxic histogram. Since the blood flow to the gerbil brain
is largely delivered by the carotid arteries, bilateral occlusion gives an almost complete anoxia as indicated in the
right-hand diagram.   However the heterogeneity of the ischemic tissue is less , the amplitude is larger and the base
of the histogram subtends only 58% of the scale.   Thus a
quantitative difference between a systemic anoxia and
low flow ischemia is indicated by the simple histogram
technique.

E.   Flavoprotein Fluorescence of Perfused and in situ Liver.

The application of the flying spot flavin fluorometer to
the evaluation of heterogeneity of redox states in the perfused liver is indicated in Figure 14.

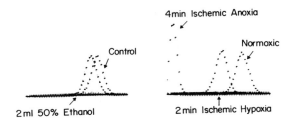

FIGURE 14. Histogram displays of metabolic changes of
Fp in rat liver in situ.

On the right are three histograms indicating the progression
from normoxia (extreme right), two minutes ischemia, and
four min. ischemia (approximately 50% shift to the left).
(The zero point of the histogram scale is set at 50% in this
particular case to provide amplifications of the histograms).
The remarkable feature here is the considerably greater homogeneity of the anoxic state of liver as measured by flavoprotein fluorescence. This might be expected, however, since
in anoxia the flavoprotein of the α-ketoglutarate and pyruvate dehydrogenases has no other metabolic pathways to participate in.
On the left is indicated the response of the Fp redox
state to injection of a high concentration of alcohol into
the stomach. After 30 min. it is seen that the histogram
shifts to the left indicating reduction. In this case,
however, there is no change of heterogeneity of the metabolic states, apparently in this case those mitochondria
metabolizing alcohol have the same heterogeneity characteristics as in the absence of alcohol.
These examples are afforded in order to give some idea
of how a two-dimensional flying spot scanner can be used
to select appropriate deviations of metabolic states by 2-D
redox scanning and micro-analytical biochemistry.

F. ^{31}P Nuclear Magnetic Resonance

THe fourth approach to be described is that of ^{31}P nuclear magnetic resonance, Figure 15.

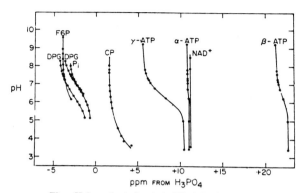

The pH-dependent chemical shift behavior of a variety of biological organic phosphates. Chemical shifts are reported relative to external 1.0 M phosphoric acid. *F6P*, fructose 6-phosphate; *DPG*, 2,3-diphosphoglycerate; *CP*, carbamyl phosphate.

FIGURE 15. Courtesy of Journal of Biological Chemistry (Ref. 27).

As shown, there is a pH dependence of several of the signals that are likely to be present in aerobic cells, particularly ATP and the sugar phosphates. Such signals have been obtained from skeletal muscle[28,29] and perfused heart.[30,31] The most prevalent signal of the anaerobic cell is inorganic phosphate and the chemical shift with decreasing pH is clearly shown by this diagram. The shift of the signal has been used to indicate intracellular pH.

In order to indicate the performance that is now obtainable from perfused organs, Figure 16 illustrates the ^{31}P nuclear magnetic resonance signals obtained from a perfused liver in the wide bore 360 megahertz (protons) NMR recently added to the Eastern Regional NMR Facility at the University of Pennsylvania.

Clearly shown in this diagram are resonances due to α, β, γ ATP and α ADP as well. The two peaks of phosphate are attributed to the pH 7.4 of the perfusate and somewhat less ($\sim$0.3 unit) for the intracellular P_i. The salient feature of the intracellular phosphate peak is its spread suggesting a heterogeneity of phosphate enviroments, most probably the cytosolic phosphate and the mitochondrial phosphate. While these signals are not well resolved under these conditions, further studies will lead to eventual resolution of the phosphate compartments of the metabolizing tissue.

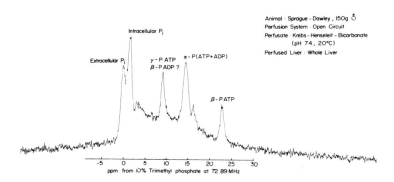

FIGURE 16. ^{31}P NMR spectrum of aerobic rat liver
(perfused)(Experiments in collaboration with
Dr. George MacDonald and Ms. M. Bond)

IV.   DISCUSSION

The ability to cope with microheterogeneity of metabolic
states of tissues and organs is in its infancy and the four
techniques described here are at the beginning of their scientific application to the manifold problems presented to the biochemist in his new departure to metabolic heterogeneity.
Recognizing the great usefulness of enzyme distribution, it has
nevertheless been essential to consider the redox ratios of key
couples of both glycolysis and respiration. In order to begin
with the problem of metabolic heterogeneity it has been essential
to develop "short cut" methods for evaluating the nature and
extent of the heterogeneity before attempting more detailed procedures. For this reason we consider the on-line direct readout
capability of the two dimensional flying spot fluorometer to be a
key starting point in investigations of metabolic heterogeneity.
The instrument is designed specifically to examine the time course
of heterogeneities through a variety of metabolic transitions and
therefore identify what we choose to term "maximal deviation
metabolic states". A similar approach can be obtained through
the use of ^{31}P NMR by observations of microheterogeneity of the
phosphate resonance or possibly the ATP and sugar phosphate
resonances. At the present time, the ^{31}P NMR method gives clear
signals from extracellular and intracellular phosphate pools for
the perfused liver, yet lacks the ability to split the intracellular compartment. The three dimensional problem of organ
metabolism is one involving the acquisition of tremendous amounts
of data either by redox scanning of successive sections of tissue
or by laborious microanalytical biochemistry. The two methods
are seen here to complement one another, the three dimensional
redox scanning is a relatively rapid method of data acquisition,
10,000 analyses can be obtained in approximately 10min. Such
redox scans identify the border zone between ischemic and anoxic

regions, for example, in model cardiac infarcts, and can be of
value as well in any other perfused or in situ organs or tissues.
Thus, preliminary observations with two dimensional redox scanning will identify tissue sections which fulfill the above mentioned criterion of "maximal deviation metabolic states" and thus
indicate the portions of the tissue on which microanalytical biochemistry is appropriate. For example, in Figure 8, all the
information on the transition from ischemic to normoxic tissues
could have been obtained with microanalysis of the regions at
200 microns on either side of the border zone.

ACKNOWLEDGEMENTS

This work was supported in part by USPHS Grants HL-18708 and
NS-10939. The help of Dr. George MacDonald is gratefully
acknowledged.

REFERENCES

1. Bergmeyer, H.U. in *Methods of Enzymatic Analysis* (Bartley, W. ed.), Academic press, New York, 1963.
2. Stuart, B., and Chance, B., *Brain Res.* 76:473-479 (1974).
3. Quistorff, B. and Chance, B., in *Oxygen and Physiological Function* (Jöbsis, F.F., ed.) Professional Information Library Dallas, Texas, 1976. pp. 100-110.
4. Reivich, M., Sokoloff, L., Gunsberg, M.D., *Proc. Third Symp. on Cerebral and Coronary Vascular Disorders and Infarcts.* 1978. In press.
5. Matschinsky, F., *this volume.*
6. Chance, B., Estabrook, R.W., Ghosh, A., *Proc. Nat'l. Acad. Sci., USA* 51:1244 (1964).
7. Chance, B., Hess, B. and Betz, A., *Biochem. Biophys. Res. Comm.* 16:182 (1964).
8. Chance, B., Williamson, J.R., Jamieson, D., and Schoener, B. *Biochem. Zeit.* 341:357-377 (1965).
9. Frankel, R., *Biochem. Biophys. Res. Comm.* 21:497 (1965).
10. Betz, A., Chance, B., Schoener, B., Elsaesser, S., *J. Biol. Chem.* 240:3170-3181 (1965).
11. Rappaprot, A.M. in *The Liver, Vol. 1* (Roullier, ed.), Ch. Acad. Press, New York and London, 1963. p. 265.
12. Prigogine,I., in *Thermodynamics Theory of Structure, Stability and Fluctuations,* (Glansdorff, P. and Prigogine, I., eds.) Wiley, Interscience, New York, 1971.
13. Leao, A.A.P.,*J. Neuro. Physiol.* 7:359-390 (1944).
14. Mayevsky, A., and Chance, B., *Brain Res.* 98:149-164, 1975.

15. Tamura, M., Oshino, N. and Chance, B., in *Oxygen Transport to tissue III* (Silver, I.A., Erecinska, M. and Bicher, H.I. eds.) Plenum Press, New York, 1979. pp. 85-101.

16. Chance, B., Schoener, B., and Schlinder, F. in *Oxygen in the Animal Organism* (Dickens, F. and Neil, E., eds.) Pergamon Press, Oxford, 1965. pp. 367-392.

17. Chance, B., and Williams, G.R., *J. Biol. Chem. 217*:409-427 (1955).

18. Chance, B. and Baltscheffsky, H., *J. Biol. Chem. 233*:736 (1958).

19. Sugano, S., Oshino, N. and Chance, B., *Biochim. Biophys. Acta 347*:340-358 (1974).

20. Chance, B., Lee, I.Y. and Oshino, N., *Fed. Proc. 35(3)*525 (1975). Abstr. 1757.

21. Chance, B., Takada, H., Nakase, Y., Itsak, F. *Fed. Proc. 38* 1978 (in press).

22. Ouistorff, B. and Chance, B. in *Oxygen Transport to Tissue III* (Silver, I.A., Erecinska, M. and Bicher, H.I., eds.) Panum Pub'l., New York. 1978.

23. Chance, B., *Suppl. to Cir. Res. 38-9* (Wildentahl, K., Morgan, H.E., Opie, L.H. and Srere, P.A., eds.) 1976. pp. I69-I71.

24. Hearse, D.J., Opie, L.H., Katzeff, I.E., Lubbe, W.F., van der Werff, T.J., Peisach, M., and Boulle, G., *Am. J., Cardiology 40*:716-726 (1977).

25. Barlow, C.H. and Chance, B., *Science 193*:909-910 (1976)

26. Chance, B., Barlow, C., Nakase, Y, Takeda, H., Mayevsky, A., Fischetti, R., Graham, N. and Sorge, J., *Am. J. Physiol.*, submitted March 1978.

27. Moon, B. and Richards, J.H., *J. Biol. Chem. 248*:7276-7278 (1973).

28. Dawson, J., Gadian, D.G. and Wilkie, B.R., *J. Physiol. 258* 823-833 (197).

29. Burt, C.P., Glonek, T. and Bárány, M., *Science 195*:145-149 (1977).

30. Gadian, D.G., Hoult, D.I., Radda, G.K., Seeley, P.J., Chance, B. and Barlow, C.H.B., *Proc. Nat'l. Acad. Sci, USA 73*:4446-4448 (1976).

31. Jacobus, W.E., Taylor, IV, G.J., Hollis, D.P., Nunnally, R. L., *Nature 265*:756-758 (1977).

THE INTRALOBULAR DISTRIBUTION OF OXIDIZED
AND REDUCED PYRIDINE NUCLEOTIDES IN THE LIVER
OF NORMAL AND DIABETIC RATS

Franz M. Matschinsky
Carol S. Hintz

Department of Pharmacology
Washington University
St. Louis, Missouri

Diabetes Research Center
University of Pennsylvania
Philadelphia, Pennsylvania

Klaus Reichlmeier

Sandoz Institute of Basic Medical Research
Basel, Switzerland

Bjoern Quistorff
Britton Chance

Johnson Research Foundation
University of Pennsylvania
Philadelphia, Pennsylvania

I.   INTRODUCTION

An important design feature of the liver as a biochemical
factory is the lobular arrangement of the parenchymal cells
(1-3). This is vividly illustrated by an example from the work
of Rappaport (3) (Figure 1). The acinus rather than the classical lobule as outlined by Kiernan (1) is the functional unit
of the liver in Rappaport's view. He describes the liver aci-

Copyright © 1978 by Academic Press, Inc.
All right of reproduction in any form reserved.
ISBN 0-12-660550-5

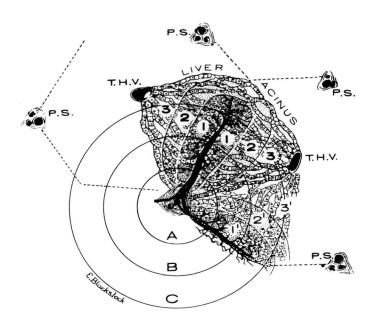

FIGURE I. The blood supply of the simple liver acinus
           and the zonal arrangement of cells.

       The acinus occupies adjacent sectors of neighbor-
ing hexagonal fields. Zones 1, 2, and 3, respectively,
represent areas supplied with blood of first, second,
and third quality with regard to oxygen and nutrients.
These zones center about the terminal afferent vascular
branches, terminal bile ductules, lymph vessels, and
nerves and extend into the triangular portal field
from which these branches crop out. Zones 1', 2', and
3' designate corresponding areas in a portion of an
adjacent acinar unit. In zones 1 and 1' the afferent
vascular twigs empty into the sinusoids. The circles
B and C indicate peripheral circulatory areas as commonly described around the "periportal" area A.
P.S. = portal space; T.H.V. = terminal hepatic venules.
From Rappaport et al. (3)

nus as follows: "The simple liver acinus is a small parenchymal mass, irregular in size and shape, arranged around an
axis of a terminal portal venule, hepatic arteriole, bile
ductule, lymph vessels and nerves which grow out together from

a small triangular portal field. The simple liver acinus lies between two (or more) terminal hepatic venules (central veins) with which its vascular and biliary axis interdigitates. In a two dimensional view it occupies sectors only of two adjacent hexagonal fields." Blood flow in sinusoids of functional units is apparently concurrent and there may be little opportunity within the unit structures for diffusible materials to short circuit the vascular pathway (4). This arrangement is ideal for the liver functions of storage and supply of fuels. As a result of these structural features lobular concentration gradients of diffusible substances can be expected to exist along the sinusoids and the columns of liver cells. Profiles of diffusible substrates (e.g. FFA and oxygen) and of products (e.g. ketone bodies and CO_2) of liver metabolism are believed to decline and rise, respectively, along the length of the sinusoids. The design of the hepatic microcirculation is complemented by the structural, biochemical, and pharmacological diversity of the parenchymal cells of zones 1, 2, and ·3 of the acinus [see (3)]. With staining histochemical methods greater succinic dehydrogenase (5), cytochrome oxidase (6) and lactic dehydrogenase activities (7) were demonstrated in zone 1 as compared to zone 3. Glutamic dehydrogenase (7), β- hydroxy butyric dehydrogenase (7,8) and isocitric dehydrogenase (7) were, however, found to be more active in zone 3 of the acinus. This general picture of enzyme distribution has been confirmed by results obtained with quantitative histochemistry (9,10). But the results of staining histochemistry and quantitative histochemistry do not agree in all instances. For example, differences of opinions still exist about the distribution of glycogen. Whereas most investigators using some version of a staining technique maintain the view that glycogen is distributed unevenly within a lobule (10) there is little evidence for this concept from quantitative studies (11).

The existence of intralobular fuel and oxygen gradients and the heterogeneity of the enzymatic complement of hepatic parenchymal cells imply that gradients of the redox and of the phosphate potentials might exist within the lobule. The present studies were undertaken to explore this possibility. The emphasis of this report is on the development and use of quantitative histochemical techniques to measure the intralobular distribution of $NADP^+$, NADPH, NAD^+ and NADH. The levels of these cofactors can be measured by specific highly sensitive methods and serve as indicators of the redox potential (12). These quantitative data are compared with results of redox potential measurements with a biophysical procedure discussed in more detail elsewhere in this symposium.

II. METHODOLOGY

A. Quantitative Histochemical Analysis
of Pyridine Nucleotides

About 10 years ago a method was described for measuring oxidized and reduced pyridine nucleotides at the microscopic level (14). This method is now applied systematically to liver tissue, with improvements.

Rats weighing 250-300 g were anesthetized with pentobarbital (30 mg/kg i.p.). The liver was exposed and one lobe was frozen between metal blocks cooled with liquid nitrogen. One of these blocks was made of brass fitted with an array of grooves to hold the frozen piece of liver tissue in place, once the brass block was fixed in the microtome for sectioning (see below). The other block was made of aluminum and had a sharp circular cutting edge, 2mm high and of a diameter smaller than the diameter of the brass block. As a result a 2 mm high circular pellet of liver tissue with a flat surface and with a radius of about 1 cm was obtained fixed to a brass holder.

The liver pellet was trimmed to a small square area (5X5 mm) and cryostat sections were cut parallel to the surface. The temperature was maintained at -25 to -27° C. The sections were kept in order in the holes of an aluminum rack and every fourth section was placed on a glass slide and stained for succinoxidase (3). Sections were freeze-dried save the stained ones. Microscopic samples were dissected from areas of the portal tracts (from zone 1 according to Rappaport's nomenclature) and from areas surrounding the central vein (Rappaport's zone 3). This was done using camera lucida drawings of adjacent sections stained for succinoxidase as a guide (for more detail see result section). The samples were weighed with the quartz fiber balance (15) and transferred to an oil well rack made of Teflon (16), and were suspended in small droplets of 0.03 N NaOH with 1 mM cysteine (for details see Table I). The droplets were covered with mineral oil and were then treated either by heating for 20 min at 70° C (for measuring reduced pyridine nucleotides) or kept at 25° C for no longer than 3 min (for measuring total pyridine nucleotides). NADH, NADH plus NAD^+, NADPH, NADPH plus $NADP^+$ were then measured with the method of enzymatic cycling which is specific for NAD (17) or NADP (15). For that purpose the appropriate reagent was added to the alkaline droplet (for details see Table I). After completion of the cycling step (usually one hour) the reaction was stopped by alkalinization

TABLE I. Enzymatic Analysis of NAD
and NADP in Microscopic Liver Samples

Substance Measured	Step (1) Tissue Extraction[a]	Step (2) Cycling[a]	Step (3) Indicator Reaction[a]	Sensitivity (femto moles)
NADH	0.5 µl 1mM cysteine HCl in 0.03 N NaOH; 20 min at 70° C.	1 µl cycling reagent[b]; 1 hr at 25° C; stop cycling with 0.5 µl 0.35 N NaOH and 10 min at 100° C.	50 µl malate reagent[c]; 50 µl malate reagent[c]; stop reaction with 50 µl 0.6M PO₄ buffer, pH 11.6 and heating for 20 min at 75° C. NADH measured by alkali enhanced fluorescence.	3-15
total NAD	0.5 µl 1mM cysteine HCl in 0.02 N NaOH; 3 min at 25° C.	5 µl cycling reagent[b]; 1 hr at 25° C; stop reaction with 1 µl 0.5 N NaOH and 10 min 100° C.	1 ml malate reagent[c]; 50 min at 25° C; measure native fluorescence of NADH.	30-210
NADPH	0.5 µl 1mM cysteine HCL in 0.03 N NaOH; 20 min at 70° C.	5 µl cycling reagent[d]; 1 hr at 25° C; stop cycling with 1.5 µl 0.33 N NaOH and 10 min at 100° C.	1 ml 6-P-gluconate reagent[e]; 45 min at 25° C; measure native fluorescence of NADPH.	25-120
total NADP	0.5 µl 1mM cysteine HCl in 0.02 N NaOH; 3 min at 25° C.	5 µl cycling reagent[d]; 1 hr at 25° C; stop cycling with 1.5 µl 0.33 N NaOH and 10 min 100° C.	1 ml 6-P-gluconate reagent[e]; 45 min at 25° C; measure native fluorescence of NADPH.	25-120

a) Steps (1) and (2) are performed under mineral oil in an oil well rack (16) and step (3) in pyrex glass tubes, 10 X 75 mm.

b) The composition of the cycling reagent was 0.2 M Tris-HCl, pH 7.95, 0.03% bovine serum albumin, 3 mM mercaptoethanol, 3 mM oxalacetate, 450 mM ethanol, 41 µg/ml malic dehydrogenase, 445 µg/ml alcohol dehydrogenase [see (17)].

c) The composition of the malate indicator reagent was 50 mM 2-amino-2-methyl-1-propanol-HCl buffer, pH 9.9, 10 mM glutamate, 100 µM NAD⁺, 5 µg/ml malic dehydrogenase, 2 µg/ml glutamic-oxalacetic-transaminase [see (15)].

d) The composition of the cycling reagent was 100 mM Tris-acetate buffer, pH 8.0, 5 mM α-ketoglutarate, 1 mM glucose-6-P, 10 mM (NH₄)-acetate, 100 µM ADP, 15 µg/ml G-6-P dehydrogenase, 200 µg/ml glutamic dehudrogenase [see(15)].

e) The composition of the indicator reagent for 6-P-gluconate was 40 mM Tris-HCl, pH 8.37, 0.1 mM EDTA, 30 mM (NH₄)-acetate, 5 mM MgCl₂, 30 µM NADP⁺, 0.5 µg/ml 6-P-gluconate dehydrogenase [see (15)].

For NADH and NADPH measurements the corresponding reduced pyridine nucleotides served as standards. For measurement of total NAD the standard was NAD⁺, and for total NADP analysis the standard was NADPH because of the preponderance of NAD⁺ and NADPH in tissue, respectively.

and brief boiling and the final product was measured enzymatically [malate for NAD and 6-P-gluconate for NADP (Table I)].

B.   The Principle of Low Temperature Fluorescence Scanning

The indirect fluorometric redox potential measurements are based on the following biochemical principle (13,18): oxidized flavoproteins (FP_{ox}) and reduced pyridine nucleotides (PN_{red}) emit fluorescent light at 550 and 450 nm, when irradiated with UV light at 436 or 366 nm, respectively.

The ratio of FP_{ox} fluorescence/PN_{red} fluorescence is, therefore, considered a sensitive indicator of the redox state of certain flavoprotein and pyridine nucleotide-dependent enzyme reactions. It is also believed that the recording of this fluorescence ratio is largely independent of interference by various tissue chromophores, most importantly cytochromes and hemoglobin. The fluorescence is greatly enhanced when the temperature is lowered, i.e. about 10-fold for a delta of 100° C. Therefore, the measurements are made on tissue blocks immersed into liquid nitrogen. Fluorescence of the two redox indicators (FP_{ox} and PN_{red}) is measured with a time sharing fluorometer and high spatial resolution is gained by employing a micro light guide for scanning. This light guide consists of six fibers surrounding a central fiber, the former being used for exitation and the latter for emission measurements. The diameter of these fibers is 80 µ. The spatial resolution of the system is approximately equal to the fiber diameter. Data are acquired with a PDP-11 computer that drives the micro light guide in a rapid scan across the frozen tissue, usually an array of 2,500 points - 50 on each side of a square field. The computer dwells a fraction of a second at each position, enabling the FP_{ox}/PN_{red} measurement to be made and the transfer of the information to the computer memory to be accomplished. The results are then projected on a TV screen and photographed.

III.   RESULTS

A.   A Simple Procedure for Sample Identification

Identification of the classical microscopic structures in thin unstained freeze-dried liver sections proved to be difficult for us, if not impossible. This is in part due to the distortion of the structure caused by the freeze clamping. Therefore, a simple technique was applied to assist in sample

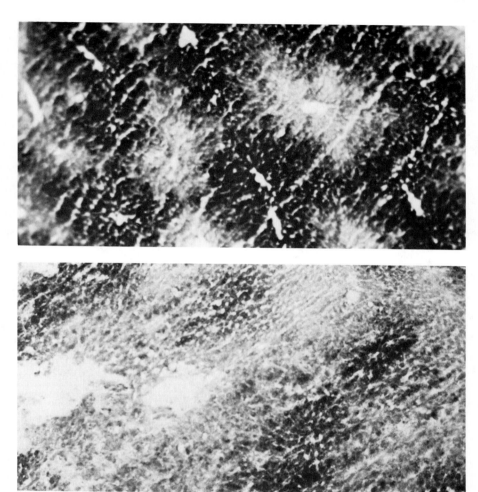

FIGURE 2.   Intralobular Distribution of Succinoxidase
as Demonstrated by Staining Histochemistry.

A 15 μ thick cryostat section was placed on a
glass slide, was air dried and then incubated for
15 min at 37° C in the following medium: 100 mM
Na^+ phosphate buffer, pH 7.6; 50 mM Na^+ succinate;
1 mM K^+ cyanide; and 1.4 mM Nitro-Blue Tetrazolium.
The sections were then fixed with 10% formalin in
0.9% NaCl. Heavily stained areas are identified as
zone 1, lightly stained areas as zone 3.   The sample
of the lower panel was freeze clamped, that of the
upper was not.

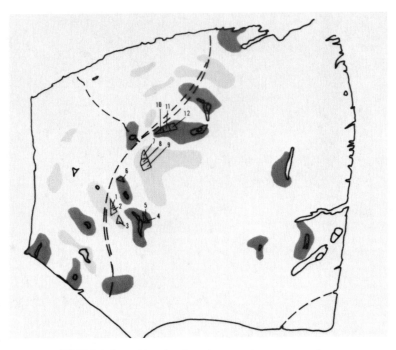

FIGURE 3.   Typical Dissecting Record

The outline of the stained section and of certain
histological landmarks are recorded with heavy black
lines.   Zone 1 (high succinoxidase activity) is indicated by dark gray shading, zone 3 (low succinoxidase
activity) by light gray shading.   The heavy dotted
lines indicate fissures in the section.   The dissecting patterns of an adjacent unstained section are
projected and indicated by thin black lines.   In this
section 12 samples were obtained.   The sample weights
were between 32 and 75 ng.   Some of the data presented
in Table II were obtained from the section depicted
here.   The remainder was taken from the other adjacent
unstained section.

identification (19).   Every fourth cryostat section was placed
on a glass slide and was stained for succinoxidase (7) (Fig 2).
The enzyme is concentrated in zone 1 of a simple acinus (see
Fig 1).   Therefore, heavier formazane deposits identify areas
of zone 1 and relatively light areas of zone 3.   A mirror im-
age of this result was obtained when the sections were stained

for glutamic dehydrogenase (not shown), consistent with published results (7). A camera lucida drawing was made of the stained section and with the help of this drawing, samples of known composition were dissected from adjacent unstained sections from zones 1 and 3 (Fig 3). With this approach the precise location of each sample is recorded.

TABLE II. REPRODUCIBILITY OF NADH MEASUREMENTS
IN MICROSCOPIC LIVER SAMPLES

Zone 1	Zone 3
mmole/kg dry tissue	
.320	.225
.335	.225
.317	.224
.296	.217
.345	.263
.265	.174
.238	.140
.263	.193
.250	.189
.257	.186
.239	.185
.263	.211
.183	.274
.287	.445
.324	.210
.301	.231
.290	.233

	Zone 1	Zone 3
Mean	.281	.225
$\pm$SD	$\pm$.042	$\pm$.065

Two groups of 17 samples each were dissected from zones 1 and 3 of freeze-dried liver sections and were analyzed for NADH. There is a statistically significant difference of 20% of NADH levels between zones 1 and 3, $p \leq 0.001$.

TABLE III. Stability of Reduced Pyridine
Nucleotides of Normal Liver Under
Dissecting Room Conditions

Dissecting Time	NADH		NADPH	
	Zone 1	Zone 3	Zone 1	Zone 3
T_1 (½ hr)	.329+.041	.191+.039	1.64+.15	1.48+.07
T_2 (1 hr)	.343+.053 (104.3)	.218+.029 (114.1)	1.56+.30 (95.4)	1.45+.05 (98.0)
T_3 (3¼ hr)	.285+.024 (86.6)	.181+.017 (94.8)	1.43+.20 (87.4)	1.46+.09 (98.4)

Groups of five samples each were dissected and exposed to dissecting room air (50% humidity and 25° C)
for various lengths of time and were then analyzed for
NADH or NADPH. The results obtained at the earliest
time point (½ hr of air exposure) are used as reference
values. It is assumed that there were no losses during
that early phase, since the results agree with data obtained by many others with bulk extraction of the tissue (21). Results are given in terms of mmole/kg dry
tissue (Mean+SD). For T_2 and T_3 the relative NAD(P)H
contents are also recorded as percent of the level
found at T_1 (in parentheses).

B. Stability of NADH and NADPH During Sampling

It has been noted previously (14) that reduced pyridine
nucleotides might be oxidized during the process of microdissection of dried tissue. To test whether this was so, freeze
dried sections were exposed for various lengths of time to 50%
humidity at 25° C and were then analyzed for NADH or NADPH
(Tables II and III). It has also been observed that extraction of dry tissue with dilute alkali (0.03 N NaOH) was successful only when sample size did not exceed a critical value
(20). It became apparent that samples equal to or smaller
than 100 ng gave reliable data. The reproducibility was acceptable with standard deviations between 15-30%.

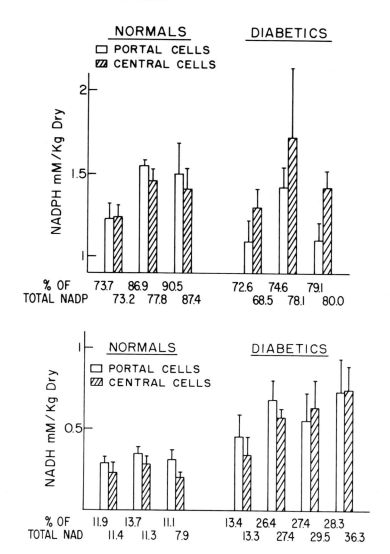

FIGURE 4. Intralobular Distribution of Pyridine
Nucleotides in Livers of Normal and
Diabetic Rats

The means ±SD of 10 or more samples are recorded
in each bar. Diabetes was induced by injecting 70 mg
of streptozotocin/kg body weight. The liver tissue
was sampled four days later following the demonstration of severe hyperglycemia (19–24 mM). Animals were
in the fed state.

TABLE IV. Intralobular Distribution of NADH
and of the Sum of NAD$^+$ plus NADH in Normal
and Diabetic Rat Liver

	NADH		Total NAD	
	Zone 1	Zone 3	Zone 1	Zone 3
	NORMAL LIVER			
Tissue Level	.31+.05 (41)	.24+.06 (49)	2.54+.40 (46)	2.28+.43 (49)
NADH as % of Total	12.1	10.4	--	--
Zonal Diff. % of Zone 1	-23.3		-10.5	
p-value	≤0.001		≤0.001	
	DIABETIC LIVER			
Tissue Level	.64+.21 (66)	.58+.22 (56)	2.85+.46 (47)	2.23+.36 (48)
NADH as % of Total	22.3	25.8	--	--
Zonal Diff. % of Zone 1	-9.6		-21.7	
p-value	≤0.001		≤0.001	

Three animals were analyzed in each group (i.e.
Normals vs. Diabetics). Tissue levels of pyridine
nucleotides are given in terms of mmole/kg dry tissue.
Means+SD are recorded. The total number of samples
analyzed is given in parentheses. The statistical
analysis for individual livers showed similarly high
significance of differences as recorded here for the
comparison of all samples analyzed.

TABLE V. Intralobular Distribution of NADPH
and of the Sum of NADP$^+$ Plus NADPH in
Normal and Diabetic Rat Liver

	NADPH		Total NADP	
	Zone 1	Zone 3	Zone 1	Zone 3
	NORMAL LIVER			
Tissue Level	1.44+.18 (36)	1.39+.13 (35)	1.70+.19 (45)	1.72+.18 (47)
NADPH as % of Total	84.5	79.1	--	--
Zonal Diff. % of Zone 1	-3.6		-0.9	
p-value	≤0.001		0.9	
	DIABETIC LIVER			
Tissue Level	1.20+.19 (30)	1.47+.31 (31)	1.59+.28 (43)	1.94+.34 (45)
NADPH as % of Total	76.0	76.0	--	--
Zonal Diff. % of Zone 1	+18.1		+18.1	
p-value	≤0.001		≤0.001	

For more details see legend to Table IV.

C. Intralobular Distribution of Pyridine Nucleotides
in Normal Livers (Fig 4, Tables IV and V)

The pyridine nucleotides are distributed nearly evenly
throughout the liver lobule. But in the NAD system a very
shallow gradient of total NAD with a tendency to fall in the
direction of the central vein appears to exist. The difference between levels of zones 1 and 3 is not more than 10%.
The NADH profile follows this trend and the porto-central dif-

ference is 23%. These differences are significant statistically. From 8-14% of the NAD is reduced. In the case of the
NADP system there are no concentration differences between
zones 1 and 3 and as much as 73-91% of the NADP is in the reduced form. The absolute levels and the degree of reduction
found here with a micro analytical method are similar to those
obtained in classical macroscale studies of pyridine nucleotides in liver (21).

D.   Intralobular Distribution of Pyridine Nucleotides
     in the Liver of Severely Diabetic Rats
          (Fig 4, Tables IV and V)

The total NAD content and its intralobular distribution
are not affected by severe insulin deficiency of 4 days duration induced by streptozotocin. However, the NAD system is
more reduced in diabetics than in controls. The NADH levels
doubled in liver tissue of diabetics. It also seems that the
distribution of $NADP^+$ and of NADPH were altered somewhat by
streptozotocin treatment. The levels of total NADP and of
NADPH of zone 3 were 18% higher than the corresponding values
found in zone 1. These differences had statistical significance. The degree of reduction of the NADP system was, however, not changed.

These results with diabetic tissue must be interpreted
cautiously, because streptozotocin, which is used here to dis-
troy the pancreatic β-cells, might have affected the pyridine nucleotide levels independently of its diabetogenic action. The data illustrate, however, that the approach enables
the biochemist to detect small circumscribed alterations of
the pyridine nucleotide system at the microscopic level. The
preferential rise of NADP in zone 3 in the diabetic state may
have pathophysiological significance.

E.   Heterogeneity of the Redox State of Freeze
     Trapped Liver as Observed with Low Temperature
          Fluorescence Scanning (Fig 5)

Results obtained by application of the light guide scanner
to the surface of freeze-clamped liver at a series of parallel
planes 50 μ apart are shown here to illustrate the biophysical
approach to the problem. The data consist of about 40,000
data points taken over a square 6 mm on a side. The light
areas correspond to high FP_{ox}/PN_{red} ratios (oxidized zones)
and the dark areas to low ratios (reduced zones). The extent
of heterogeneity is large and might correspond to different

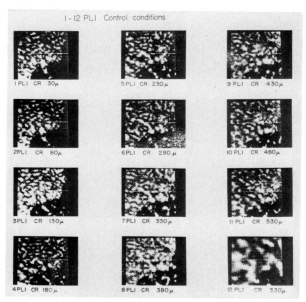

FIGURE 5.   Heterogeneity of the Redox State of
Freeze Trapped Perfused Rat Liver.

A serial display of cross sections 50 µ apart, from
30-530 µ depth, is presented. A 6X6 mm scan area was
used which resulted in 3,600 points per scan. The single
elements are 0.01 mm^2. The FP_{ox}/PN_{red} ratios (CR) are
recorded, white representing a relatively oxidized and
black a relatively reduced area.

metabolic states in various portions of the liver. The spatial
pattern of the metabolic inhomogeneity appears to follow the
architecture of the lobule. Preliminary microscopic controls
suggest that the relatively oxidized areas correspond to the
portal triads and zone 1, whereas the more reduced areas correspond to zone 3 of the acinus. Virtually identical results
were obtained with livers freeze-clamped <u>in vivo</u> using fed
rats briefly anesthetized with pentobarbital.

IV. DISCUSSION

The two sets of data, i.e. the results obtained by direct
chemical analysis of well-defined microscopic liver structures
on one hand and those recorded by indirect biophysical methods
on the other, appear contradictory. The biophysical results

seem to suggest that redox potential gradients exist within
the liver lobule with a higher degree of reduction in zone 3
as compared to zone 1. The chemical analytical results suggest that the redox potential is equal throughout the liver
lobule.

In order to resolve the dilemma, the advantages and the potential shortcomings of the two approaches have to be compared
and assessed.

The results of the microchemical determinations are more
easily evaluated than those obtained by the biophysical approach. The specific nature of the enzymatic fluorometric
assay, the fortunate outcome of the storage experiments and
the favorable comparison with corresponding whole tissue data
accumulated by other investigators indicate that the measurements are reliable. Most importantly, reduced pyridine nucleotides seem to be reasonably stable during the process of sampling and seem to survive the mild extraction process used
here. The small, but clearly demonstrable gradient of NAD is
consistant with numerous histochemical data (3,5,6-10) which
suggest that zone 1 of the hepatic acinus is metabolically
more active than zone 3. The constancy of the NAD^+/NADH and
$NADP^+$/NADPH ratios across the lobule is not unreasonable physiologically, since under normal conditions the oxygen tension
might be maintained sufficiently high to assure saturation of
cytochrome oxidase in all 3 metabolic zones of the liver acinus. However, the interpretation of the data is clouded by
the uncertainties about the degree of binding of pyridine nucleotides to cellular components (22-24). The present data
represent, therefore, merely a rough estimate of the redox
potential of zones 1 and 3 and more sophisticated approaches
have to be used to obtain information on the intralobular distributions of the free fractions of pyridine nucleotides. Such
measurements would seem feasible.

Great efforts have been made to validate the biophysical
procedure for measuring redox potentials by surface fluorescence (13,18,25). The low temperature fluorescence scanner of
FP_{ox}/PN_{red} ratios has been designed to overcome some of the
difficulties encountered in the past (13,18). It is assumed
that the ratio method is largely independent of the fluoro-
chrome concentrations and that it is less susceptible to interference by hemoglobin or tissue pigments than selected monito-
ring of reduced pyridine nucleotides or oxidized flavoproteins.
The method is extremely sensitive to small opposite level
changes of the two members of the redox couple FP_{ox} and PN_{red}.
But this increased sensitivity also increases the susceptibi-
lity to interference. The technique is attractive because

data acquisition is comprehensive and rapid. The results gathered to date indicating the presence of a redox potential gradient across the liver lobule have considerable biochemical implications. The most plausible explanation might be that the cells in zone 1 and 3 are biochemically different and that peculiar features of the energy metabolism of these two cell populations determine the redox potential differences.

It is not possible at this stage of the investigations to resolve the discrepancies of results obtained with the two methods. The opposite results in liver are particularly puzzling since in another tissue the two methods provided comparable data (13). It was found that the redox potential gradient that characterizes the border zone between infarcted and normal tissue of the rabbit heart manifests itself equally well with both techniques. One possible explanation for the opposite outcome in liver is that the results of the quantitative histochemical approach may have become biased due to limiting the sampling to zones 1 and 3 so that the heterogeneity of the redox potential, manifest in the comprehensive picture obtained by the fluorescence scanner, may have been missed. It is, therefore, essential to carry out parallel studies with both techniques on the same tissue blocks focusing on the same lobules and the same groups of cells. Such point by point comparisons of results seems feasible.

The topic is of importance for many questions of the physiology, pathophysiology and toxicology of the liver and deserves vigorous research.

ACKNOWLEDGMENTS

This study was supported by United States Public Health Service Grant AM-10591 and by Diabetes Research Center Grant AM 19525. Franz M. Matschinsky is an Established Investigator of the American Diabetes Association.

REFERENCES

1. Kiernan, F., Phil. Trans. Royal Soc. London, 123, 711 (1833).
2. Elias, H., in "The Liver," vol. 1, ed. Ch. Roullier, Acad. Press, New York and London (1963) 41.
3. Rappaport, A.M., in "The Liver," vol. 1, ed. Ch. Roullier, Acad. Press, New York and London, (1963) 265.

4. Goresky, C.A., in "Regulation of Hepatic Metabolism,"
    Alfred Benson Symposium VI, ed. F. Lundquist and N. Tygs-
    trup, Academic Press, New York (1974) 808.
5. Novikoff, A.B., and Essner, E., Am. J. Med. 29, 102
    (1960).
6. Burstone, M.S., J. Histochem. Cytochem. 7, 112 (1959).
7. Pette, D. and Brandau, H., Enzym. Biol. Clin. 6, 719
    (1966).
8. Novikoff, A.B., J. Histochem. Cytochem. 7, 240 (1959).
9. Shank, R.E., Morrison, G., Cheng, C.H., Karl, I.,
    Schwartz, R., J. Histochem. Cytochem. 7, 237 (1959).
10. Sasse, D., Kohler, J., Histochemie, 18, 325 (1969).
11. Welsh, F.A., J. Histochem. Cytochem. 20, 112 (1972).
12. Hoek, J.B., Tager, J.M., Biochem. Biophys. Acta, 325, 197
    (1973).
13. Chance, B., see this symposium.
14. Matschinsky, F.M., J. Neurochem. 15, 643 (1968).
15. Lowry, O.H. and Passonneau, J.V., A Flexible System of
    Enzymatic Analysis, Academic Press, New York (1972).
16. Matschinsky, F.M., Passonneau, J.V., Lowry, O.H., J.
    Histochem. Cytochem., 16, 29 (1968).
17. Kato, T., Berger, S.J., Carter, J.A., Lowry, O.H.,
    Anal. Biochem., 53, 86 (1973).
18. Quistorff, B., Chance, B., Fed. Proc. 36, 1358 (1977).
19. Godfrey, D.A., Matschinsky, F.M., J. Histochem. Cytochem.
    24, 697 (1976).
20. Trus, M., unpublished observation.
21. Burch, H.B., Dippe, P., J. Biol. Chem. 239, 1898 (1964).
22. Bucher, T., Klingenberg, M., Angew. Chemie, 70, 552 (1958).
23. Veech, R.L., Eggleston, L.V., Krebs, H.A., Biochem. J.
    115, 609 (1969).
24. Veech, R.L., see this symposium.
25. Chance, B., Mayevsky, A., Goodwin, D., Mela, L., Micro-
    vasc. Res., 8, 276 (1974).

DISCUSSION

J. KATZ: I would like to ask a question of Dr. Matschinsky.
Did you measure the activity of succinate dehydrogenase or
just the levels of reduced pyridine nucleotides; the DPNH
and TPNH. Maybe I didn't get you.

F. MATSCHINSKY: You didn't get me. The slide which I showed you was a stained section used to guide us in the microdissection. I have not the slightest idea whether this
represents the actual activity of succinate dehydrogenase.

J. KATZ: You show a very sharp boundary on the slide between the periportal succinic dehydrogenase zone (which is blue), and the unstained perivenous zone. Nolte and Pette (J. Histochem. Cytochem. 20, 507, 1972) have measured succinate dehydrogenase in the periportal and perivenous zones of the liver lobule and report the activity of the dehydrogenase in the periportal zone to be 1.5 times that in the perivenous area. This is not much of a difference. I see a discrepancy between the histochemical distribution, which is nearly all or nothing, and the enzyme assays which only show a moderate difference.

F. MATSCHINSKY: I have been wondering about this discrepancy myself. In this study, the staining histochemistry was used merely as an indicator of the location of the sample. We have complementary staining results with glutamate dehydrogenase which show the opposite distribution. It is well known that glutamate dehydrogenase is higher in the central than the portal area. From these studies we are sure that the samples we get are of portal or central origin. That is the point I wanted to make. I don't want to get into the value or lack of value of staining histochemistry. That is a very muddy area as you very well know.

J. LOWENSTEIN: It seems to me that Dr. Chance's evidence for microheterogeneity in the redox state of pyridine and flavin nucleotides might be explained in terms of oscillations of metabolite concentrations in individual cells. The oscillations in different cells would have to be non-synchronized or at most partially synchronized. Would you comment Dr. Chance?

B. CHANCE: Fascinating idea and indeed verified by microfluorometry of individual yeast cells. But there is a clear synchronizing signal in yeast, and in slime mold as well. In the brain cortex the neurons are synchronized in spreading depression. Thus most of the metabolic oscillations known are self-synchronizing, but of course this is how they are observed.

J. LOWENSTEIN: Conditions that prevail in mammalian cells are different and would tend to run the synchrony. For example in muscle not all cells are contracting at the same moment and in brain not all cells are firing at the same time and that would tend to lead to asynchronous oscillations.

B. CHANCE: Yes, an asynchronous oscillation in a tissue
would be difficult to observe by any other approach than the
histogram display that we use. Perhaps synchronizers, such
as substrates, functionally active, would decrease the
apparent heterogeneity. Again, it's a good idea.

S. BESSMAN: I have a question that is just a technical one.
The size of a liver lobule is a millimeter or 2 millimeters
thick. If you freeze-clamp it, and if you are going to retain the architecture without making a hash of it, then I
think it is going to take more time which permits changes
in the concentration of intermediates than one would think
would occur with freeze-clamping. In other words, the
question is how can you get away from the problem of heat
exchange and still retain the architecture of the system.

B. CHANCE: Well, a cold block (-196°) is laid upon the
liver lobe and the freezing gradient moves at about 12
microns per millisecond initially and slower after about
50 μ. Within 1 millimeter travel you have fairly valid
freezing since 1 or 2 seconds is satisfactory for maintaining aerobiosis in the tissue. Now, if you do a redox scan
through such a tissue, of course the initial 50 μ layer
may be disturbed. In fact you saw that in the heart redox
scan. From 200 microns onwards the profiles are very clear
and consecutive. Ice-crystal formation could be another
disturbance in these sections but they are usually too small
to affect the mitochondrial signals.

COMPARTMENTATION OF GLYCOLYSIS IN ESCHERICHIA COLI

Vivian Moses

Department of Plant Biology and Microbiology
Queen Mary College, University of London
London, England

I.   INTRODUCTION

One cannot fail to be impressed and intrigued by the
complexity of metabolism, particularly when one realises how
small is the volume in which so much takes place. It has
been estimated that an individual growing bacterial cell, in
a volume of perhaps 10^{-12}ml., may contain at any one time a
million protein molecules catalysing a variety of chemical
interactions approaching a thousand in number. Instinctively
one feels that such a system is "highly organised" but the use
of this term is not really very informative unless an attempt
is made to define the many sorts of organisation which may be
applicable. At the very least two main categories present
themselves for consideration. One is to suppose that the
whole complex of biochemical events is interrelated through a
comprehensive network of mutual interactions so that a per-
turbation in one area will have its ramifications throughout
the system as a readjustment takes place to meet it. The
other, and it is not exclusive of the first, imagines a
hierarchy of organisational states in which local interactions
and equilibrations may take place without immediately involving the whole system. The consequences of the local adjust-
ments would, of course, have their repercussions on neighbouring activities but only, perhaps, at a limited number of
points of interaction. This second organisational state is
one of the possible forms of compartmentalised arrangement;
but merely recognising the existence of the organisation does
not ipso facto reveal anything about its physical or chemical
basis.

Copyright © 1978 by Academic Press, Inc.
All right of reproduction in any form reserved.
ISBN 0-12-660550-5

Our own studies of glycolysis as an organised pathway have developed slowly over nearly two decades. It was largely fortuitous that glycolysis was chosen as a pathway worth studying, although the fairly early decision to concentrate attention onto simple bacteria was a rational and considered one. Glycolysis is a pathway of central and ubiquitous metabolic importance, well understood experimentally, and a major route among heterotrophes for the catabolism of substrate molecules. Even more to the point (and, as we all know, progress in science works like this) my first collaborator in this venture, Karl Lonberg-Holm, had based his Ph.D. work on an investigation of glycolysis in ascites tumour cells and was very skilled in its study.

The concept of metabolic compartmentation was not unknown when we started and it had from time to time been invoked in several studies to explain data which could not be readily understood in any other way; some of these earlier studies have been reviewed by a number of authors (1, 2, 3). But ten or fifteen years ago most people, even those who brought it in to aid comprehension of their own results, often felt rather uncomfortable about relying on compartmentation explanations, feeling that it was a sort of explanation to be used when all else had failed and the imagination had run dry, and as such was not really very satisfactory. It seemed to us at that time worth while to try to investigate metabolic compartmentation on a more systematic basis and to try to design experiments to test the possibility of its importance rather than to fall back on it when one could think of nothing else.

II. A TEST SYSTEM FOR COMPARTMENTATION

It proved possible to design a theoretical test system but its success in any real context was a gamble: a positive result would be highly suggestive of compartmentation, but a negative finding would be totally equivocal. The method was to study the fate of metabolic substrates in living cells as a function of their biochemical origin. It was reasoned that if metabolic compartmentalisation occurred then access to one compartment might be possible for the substrate derived from one source but not from another, the reverse being true for access into another compartment. In a practical sense one would incubate cells in several identical reaction mixtures containing the range of substrates under test. At an appropriate time labelled substrates in tracer amounts would be added to the various reaction vessels in such a way as to cause no perceptible change in chemical milieu, so that chemically and physiologically each reaction vessel would remain identical with all the others. The labelling patterns would, of course, be different and would be designed to reveal the metabolic fate of a labelled substrate in the presence of another unlabelled substrate and to compare this with the obverse situation in which the second substrate was labelled and the first was not. If the correct choice of substrates were made in testing a possibly compartmented system potentially producing different products, it might be possible to observe the metabolism of one substrate to give predominantly one product while the other substrate gave another. In the context of glycolysis alternative substrates might be free glucose compared with glucose derived by disaccharide or polysaccharide hydrolysis, or perhaps glucose 6-phosphate formed in vivo from free glucose contrasted with glucose 6-phosphate added to the system directly. It would, of course, be necessary to select substrates for comparison which were readily able to enter the cells and were capable of being metabolised.

III. GLYCOLYSIS IN EHRLICH ASCITES TUMOUR CELLS

For the first test of the approach we made use of Ehrlich ascites tumour cells. Since they grow in the relative homoeostatic chemical environment of the mouse abdomen it was felt that in common with other metazoan cells, as distinct from free-living unicellular organisms, they might be fairly non-selective in allowing the passage of metabolic intermediates across the cell membrane and thus permit the simultaneous uptake of several substrates.

In the event, six parallel and biochemically identical incubation vessels containing ascites cells each received six substrates simultaneously: glucose, fructose, glucose 6-phosphate, 6-phosphogluconate, 3-phosphoglycerate and L-lactate; in each vessel one only of these was labelled with ^{14}C. Samples were taken from each reaction vessel in the period from 3 sec. to 45 min. after adding the labelled substrates, product compounds were separated by two-dimensional paper chromatography and measurements made of their ^{14}C contents. The specific radioactivity of each substrate being known it was possible to determine the rate of formation of each product molecule from each substrate in the presence of all the other substrates. A comparison of the ratios between the yields of product substances was made to elucidate possible compartmental behaviour (4).

The metabolism of 6-phosphogluconate was very slow indeed and no useful information was obtained. A series of interesting conclusions could be drawn from the product yields with time from the other substrates. Among these was the fact that the overall conversion of glucose carbon was some 300 times greater than that of fructose carbon, yet more citric acid was formed from fructose than from glucose carbon in the earlier part of the experiment. Other differences in the contribution of glucose and fructose to lactate, malate, glutamate and alanine confirmed that glucose and fructose are metabolised separately at least to some extent. Another unexpected conclusion was that the metabolism of glucose 6-phosphate fed directly to the cells was not identical with the fate of glucose 6-phosphate produced within the cells from free glucose added to the medium. Furthermore, the metabolism of glucose 6-phosphate, 3-phosphoglycerate and L-lactate all showed distinctive characteristics demonstrating a considerable lack of equilibration. One was led to conclude that, whatever the mechanism, compartmentation of some sort existed in the system.

There were considerable experimental difficulties associated with using ascites tumour cells and it was not possible to meet all the criteria for steady-state metabolism without metabolic transient effects which were necessary for a satisfactory study of compartmentation. But accepting nevertheless that the data were indicative of compartmentation there were at least three levels of complexity at which this might operate and which were not readily distinguishable in this system: (a) a non-homogeneous cell population, with some cells preferentially using one substrate while others used another: this might have been due either to a structural or a physiological difference between them; (b) compartmentation effected by membrane separation, e.g. the inside of an organelle versus the cytosol; (c) channelling at the molecular level based on protein-protein interactions and multi-enzyme complexes.

IV. CARBOHYDRATE METABOLISM IN ESCHERICHIA COLI

In an attempt to overcome some of these limitations and to make use of more easily controlled biological material, we turned out attention to bacteria, and in particular to carbohydrate metabolism in Escherichia coli. These bacteria are simple in structure compared with animal and plant cells, the only membrane they possess being the plasma membrane itself. Reactions occurring within the limits of the plasma membrane

take place either on that membrane surface or in the cytoplasm.
Bacterial cultures are, of course, derived within a few hours
if need be from a single cell, and one may have a high degree
of confidence that all the cells are similar, or very nearly
so, both structurally and physiologically. If such cells
were to show compartmentalised metabolism for whole pathways
this would indicate either an organised array of co-operating
enzymes on the membrane surface or some sort of soluble enzyme
complex acting as an integrated system and not releasing
metabolites between one reaction and the next. Furthermore,
the well-understood genetics of this organism allowed the
possibility of testing the behaviour of strains defective in
specified portions of the metabolic sequence.

A.   Compartmentation of Glycolysis

Our first investigation of glycolysis in E. coli used non-
growing cultures induced for the lactose and galactose enzymes,
and constitutive for glucose metabolism. Four identical cultures of washed, resting cells, treated with chloramphenicol
to prevent further enzyme synthesis, were incubated simultaneously with glucose, galactose and lactose. After a period
for equilibration and attainment of a steady state, tracer
quantities of the substrates labelled with ^{14}C were added to
each of the cultures as follows: (a) {G-^{14}C}-D-glucose;
(b) {G-^{14}C}-D-galactose;   (c) { (G-^{14}C) glucose}lactose;
(d) { (G-^{14}C) galactose}lactose (5). As in the earlier experiments with ascites cells, samples were taken at intervals for
later analysis of ^{14}C incorporated into metabolic intermediates with time, and measurements were also made of the
rates of removal of the three substrates from the medium.   In
subsequent experiments similar protocols were employed with
cells in which the lactose enzymes or the galactose enzymes,
or both, were repressed and which were therefore unable to
metabolise those sugars.

The uptake of the substrates was very unequal and prefer-
ences were shown. With both the galactose and lactose enzymes
functional, nearly 80% of all the carbohydrate used was
galactose, about half of that coming from lactose hydrolysis
and half from the free sugar in the medium. With the lactose
operon repressed half the previous supply of galactose was
unavailable, and this was replaced, not by increasing the uptake of free galactose from the medium, but by increasing the
uptake of glucose. There was no increase in the utilisation
of glucose derived from lactose since lactose hydrolysis was
blocked. One was led to believe that the route from external
galactose to intermediary metabolism was already fully

saturated when lactose hydrolysis was operative and could carry no additional material to compensate for the shortage of galactose from lactose when the lactose enzymes were absent. Galactose permease might have been the limiting factor.

When it was available, glucose from lactose hydrolysis was used in preference to external free glucose. If the galactose operon was not induced no metabolism of galactose was possible from either source. In those conditions glucose from lactose was the substrate of choice although if that were unavailable free glucose could be used. These data strongly suggested a lack of mixing between the intermediary metabolites from hexoses entering metabolism by different portals, and this in turn implied a compartmented organisation.

Comparison of the temporal labelling patterns of metabolic products confirmed this view. Among the most striking were the kinetics of labelling in citrate, succinate and glutamate. The picture that emerged was one in which free glucose and free galactose taken up from the medium contributed to a common pool of metabolites including the citric acid cycle inter-mediates. A different pool of metabolites received its carbon from glucose and galactose resulting from the hydrolysis of lactose. Since β-galactosidase is located within the cell, and catalyses the hydrolysis of free lactose, the glucose and galactose produced from that hydrolysis were liberated in the cytoplasm as the free sugars. The monosaccharides entering the cell via the appropriate permease would have been released as phosphate esters, so the origin of the metabolic channelling may be located at the level of sugar phosphates rather than free monosaccharides. The observation of kinetic differences involving citrate, succinate and glutamate suggests that the channelling continues into the tricarboxylic acid cycle.

B.   Amino Acid Synthesis

Interesting and suggestive though these conclusions were it was felt that they were sufficiently novel to warrant con-firmation in further experiments. The first studies with E. coli were very elaborate and time-consuming, and in many ways difficult to perform because of the low levels of radio-carbon incorporated into each product compound in each sample. There was still, to some degree, the problem of the steady-state. In order to use cells with a specified phenotype in the presence of substrates acting as inducers it was, of course, necessary to prevent further protein synthesis with chloramphenicol. This, however, unbalanced the overall metabolic picture: cells would normally be conducting their catabolic activities, including glycolysis, in concert with anabolism, of which protein synthesis is the most important quantitative manifestation. Although the bacteria had been allowed to metabolise the mixture of unlabelled glucose, galactose and lactose for 15 min. before the tracer substrates were added, this may not have produced a true steady state of metabolism. It therefore seemed appropriate to extend multi-substrate studies to actively growing cells in experiments lasting several generations. The experimental technique was greatly simplified, and the levels of radioactivity in the samples enhanced, by observing the incorporation of ^{14}C from substrates into protein amino acids. The latter accumulate as the cell population in the culture grows and it becomes a simple matter to hydrolyse samples of the total cellular protein and to separate individual amino acids for radio-activity measurements.

The experiments were performed using two pairs of competing substrates (6). To permit correlation with the earlier work of McBrien and Moses (5) one pair was galactose and lactose, the label being present either as {G-^{14}C}galactose or {(G-^{14}C)galactose}lactose. The cells were allowed to grow experimentally for 3-4 doublings before being harvested, while samples of the supernatant medium were obtained at intervals for measurement of the rates of substrate utilisation. It was found that with each sugar as the sole substrate growth on galactose was slower and the yield less. When both substrates were present together the yield was higher than with either alone, indicating complementarity. The detailed investigation of radiocarbon incorporation into individual amino acids with both substrates present showed that glucose and galactose carbon were distinguished metabolically. Cysteine, threonine and histidine were derived almost entirely, and lysine mainly, from galactose. It was concluded that a pentose phosphate pathway and a glycolytic sequence as far as oxaloacetate must exist which could accept carbon skeletons from galactose but not from glucose.

Galactose carbon derived from lactose was used preferentially for amino acid synthesis except for cysteine, threonine and proline. Since the favouring of lactose-galactose affected amino acids originating both in the tri-carboxylic acid cycle and more directly from glycolysis, the discrimination against free galactose as a precursor must have taken place before its entry into glycolysis. Two metabolic compartments are indicated: one of them would accept carbon from galactose (either from the free sugar, or from lactose) more readily than glucose carbon, while the other would favour either galactose or glucose derived from lactose compared with free galactose. Histidine carbon came almost exclusively from the galactose moiety of lactose when both lactose and

galactose were present together, suggesting that the hexose
monophosphate pools derived from the galactose moiety of
lactose were distinct from those both from the glucose moiety
of lactose and from free galactose. A role for galactose
carbon separate from glucose carbon was further supported by
the sparing effect free galactose exerted on the utilisation
of the galactose moiety from lactose, but not on the glucose
moiety.

The other pair of substrates was maltose and glycerol.
Here the intention was to observe the utilisation of glycerol
carbon, feeding into glycolysis midway along the sequence at
the level of triose phosphate, when the glycolytic enzymes
were already being used for the metabolism of maltose carbon.
(Maltose rather than glucose was used as the source of hexose
in order to avoid possible catabolite repression effects.)
Again the cells were grown exponentially for 3-4 doublings
with glycerol and maltose, alone or in combination, as the
substrates, and with label supplied either as {G-^{14}C}glycerol
or {G-^{14}C}maltose. Both substrates gave similar growth rates
and growth yields; when present together maltose was the
preferred precursor for alanine, valine, histidine and proline.
Presumably it was preferred for histidine because it is closer
to the source of the pentose phosphate cycle. It is more
interesting that maltose should contribute preferentially to
alanine and valine (via a pyruvate pool) but contribute
equally with glycerol to the amino acids emanating directly
from the tricarboxylic acid cycle except for proline. This
requires that maltose and glycerol contribute to different
pyruvate pools by virtue of their metabolism through different
glycolytic pathways which converge in the tricarboxylic acid
cycle. Thus the question of competition between glycerol and
maltose carbon at triose phosphate does not arise; each enters
a different glycolytic compartment.

Among the tricarboxylic acid cycle amino acids proline
represents a special case. Proline is formed from glutamic
acid. The label in protein glutamic acid derived equally
from glycerol and maltose, whereas the label in proline
residues in protein came preferentially from maltose. This
result suggested that the glutamate pool providing glutamic
acid for incorporation into protein is different from that
pool of glutamate acting as a precursor for proline biosynthesis.

The studies on the contribution of competing substrates to
the carbon skeletons of amino acids were in general agreement
with the earlier investigations on the metabolic intermediates of glycolysis and the citric acid cycle. Metabolic compartmentation began to appear as a real phenomenon in E. coli
and it was felt by then that a sufficiently sound basis for it
existed to warrant studies on its physical meaning.

C.   Intracellular Localisation of
Glycolytic Enzymes

A series of studies carried out over several years has yielded a body of evidence for the existence of a physical particle associated with the channelling of metabolism (7, 8, 9, 10, 11).   They all sought the characterisation of a possible complex of glycolytic enzymes from E. coli and, recognising its potential fragility, all used mild techniques to disrupt the cells.   Generally, sphaeroplasts were prepared, using either the penicillin or the EDTA-lysozyme technique, and these were ruptured osmotically (with a minimum dilution of the intracellular cytoplasmic content), mechanically or by freezing and thawing.   Some studies were also performed with bacteria disrupted in the French pressure cell.   The attachment of glycolytic enzymes to various membrane fractions was studied and measurements were made of the ease with which they were solubilised.   The behaviour of the enzymes under conditions of differential and density gradient centrifugation was examined and experiments were carried out on the elution patterns from gel exclusion columns in a search for a possible complex.

Differential centrifugation of the lysed sphaeroplasts sedimented 50-70% of the glycolytic activities in P-1, a low speed pellet (1000 g(av.) for 15 min.).   Lysed sphaeroplasts tend to form empty membrane vesicles, showing full semipermeable characteristics, and because of the high concentration of lysozyme which we employed they clump into large masses and sediment at low centrifugation speeds.   Electron microscopic examination of the P-1 pellets showed them to contain only lysed sphaeroplasts, which were essentially devoid of cytoplasmic contents and consisted of membrane attached to fragments of partially degraded cell wall.   A convenient marker for cell membrane is NADH oxidase and measurement of this enzyme in our preparations showed about 80% in P-1, with the rest in a subsequent pellet (P-9) obtained by centrifuging the supernatant from P-1 (i.e. S-1) at 9000g (av) for 15 min.

The nature of the attachment of the glycolytic enzymes to cell membrane fractions is critical to an understanding of their role there.   Were they normally localized in the "soluble cytoplasm" and present in P-1 solely because of entrainment of portions of the supernatant fluid in membrane vesicles, their presence in a membrane fraction would have little or no physiological significance.   However, entrainment can be revealed by repeated washing, since once a vesicle is broken all the entrapped enzymes are liberated, and the quantities of the released enzymes would be similar to the gross proportions in which they were initially present in the membrane fraction. In practice repeated washing liberated enzyme activities at different rates. Two enzymes of the pentose phosphate pathway, glucose 6-phosphate dehydrogenase and 6-phosphogluconate dehydrogenase were included in these measurements since they would not be expected to be part of a glycolysis complex, and their washout behaviour might enable entrapped enzymes to be distinguished from those more specifically bound to membrane. Indeed, these two enzymes were removed very readily (more readily than any enzyme of glycolysis) by suspending the pellet P-1 in buffer and resedimenting it. The glycolysis enzymes were washed out differentially: glyceraldehyde 3-phosphate dehydrogenase was removed most easily, followed by phosphoglucose isomerase and triose phosphate isomerase while phosphofructokinase was retained most tenaciously.

The presence of enzymes in the membrane fraction was sensitive to the mode of sphaeroplast preparation and to their subsequent treatment. Breaking them by passage through a French pressure cell markedly altered the distributions of some activities, particularly glyceraldehyde 3-phosphate dehydrogenase and phosphoglucose isomerase, and resulted in higher proportions being found in the final supernatants. For triose phosphate isomerase there was redistribution into pellets sedimenting at higher speeds, while phosphofructokinase showed marked inactivation. The distribution of enzymes among the various pellets and supernatants depended also on the pH and ionic composition of the lysis fluid; for example, lysis at pH 8.0 resulted in 95% of the glyceraldehyde 3-phosphate dehydrogenase activity being retained in the pellet P-1 compared with 63% from lysis at pH 7-2. Phosphofructokinase activity overall was reduced by lysis at pH 8.0, but what activity was present was tightly bound to the membrane fraction with none at all present in the final high-speed supernatant. Passage of the lysed sphaeroplast preparation through the French pressure cell had little effect on the activity of most of the enzymes studied, but did cause considerable inactivation of phosphofructokinase: 65% of the activity was lost after one passage through the press with 87% after three passages. These results suggest that binding of the enzymes to membrane fractions is not haphazard and nonspecific, but may have real physiological significance, a conclusion substantiated in studies of the ability of these preparations to catalyse the complete sequence of glycolysis.

The total lysate and the pellet P-1, but not the supernatant S-1, were capable of converting glucose to pyruvate,
thereby demonstrating that all the enzymes of glycolysis were
present. The specific catalytic activity of the pellet was
about twice that of the lysate. The lack of measurable
pyruvate formation in the supernatant S-1 was unexpected. Of
six glycolytic enzymes specifically measured in the total
lysate an average of 60% was present in the pellet P-1
(ranging from 75% for glyceraldehyde 3-phosphate dehydrogenase
to 43% for phosphoglucose isomerase), leaving about 40% in the
supernatant S-1. The total protein concentration, and hence
the total activity of each glycolytic enzyme, was high enough
in S-1 for some product to have been expected. The fact that
none was observed suggests either that an unmeasured factor
was missing or that an essential organisational aspect,
present in P-1, was absent in S-1. Dilution of P-1 of course
reduced the total activity per unit volume of reaction mixture,
but more interestingly reduced it to a greater degree than
warranted by the extent of dilution; thus dilution reduced
the specific catalytic activity, presumably as a result of
some loss of catalytic components from the membranes to the
supernatant where, as we have just noted, they are effectively
inactive as a coherent pathway at the prevailing concentrations. This is precisely a property expected of a complex
enzyme system in which dilution results in disaggregation of
the component entities of the organised structure. High
protein concentration per se does not appear to be important
for maintenance of the organisation: an eight-fold dilution
of the pellet P-1 still retained throughput glycolytic
activity although its total protein concentration was only one
quarter that of the inactive supernatant S-1.

We have not yet sufficient information to decide whether
two species of the glycolytic enzymes coexist in the sense of
one species being membrane-bound and the other free in the
cytosol. Our data so far is consistent with enzyme activities
present in the soluble supernatants being derived from enzyme
molecules detached from the membranes during their preparation,
but does not exclude other interpretations. Thus, while we
have evidence of glycolytic activity being associated with
membranes we do not yet know whether this is related to the
functional compartmentation in living bacteria described
earlier.

D. A Multi-Enzyme Glycolysis Complex

Whether the glycolytic enzymes are normally resident on
the membranes or in the cytosol it should be possible to
isolate a complex of enzymes if one exists as a functional

unit; attempts have been made to do this from the supernatant
of sphaeroplast lysates. The molecular weights of all the
glycolytic enzymes in E. coli are not known with certainty;
using data from Mowbray and Moses (7) and from Gorringe (8)
it can be calculated that a glycolytic complex containing one
molecule of each enzyme would have a molecular weight of
between 1.0 and 1.6 million. In a lysate one might reasonably
expect to find the individual enzymes in both the complexed
and uncomplexed states. Separatory techniques should therefore
yield two molecular weight fractions showing activity for each
enzyme, one at a high value corresponding to a complex and the
other at a low value indicative of the molecular weight of the
uncomplexed molecule.

The supernatant obtained after sedimentation of the pellet
P-1 was concentrated by ultrafiltration and a sample applied
to Agarose A-1.5M covering the molecular weight range 5×10^4
to 1.5×10^6. Two peaks of activity were obtained for several
of the enzymes. In each case most of the activity was eluted
in fractions corresponding to the molecular weight of the
enzyme itself, but a proportion of each activity was also
recovered from a fraction with a molecular weight of 1.15×10^6.
The enzymes in the high molecular weight fraction showed a high
degree of co-chromatography. A similar distribution of
glycolytic enzymes was obtained by using ultrafiltration to
concentrate a solution of enzymes released by washing the
pellet P-1, again with a clear distinction between the high
and low molecular weight activities. These results lend
support to the idea that the enzymes exist normally in a complexed form, perhaps membrane bound; washing, or dilution,
would cause dissociation of the complex which could be reformed
to a degree by reconcentration. It was possible to confirm
the pattern of dissociation and association resulting from
dilution and concentration. If the eluted fractions containing all the low molecular weight enzymes were pooled,
concentrated and reapplied to the column, some of the activity
was recovered in a high molecular weight form. Similarly, if
the high molecular weight fractions were recycled through the
column, much of the activity reappeared with a low molecular
weight.

The high molecular weight complex displayed crypticity
for some of the enzyme activities. Triose phosphate isomerase
activity could not be demonstrated in the complex by direct
assay and that of phosphoglucose isomerase was very low.
There was no doubt that they were present: recycling of the
complex through the column resulted in measureable activities
for these enzymes at low molecular weight, and the complex
itself was able to catalyse the production of pyruvate from
glucose. We therefore concluded that, as a result of

shielding, some of the enzymes in the complex are unable to use substrates in free solution although the same substrates can be accepted when generated by a neighbouring enzyme. This, of course, is the very essence of molecular channelling and, as we shall see later, similar effects were obtained in experiments with labelled substrates.

The complex had a physical form. Electron microscope studies of negatively-stained preparations showed fields of circular (or spherical) particles with a diameter of about 30 nm. Their uniform appearance suggested a specific association. Their size was appropriate for a protein particle with a molecular weight rather more than 1 million. Washing the particles on the formvar grids before fixing suggested an aggregation of between seven and thirteen smaller units, which again fits roughly with the number of enzymes in the glycolytic sequence.

The complex was able to convert glucose to pyruvate much more effectively than a mixture of the low molecular weight glycolysis enzymes at equivalent concentration. At a protein concentration of 0.20 mg./ml. the collection of individual enzymes produced no detectable pyruvate (measured as lactic acid). The complex, at a protein concentration of 0.13 mg./ml., generated lactic acid at a rate of 3.2 µg./min./mg.protein. Concentration of the pooled individual enzymes by ultra-filtration to 0.48 mg.protein/ml. then gave a yield of lactate of 1.97 µg./min./mg. protein; complex formation thus appears to be quite sensitive to the concentration of the individual enzymes, but this has not yet been studied in detail.

Finally, it has been found that the complex acts as a metabolic compartment. Labelled glucose or glucose 6-phosphate was supplied to the complex together with cofactors, glutamic acid and alanine amino transferase; the labelled alanine produced was isolated by paper chromatography. The very production of alanine demonstrated the presence in the complex of all the glycolysis enzymes. The yield of labelled alanine was also measured in the presence of unlabelled glycolytic intermediates added to the reaction mixtures in such concentrations that had they been able to act as alanine precursors the specific radioactivity of the alanine would have been greatly reduced. Three intermediates were investigated: fructose 1,6-diphosphate, 3-phosphoglycerate and phosphoenolpyruvate. Each added intermediate reduced the specific radioactivity of alanine to some extent, with fructose 1,6-diphosphate having the least effect and phosphoenolpyruvate the most. But the concentrations of the unlabelled intermediates were several times higher than the maximum concentrations possible for those same metabolites generated from labelled glucose or glucose 6-phosphate. When an appropriate allowance was made

for that it became clear that the labelled intermediates
derived from hexose were highly favoured for alanine formation.

   With this system we feel we have now reached a stage of
partial understanding. The glycolytic enzymes are able to
form a high molecular weight complex which converts glucose
to pyruvate in a slightly leaky compartment. It is not yet
known how specific the association is between the glycolytic
enzymes, nor whether the complex exists in the living cell in
the form in which we have observed it. It may be present
free in the cytosol or attached to the membrane. Alternatively, the individual enzymes may in vivo normally be bound
to the membrane in a structured array, but, on being concentrated in solution in the absence of membrane, may bind with
one another to give a structure not normally found in the
cell, but reminiscent of one that is. The role of the complex
has yet to be related directly to the metabolic compartmentation found in a behavioural sense in the living bacteria,
yet it is not unlikely that they are different facets of the
same phenomenon.

                V.   CONCLUSIONS AND INTERPRETATIONS

   Some calculations have suggested that the frequency of
enzyme-substrate encounters by free diffusion in an aqueous
medium is quite sufficient to account for the observed rates
of metabolism and of growth in cells as small as those of
E. coli. One might ask what advantage would then ensue from
the compartmentation of metabolism. A possible answer might
lie in the matter of solvation. Atkinson has pointed out
that the presence in cytoplasm of so many solutes may limit
the availability of water as a solvent and force metabolite
concentrations to be lower than they would need to be to
saturate protein binding sites (12). By the formation of
enzyme complexes the need for solvent water for metabolic
intermediates might be markedly reduced. It has been shown
by Sols and Marco that many glycolytic and other intermediates
in eukaryotic cells are protein-bound, which is consistent
with their being confined to metabolic channels (13). Such
binding might also explain the observation made by Ling and
Cope that the diffusion co-efficients for small molecules
within cells may be very much smaller than values calculated
for the same substances in free solution (14); there may
actually not be sufficient time for enzymes and substrates to
encounter one another by diffusion to the extent necessary to
satisfy observed reaction rates. Interaction would presumably

be made more likely and more rapid by the generation of substrates in the immediate vicinities of the catalytic sites at
which they react.

Lastly, there may be an advantage of compartmentation for
the control of metabolism. A useful analogy is that of an
urban motorway. Most streets in a city interconnect with one
another, and traffic may move in all conceivable directions.
Progress is, however, slow, routes are indirect and congested,
and the rapid movement of bulk loads between distant points
is difficult. A motorway is superimposed on the network of
city streets and interacts with them at infrequent and well-
defined access points. A vehicle once entered upon a motorway
cannot readily be diverted by frequent intersections, but
must travel a long distance before it may escape and that it
may do at relatively high speeds. The mass movement of bulk
goods becomes fast and efficient. A metabolic compartment
may be just like that in relation to the overall network of
cellular metabolism. Glycolysis, being one of the very central pathways for the metabolism of primary energy-yielding
substrates, and requiring the conversion of large amounts of
material from hexose to pyruvate, may be an ideal candidate
for a compartmentalised organisation. For a small cell
devoid of internal membranous architecture the only way to
achieve this might be by interactions at the molecular level
between enzyme molecules engaged in a common co-operative
series of actions.

REFERENCES

1. Moses, V., in "Die Zelle: Struktur und Funktion" (H.
   Metzner, ed.), 2nd ed., p. 260, Wissenschaftliche
   Verlagsgesellschaft, Stuttgart, 1971.
2. Srere, P.A., and Mosbach, K., Ann. Rev. Microbiol. 28:61
   (1973).
3. Oaks, A., and Bidwell, R.G.S., Ann. Rev. Plant Physiol.
   21:43 (1970).
4. Moses, V. and Lonberg-Holm, K.K., J. Theoret. Biol.
   10:336 (1966).
5. McBrien, D.C.H. and Moses, V., J. Gen. Microbiol. 51:159
   (1968).
6. Macnab, R., Moses, V., and Mowbray, J., Eur. J. Biochem.
   34:15 (1973).
7. Mowbray, J. and Moses, V., Eur. J. Biochem. 66:25 (1976).
8. Gorringe, D.M., Ph.D. Thesis (University of London) (1977).
9. Gorringe, D.M., and Moses, V., Biochem. Soc. Trans.,in
   the press (1978).

10. Gorringe, D.M., and Moses, V., Biochem. J., in prepara-
     tion (1978).
11. Gorringe, D.M., and Moses, V., Biochem. J., in prepara-
     tion (1978).
12. Atkinson, D.E., Curr. Top. Cell. Regul. 1:29 (1969).
13. Sols, A., and Marco, R., Curr. Top. Cell. Regul. 2:227
     (1970).
14. Ling, G.N., and Cope, F.W., Science (Wash. D.C.) 163:1335
     (1969).

DISCUSSION

R. WELCH: I have a question to Dr. Moses regarding the
stability of what may be called the "glycosome" (cf.
Opperdoes, F. R. and Borst, P., FEBS Letters 80, 360, 1977).
Do you find metabolic effector substances which may enhance
or weaken the stability of this complex? For example, in
muscle, Clark and Masters (Biochim. Biophys. Acta 358, 193
(1974)) showed that positive effectors tend to enhance
structuralization whereas negative effectors tend to promote disaggregation. So, do you find that substances like
ATP, ADP, or fructose-phosphates influence the stability
of your "glycosome"?

V. MOSES: We haven't looked so I can't give you an answer.
The only thing I can say about the stability of the complex
is that the material comes off a column and is stable long
enough to exist in this diluted solution so that it doesn't
fall to pieces immediately and can be measured. But we have
done no tests on the effect of environmental effectors on
the stability of the complex.

C. deDUVE: I was very interested in Dr. Moses' presentation
since I wrote a paper a few years ago in which I asked the
question: "Is there a glycolytic particle?" (In: "Structure
and Function of Oxidation. Reduction Enzymes", A. Akeson
and A. Ehrenberg, eds., Oxford: Pergamon, pp. 715-728,
1972), and my answer was "No". Now my paper concerned rat
liver, not E. Coli. One of my arguments was that the
stoichiometry was all wrong. How is it in E. Coli?

V. MOSES: Again, I think the studies are at too early a
stage to be really very conclusive. As far as we can tell
there is a single representative of each enzyme. Now, what
we don't know is what would happen if one tried to form such
particles out of a mixture of soluble enzymes of varying portions. This we have never done. We have only used wild-type

E. coli lysates which contain whatever proportion of enzymes the extract contains and the particle I have described is the one that comes out of it. If one were to use some other proportion of enzymes to start with, would one always get a constant proportion of enzymes in the particle or not? That we don't know yet but it is a very critical thing to establish whether this complex has any real validity or is simply an artifactual conglomeration.

R. DAVIS: Dr. Moses, I wonder about cell heterogeneity in some of the earlier experiments you described where you have different pathways of utilization using given precursors of glycolysis. Is heterogeneity excluded by your data?

V. MOSES: I think it is fairly well excluded, in particular in the experiments on amino acid biosynthesis. In those experiments we had a much better steady-state of growing cultures which were in no way inhibited. In the earlier work we had to use chloroamphenicol as an inhibitor since we were using inducers as substrates in a system where we didn't want any induction. So, yes, you could argue that there may be some uncertainty about a steady-state in the inhibited cells. However, I think that having done this sort of investigation in a variety of ways, coming up every time with more or less the same conclusion, one feels fairly happy that it is a real physiological phenomenon not to be explained simply on the grounds of a heterogeneous population.

B. CHANCE: Have you pondered the "go-fast" or "M-4" motorway idea on a kinetic basis? In most enzymatic reactions, the enzyme is essentially stationary and the reaction rate is determined by the diffusion of the substrate molecule. You have to have substrate diffusion gradients in a "go-fast" scheme. On this basis you may decide whether your idea has merit or not? Do you love it?

V. MOSES: Yes, of course, I love it. It is mine. Well not mine, it is ours. One has this relationship to one's ideas, as you may have noticed. I just can't comment on your observation as these sorts of considerations are not within my experience. I will think about it, however.

J. BLUM: There is a paper in a recent issue of the Journal of General Physiology (Volume 69, pg. 605-632, 1977) showing that some glycolytic enzymes are located on the membrane of red blood cells in such a way to cause a compartmentation of ATP in the membrane. It occurs to me that perhaps some

of the differences you find in the labeling patterns of
glucose, galactose, and those sugars derived from lactose,
might be a reflection of the compartmentation of ATP rather
than the existence of the glycolytic complex you find, even
assuming that it exists in the cell.

V. MOSES: I accept that, but then would you like to interpret
the significance of the complex?

J. BLUM: No, that is not the issue I was raising. It may
exist but not be a functionally different compartment. The
relative labeling and accessibility to some of these enzymes
may be determined by events at the membrane even if the complex exists as such in the cytosol.

V. MOSES: Yes, I think I would agree with that. What you
are saying is that the compartmentation may be of the adenine nucleotides. Yes, I certainly wouldn't deny that possibility, because what I presented at that stage of the talk
was behavioral data which would be subject to interpretation
on a variety of bases.

S. BESSMAN: I just wanted to say that Dr. Kanter in our
laboratory showed that the glycolytic system in its entirety
is attached to the membrane of the red cell. He showed this
by demonstrating that complete glycolysis occurs using the
membrane which has been badly mistreated according to the
ways they said removed enzymes from the membrane. Just as
Dr. Moses showed, we are able to show you couldn't detect
any of the glycolytic pathway at the same time that you
could convert glucose-6-phosphate to lactate by these
membranes.

MECHANISMS FOR THE INTRACELLULAR
COMPARTMENTATION OF NEWLY
SYNTHESIZED PROTEINS

Günter Blobel

Department of Cell Biology
The Rockefeller University
New York, New York 10021

Following their synthesis on either free or membrane-
bound ribosomes, proteins have to follow distinctly different
intracellular pathways in order to reach their characteristic
localization in various compartments. One of the obligatory
steps in some of these pathways is the crossing of intracellular membranes. Since the lipid bilayer of membranes is impermeable to charged molecules, such as proteins, it is evident that complex mechanisms must exist in order to achieve
this transfer. Based on what is presently known about this
phenomenon, the following general rules can be formulated:
transfer of proteins across intracellular membranes should be
(1) vectorial, i.e., it should proceed from the site of the
membrane which faces the protein synthetic machinery;
(2) irreversible, i.e., transfer back into the opposite direction should not occur; (3) selective, i.e., only specific
proteins should cross specific membranes; and (4) conservative, i.e., during crossing of the protein through the membrane the permeability barrier to other solutes should be
conserved.

Copyright © 1978 by Academic Press, Inc.
All right of reproduction in any form reserved.
ISBN 0-12-660550-5

Recent experiments in which synthesis and transfer of proteins across membranes has been achieved in vitro have provided some clues as to the mechanisms involved. From the examples which have so far been analyzed the following principles have emerged. Proteins to be transferred across intracellular membranes are initially synthesized as larger molecules with an additional sequence, referred to as "signal" sequence, which is anywhere from 15 to 45 amino acid residues long. The signal sequence is presumably recognized by specific integral membrane proteins that are restricted in their localization to certain intracellular membranes. Interaction of the signal sequence with these receptor proteins presumably leads to formation of a pore in the membrane through which the protein can pass. In most cases the signal sequence is removed either shortly before, during, or shortly after passage of the protein by specific endoproteolytic enzymes referred to as signal peptidases. After passage of the protein is completed, the pore is presumably disassembled, to be reassembled again only by the signal sequence of another protein molecule. Thus the lifetime of the cyclically reassembled and disassembled pores would be synchronized with the duration of transfer of a single protein molecule across the membrane. In this way transfer would be "conservative" (see above).

From the experimental evidence so far accumulated, two distinctly different formulas can be discerned for the transfer of proteins across membranes. These two formulas differ primarily in the timing of transfer with respect to protein synthesis. In the "cotranslational" formula, transfer is tightly coupled to translation and proceeds while the protein is being synthesized on membrane-bound ribosomes. In the "posttranslational" formula, transfer occurs after chain completion and does not depend on a ribosome-membrane junction. In the following, a brief review will be given of what is presently known about these two formulas. The intent is not to cover the data in detail. Rather, the aim is to analyze the available data conceptually and to provide the reader thus initiated with a key to some of the pertinent literature.

Cotranslational transfer

The signal hypothesis (1) has been proposed as a scheme for a cotranslational transfer of secretory proteins across the endoplasmic reticulum membrane via a ribosome-membrane junction (see Fig. 1).

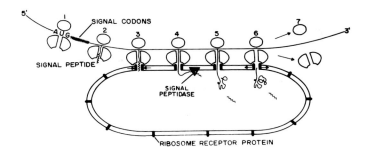

FIG.1. Schematic illustration of the signal hypothesis for the cotranslational transfer of secretory proteins across the endoplasmic reticulum membrane (taken from ref. 2).

A detailed description of this hypothesis as well as of some of the evidence for it has been given previously (2). Among the most compelling data in support of the signal hypothesis are those which were obtained from "in vitro reconstitution" experiments (3-8). mRNA's for various secretory proteins were translated in a cell-free, protein-synthesizing system in vitro either in the presence or the absence of microsomal membranes from dog pancreas. The latter were prepared by subjecting isolated rough microsomes to procedures which remove the bulk of the membrane-bound ribosomes but presumably leave the putative ribosome receptor proteins intact and exposed on the outside of the microsomal membrane vesicles. While translation of various mRNA's for secretory proteins in cell-free systems in the absence of membranes resulted in the synthesis of molecules larger than mature secretory proteins (referred to as "presecretory" proteins), tranlation in the presence of microsomal vesicles yielded molecules identical in size to mature secretory proteins or their "pro" forms. Thus translation of these mRNA's in the presence of microsomal membranes resulted in cleavage ("processing") of the signal peptide portion. Most importantly, however, translation in the presence of the microsomal membrane vesicles also resulted in segregation of the "processed" chain within the lumen of the microsomal vesicles. As a result, the processed chains

were found to be resistant to proteolytic enzymes. Resistance, however, was abolished when incubation with proteolytic enzymes was done in the presence of detergents to sol-
ubilize the membrane. Thus resistance to proteolysis was not
merely an intrinsic property of the processed chain but was
due to the protection afforded by microsomal vesicles. Processing and segregation took place only when microsomal membranes were present during translation but not when added
after translation. Thus, processing and segregation are cotranslational, not posttranslational events. It was also
shown that translation of mRNA's for the α and β chains of
globin did not result in segregation of the newly synthesized
globin chains within the dog pancreas microsomal vesicles.

Taken together these data strongly suggested that the initial events in the intracellular pathway of secretory proteins, namely, synthesis and segregation, had been successfully reconstituted in vitro, and that this reconstitution
had proceeded according to the predictions made in the signal
hypothesis.

The components of the first reconstitution experiment (3)
were derived from widely different sources: the ribosomal subunits were from rabbit reticulocytes, the mRNA for the light
chain of IgG from mouse myelomas, the microsomal membranes
from dog pancreas, and the factors for protein synthesis from
mouse Ascites cells. The fact that processing and segregation of the mouse light chain occurred in this heterologous
system suggested that the various sites which in the signal
hypothesis have been proposed to interact with each other
have been largely conserved, at least among mammals. The
results of subsequent reconstitution experiments using components from widely different sources indicated that conservation and equivalence of sites may extend to most if not all
eukaryotic cells. Thus translation of mRNA for the light
chain of mouse IgG in a wheat germ cell-free system supplemented with dog pancreas microsomal membranes resulted in
processing as well as segregation of the nascent light chains
(4), indicating that plant ribosomes are able to establish a
functional junction with animal microsomal membranes.
Furthermore, translation of a mRNA for a fish secretory pro-
tein--insulin--in the wheat germ cell-free system supplemented
with mammalian (dog pancreas) microsomal membranes resulted in
processing of nascent fish preproinsulin and segregation of
fish proinsulin (5), indicating that mammalian microsomal membranes are able to recognize signal sequences of evolutionarily distant species. Furthermore, it was found that cleavage of various nascent presecretory proteins from fish (5),

cow (6), and rat (7) by dog pancreas microsomal signal peptidase was always at the correct site generating the authentic
amino termini of their "pro" forms or their secreted forms.
Correct cotranslational processing of nascent presecretory proteins has been achieved also with microsomal membranes from
Ascites cells (9) or bovine pituitary (6).

From the data of the reconstitution experiments it is
clear that the signal peptide portions of a great variety of
nascent presecretory proteins are likely to share those structurally distinct features which constitute the proper two recognition sites, one for the putative ribosome receptor proteins and one for signal peptidase (see Fig. 1). However,
from the primary structure of the signal peptide portion of
the more than 20 presecretory proteins that is now known, it
is at present not clear what these distinct features are.
The signal peptides may vary in length from 15-30 amino acid
residues. They usually contain a cluster of hydrophobic residues in the middle with some charged or hydrophilic residues
on either end. The penultimate residue of the signal peptide portion which could have provided some clues as to the
specificity of signal peptidase has been found to vary.
ALA, CYS, GLY and SER have so far been detected in this position. It is most likely, therefore, that the distinct features of the signal peptides reside in their secondary structure.

Evidence has been obtained that signal peptidase is an
endoproteolytic enzyme which removes the signal peptide portion by a single endoproteolytic cleavage (10, 11). The
enzyme has been solubilized by detergents (10, 11). It was
shown to be present only in rough but not smooth microsomes
(10). Its activity in rough microsomes is latent, indicating
that the active site is not facing the cytosol (10).

It had been anticipated in the signal hypothesis (1) that
cleavage of the signal peptide may not be an obligatory step
for cotranslational transfer of all secretory proteins. Ovalbumin appears to provide the first example for this. It has
been reported recently that ovalbumin is not synthesized as a
larger molecule (12). This finding, however, has been interpreted (12) to indicate that segregation of ovalbumin proceeds
by mechanisms different from those which were proposed in the
signal hypothesis. However, recent reconstitution experiments
to be reported elsewhere (8) have indicated that ovalbumin is
cotranslationally transferred across the dog pancreas membrane
like any other nascent secretory protein except that the functional equivalent of the signal peptide is retained in the
mature molecule.

Another variant for cotranslational transfer that has been
anticipated in the signal hypothesis (1,2) concerns synthesis
and insertion into the membranes of certain integral <u>membrane</u>

proteins. It was proposed that passage of the <u>amino</u> terminal
portion of these proteins proceeds as for secretory protein
but that cotranslational transfer of the remainder of the nascent chain is halted at some point during synthesis.

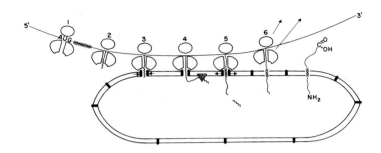

FIG. 2. Schematic illustration of a variant of the signal
hypothesis for the cotranslational insertion of a bitopic integral membrane protein into the endoplasmic reticulum membrane (taken from ref. 2).

The information for this event was proposed (2) to reside in--
or very close to--that portion of the nascent polypeptide chain
which spans the lipid bilayer. It is likely that this "stop-
transfer" sequence exhibits distinct structural features which
are common to all bitopic[1] integral membrane proteins.
        Evidence in support of cotranslational insertion into the
membrane has been obtained so far for two bitopic integral
membrane proteins, one eukaryotic and the other prokaryotic.
Both, however, are proteins which are coded for by viral nucleic acids.
        In the first case, <u>in vitro</u> synthesis and insertion of the
glycoprotein G of vesicular stomatitis virus (VSV) has been
studied. mRNA for G was translated in a cell-free wheat germ
system supplemented with dog pancreas microsomal membranes(13).

---

        [1]Based on biosynthetic considerations, integral membrane
proteins are classified as mono-, bi-, or polytopic. A comprehensive analysis of their biosynthesis and intracellular
pathway will be published elsewhere (Blobel, G. <u>et al</u>., in
preparation).

The newly synthesized protein--referred to as G_1--was observed to be core-glycosylated. Most importantly however G_1 was found to be asymmetrically inserted into the dog pancreas microsomal membranes: a distinct, but minor portion of G_1, amounting to about 30 amino acid residues in size, was removed by posttranslational incubation with proteolytic enzymes. The remaining bulk of the G_1, referred to as G_1', was resistant to proteolytic enzymes unless the membranes were solubilized with detergents. Translation of the mRNA for G in the absence of microsomal membranes yielded synthesis of an unglycosylated form of G referred to as G_0. There was no conversion of G_0 to G_1 nor was there protection of G_0 from proteolysis after posttranslational incubation of G_0 with microsomal membranes. Thus, core glycosylation as well as asymmetric insertion into the membrane are cotranslational and not posttranslational events (13). Further studies using amino terminal (14) sequence analysis of the various forms of G revealed the following: (1) G_0 contained an amino terminal "signal" peptide of 16 amino acid residues that was absent in G_1; (2) the amino terminal sequences of G_1 and G_1' were identical, indicating that G_1' was generated from G_1 by loss of a carboxy terminal fragment. Recent experiments (14) have also shown that the signal peptide of nascent G_0 is functionally equivalent to those of nascent presecretory proteins since both compete for the same sites that are present in the dog pancreas microsomal membranes. A second bitopic membrane protein that has been studied is one which is integrated, at least temporarily, into the plasma membrane of E. coli. This protein is the coat protein CP of bacteriophage f1. Synthesis of this protein in a cell-free and coupled transcription-translation system yielded synthesis of a larger molecule--preCP--which contained an amino terminal signal peptide (15, 16). Supplementation of the cell-free system with inverted vesicles derived from the inner membrane of E. coli yielded cleavage of the signal peptide and synthesis of CP. There was no conversion of preCP to CP when preCP was incubated with inverted vesicles only after translation. Preliminary experiments using posttranslational incubation with proteolytic enzymes indicated (17) that only a carboxyterminal portion of the in vitro inserted CP is accessible to proteolysis whereas the amino terminal portion, presumably protruding into the lumen of the inverted vesicles, was entirely protected.

In both instances then, representing a eukaryotic and a prokaryotic bitopic integral membrane protein, synthesis proceeds as for secretory proteins via a short-lived amino terminal signal peptide which triggers the formation of a functional ribosome-membrane junction. Unlike in the case of secretory proteins, however, transfer across the membrane is

incomplete so that the nascent chain of a bitopic integral
membrane protein becomes lodged in the membrane with the carboxyterminal portion exposed to the cytoplasm.

Posttranslational transfer

Recent work (18) on the in vitro synthesis of a polypeptide that is localized in the chloroplast stroma but is synthesized in the cytosol (the small subunit "S" of ribulose-1,5-
biphosphate carboxylase of Chlamydomonas reinhardtii) reveals
that a second formula exists for transfer of proteins across
intracellular membranes.   Translation of mRNA for S in a wheat
germ cell-free system resulted in the synthesis of a larger
form of S, pS. It was shown that this molecule is synthesized
by free ribosomes and not by membrane-bound ribosomes. A
soluble endoprotease has been detected in Chlamydomonas which
is able to cleave pS to S and a small peptide "F". By sequence
analysis it has been established recently (19) that pS contains an additional sequence of 44 amino acid residues at the
amino terminus and that the above-mentioned soluble endoprotease cleaves pS at the correct site yielding mature S. It
was proposed (18) that the F portion of pS interacts with a
receptor in the chloroplast envelope that might be located in
those portions of the chloroplast envelope which show a close
apposition of the outer and the inner chloroplast envelope
membrane. This interaction was proposed (18) to generate a
pore through which a posttranslational import into chloroplast
would proceed.
      Studies are now under way to determine which of these two
formulas is used for the compartmentation of lysosomal and
peroxisomal proteins and of those mitochondrial proteins which
are synthesized in the cytosol.

REFERENCES

1. Blobel, G., and Dobberstein, B. 1975. J. Cell Biol. 67:
    835-851.
2. Blobel, G. 1977. In International Cell Biology 1976-1977,
    eds. B.R. Brinkley and K.R. Porter, pp. 318-325. New York:
    The Rockefeller University Press.
3. Blobel, G., and Dobberstein, B. 1975. J. Cell Biol. 67:
    852-862.
4. Dobberstein, B., and Blobel, G. 1976. Biochem. Biophys.
    Res. Commun. 68:1-7.
5. Shields, D., and Blobel, G. 1977. Proc. Natl. Acad. Sci.
    U.S.A. 74:2059-2063.
6. Lingappa, V.R., Devillers-Thiery, A., and Blobel, G. 1977.
    Proc. Natl. Acad. Sci. U.S.A. 74:2432-2436.

7. Lingappa, V.R., Lingappa, J.R., Prasad, R., Ebner, K., and Blobel, G. Proc. Natl. Acad. Sci. U.S.A., in press.
8. Lingappa, V.R., and Blobel, G., in preparation.
9. Birken, S., Smith, D.L., Canfield, R.E., and Boime, I. 1977. Biochem. Biophys. Res. Commun. 74:106-112.
10. Jackson, R.C., and Blobel, G. 1977. Proc. Natl. Acad. Sci. U.S.A. 74:5598-5602.
11. Chang, C.N., Blobel, G., and Model, P. 1978. Proc. Natl. Acad. Sci. U.S.A. 75:361-365.
12. Palmiter, R.D., Gagnon, J., and Walsh, K.A. 1978. Proc. Natl. Acad. Sci. U.S.A. 75:94-98.
13. Katz, F.N., Rothman, J.E., Lingappa, V.R., Blobel, G., and Lodish, H.F. 1977. Proc. Natl.Acad.Sci.U.S.A.74:3278-3282.
14. Lingappa, V.R.,Katz, F.N.,Lodish,H.F., and Blobel, G., in preparation.
15. Model, P., McGill, C., and Kindt, T., in preparation.
16. Chang, C.N., Blobel, G., and Model, P. 1978. Proc. Natl. Acad. Sci. U.S.A. 75:351-365.
17. Chang, C.N., Model, P., and Blobel, G., in preparation.
18. Dobberstein, B., Blobel, G., and Chua, N.H. 1977. Proc. Natl. Acad. Sci. U.S.A. 74:1082-1085.
19. Schmidt, G., Devillers-Thiery, A., DesRuisseaux, H., Blobel, G., and Chua, N.H., in preparation.

DISCUSSION

R. BUTOW: Two questions for Dr. Blobel. First is whether
or not the Chlamydamonas signal peptidase will work on
secreted pre-proteins in higher eukaryotes and vice-versa.
The second question is whether you have tried reconstruction
experiments with polysomes translating the small subunit of
the chloroplast carboxylase in the presence of membrane?

G. BLOBEL: In answer to your first question: No, it does
not and we tried the reconstitution experiment which you
suggested and the result was negative. We added animal
membranes to the wheat germ system translating the messen-
ger RNA for the carboxylase and we did not find any cleavage nor did we find any segregation.

B. CHANCE: It seemed to me that you sort of "took the
fifth" on your views on membrane proteins such as cytochrome
oxidase? Was there a reason for that?

G. BLOBEL: Well, if you accept the proposed nomenclature
of bitopic and polytopic integral membrane proteins (IMPs)
we would think that bi- and polytopic IMPs, having sites
on either side of the lipid bilayer, would be important in
the sorting of monotopic IMPs. In the case of cytochrome
oxidase, or ATPase there are a number of subunits which are
synthesized in the mitochondria, probably by membrane bound
ribosomes, and they are probably inserted into the inner
mitochondrial membrane cotranslationally. We would predict that they are bitopic or polytopic in nature. The
other subunits, however, which are synthesized in the
cytoplasm are probably monotopic in nature and after they
have been transferred across the membrane, by a posttranslational formula, they will probably find their proper bi-
or polytopic partner with which they will associate to
form the holoenzyme.

INTRACELLULAR METABOLITE DISTRIBUTION
AS A FACTOR IN REGULATION
IN NEUROSPORA[1]

Rowland H. Davis

Department of Molecular Biology and Biochemistry
University of California, Irvine
Irvine, California

Richard L. Weiss

Department of Chemistry
University of California, Los Angeles
Los Angeles, California

Barry J. Bowman

Department of Human Genetics
Yale University Medical School
New Haven, Connecticut

I.   INTRODUCTION

The arginine pathway of the filamentous fungus, Neurospora, has long been a focus of genetic, enzymological and metabolic work. One of the earliest investigations in biochemical genetics was that of Srb and Horowitz (1) who described genetic blocks in the familiar ornithine-citrulline-arginine sequence. With the detection of arginase, they speculated that an ornithine cycle prevailed in the organism. Later work in various laboratories, including our own, has culminated in

[1]Supported by NSF grants GB-13398 and PCM75-16245 to R.H.D. and PCM76-07708 to R.L.W.

Copyright © 1978 by Academic Press, Inc.
All right of reproduction in any form reserved.
ISBN 0-12-660550-5

the metabolic and cytological map of the arginine pathway depicted in Figure 1. All or most of the enzymes of the pathway
prior to the appearance of citrulline are located in the
mitochondria (2). The enzymes include those of the acetylglutamate cycle, which produces ornithine, together with
ornithine transcarbamylase and a carbamyl phosphate synthetase
(CPSase-A) specific for the arginine pathway. Citrulline is
transformed, via argininosuccinate, to arginine by two cytosolic enzymes (2). The biosynthetic pathway provides not
only arginine for protein synthesis, but also, diverging from
ornithine, provides putrescine for polyamine biosynthesis.
Putrescine is made in the cytosol from ornithine which emerges
from the mitochondria (2).

    As we shall see, an ornithine cycle does not prevail to
any great extent. The prevention of this cycle, even in conditions of excess arginine, is one of the major issues discussed below. Arginine, however, can be catabolized by the
cytosolic enzymes arginase and ornithine transaminase. Urea,
produced in the arginase reaction, is degraded to CO_2 and NH_3.

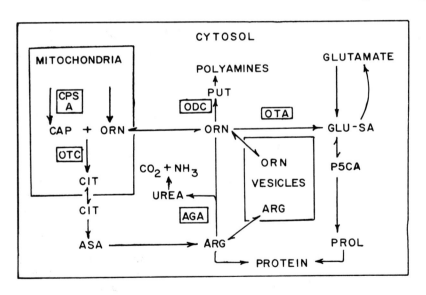

    FIGURE 1. Arginine and proline metabolism in Neurospora.
Abbreviations: (a) Intermediates: ARG, arginine; ASA,
argininosuccinate; CAP, carbamyl phosphate; CIT, citrulline;
GLU-SA, glutamate semialdehyde; ORN, ornithine; PROL, proline;
PUT, putrescine; P5CA, pyrroline-5-carboxylate. (b) Enzymes
(boxed symbols): AGA, arginase; CPS-A, carbamyl phosphate
synthetase A; ODC, ornithine decarboxylase; OTA, ornithine
transaminase; OTC, ornithine transcarbamylase.

Ornithine, the other product of the arginase reaction, is transformed to glutamic semialdehyde by ornithine transaminase. The semialdehyde can be oxidized to glutamate, or (in its cyclic form, pyrroline-5-carboxylate) it can be reduced to proline. One of our interests was to determine how ornithine reentry into the anabolic reactions is minimized in conditions favoring arginine catabolism.

Neurospora, even during growth in arginine-free medium, contains large amounts of arginine and ornithine. The pools (ca. 30 nmoles per mg, dry weight) would be about 10mM if distributed evenly in cell water (3). Such concentrations should result in catabolism of these compounds, feedback inhibition of the biosynthetic path, and maximal induction of the catabolic enzymes. As we will show, no catabolism of arginine occurs under these conditions despite the presence of substantial arginase activity. This paradox was resolved in general terms by the discovery of intracellular, membrane-enclosed vesicles which contain over 98% of the arginine and ornithine pools of cells grown in minimal medium (4). It is our thesis that these vesicles, together with the mitochondrial membrane, perform profound, dynamic roles in controlling the flow of metabolites in the pathway in "anabolic" and "catabolic" conditions (5-7). In particular, the membranes prevent arginine degradation when it is not called for; they promote it when it is called for; and they minimize ornithine cycling back through the biosynthetic path when the catabolic pathway is in operation. We shall discuss arginine and ornithine in turn, demonstrating how kinetic and "spatial" regulatory mechanisms interact to control metabolite flow.

II. ARGININE

A. Arginine Metabolism In Cells Grown In Arginine-free Medium

Several years ago, we used the ure-1 strain of Neurospora to monitor the fates of arginine in the cell (5). This strain has no detectable urease, and consequently urea accumulation could be used as an in vivo assay of the arginase reaction. The only other fates of arginine are entry into an acid soluble pool or into protein (8). When a very tiny amount of highly labelled ^{14}C-guanidino-arginine was added to a culture growing in arginine-free medium, about half of it appeared without delay in proteins (5). This happened despite the huge intracellular pool of unlabelled arginine. The remaining radioactive arginine was only slowly incorporated into protein. No label appeared in urea. The labelled

arginine was exhausted from the medium in about two minutes.
The labelled arginine which did not immediately enter proteins
appeared to be sequestered in the vesicles, and emerged at a
very low rate thereafter as a substrate for protein synthesis.
By comparing the specific radioactivity of intracellular
arginine and of new protein arginine as the label entered the
cell, we concluded that the cytosol contained no more than 1-
3% of the arginine of the cell (5). From these and other
data, we concluded that the cytosolic arginine concentration
was approximately 0.2 mM at most, the rest being in the
vesicles. Because no arginine was catabolized, we hypothe-
sized that this concentration was optimal for protein synthesis (i.e., arg-tRNA synthetase; Km = 2 x 10^{-5}M) but insuffi-
cient to satisfy the concentration requirement for arginase.

Another experiment extended the conclusions about catabolism. A culture of <u>ure-1</u> was grown for many hours in arginine-free medium, and urea accumulation was monitored. While
a small amount of urea was barely detected after inoculation,
the amount did not increase despite a 50-fold increase in
mass over 16 hours (9). This shows that arginase does not
exert its enzymic role at all in such cultures. Yet when
arginine is provided in high concentration to such a culture,
catabolism at a high rate is immediate (7,10).

These experiments led us to inquire whether the kinetic
properties of arginase included a threshhold arginine concentration below which the enzyme was inactive. Prior work with
arginase had always been performed after Mn^{++} activation, and
at the unphysiological, but optimum pH of 9.5. Assay of
crude "native" arginase, extracted and assayed without added
Mn^{++} at pH 7.5, yields a substrate-velocity curve which is
decidedly sigmoid (Figure 2). Moreover, the "native" enzyme
is about 80-fold less active at pH 7.5 than the Mn^{++}-enzyme
at the same pH (not shown). At pH 9.5, the native enzyme is
Michaelian (Figure 2), but it is still very much less active
than the Mn^{++} enzyme.

A second finding was that ornithine, the product, is even
more inhibitory to the native enzyme at pH 7.5 than it is in
the usual Mn^{++}-assay system at pH 9.5. Because the cytosolic
ornithine concentration in <u>Neurospora</u> is about 0.2mM (see
below), this is probably physiologically significant (11).

Our in vivo experiments, then, can be rationalized in
kinetic and spatial terms. The failure of arginase to catabolize endogenous arginine in arginine-free cultures is due in
great measure to three factors: the sequestration of arginine
in the vesicles; the sigmoid concentration-velocity curve of
arginase; and the inhibition of arginase by ornithine. The
"threshhold" arginine concentration of arginase is higher
than the estimated range of cytosolic arginine concentrations
for such cells.

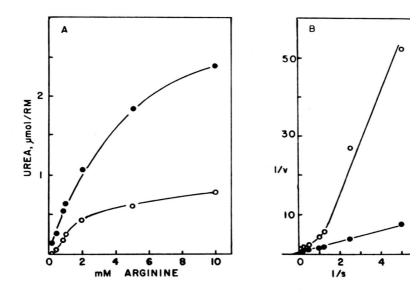

FIGURE 2. Substrate-velocity relationship of native arginase in crude extracts of a Neurospora mutant (ure-1) lacking
urease. ^{14}C-guanidino-L-arginine was incubated with crude
extract for 20 min. at 37C. Reaction mixtures were stopped
by adjusting to pH 5.0 and boiling. ^{14}C-urea released during
the enzyme reaction was measured after passing reaction mixture supernatants through AG-50W columns (Na[+]-form) at pH 5.3
to remove substrate. (A) Linear plot of data from reactions
performed at pH 7.5 (open circles) and at pH 9.5 (closed
circles). (B) Lineweaver-Burk plots of same data, using
same symbols.

B. Response of Cells to Added Arginine

When a large amount of arginine is added to cultures of
Neurospora grown in minimal medium, conditions appropriate
for catabolism are established. We have measured various
parameters following arginine administration to test the
immediacy of the cells' responses. The responses, drawn from
several experiments, are summarized in Table I, and are
described in turn. First, urea production begins immediately
and continues at a constant rate for the first hour (10).
Second, the induction of "synthetic capacity" (presumably
mRNA) for ornithine transaminase also begins immediately and
continues at a constant rate (12). We presume that arginase
synthetic capacity increases similarly, although we have not
measured it. The appearance of increased activity for both

TABLE I.   Response of Neurospora to the Addition of 1 mM
Arginine to the Growth Medium

Measured Response	Min after arginine addition		
	0	30	60
Urea (nmole/ml culture)	0	63	138
OTA synthetic capacity (units/mg protein)[a]	0.020	0.035	0.050
Arginine biosynthesis (CPM/ml culture)[b]	1015	948	987
Cellular arginine pool (nmole/mg dry weight)[c]	20	120	150
Cytosolic arginine pool (mM)[d]	0.2	15	15

[a] Cells were transferred to minimal medium at the times indicated and incubated for 90 min to allow for full expression of synthetic capacity (12).

[b] Cells were exposed to ^{14}C-glutamate for 1 hr prior to addition of arginine. At 0, 30, and 60 min after arginine addition they were analyzed for radioactivity in ornithine, soluble arginine, and protein arginine.

[c] Total, trichloroacetic-acid-soluble arginine was extracted from cells.

[d] Cytosolic arginine was measured in labelling experiments by the discrepancy of specific radioactivities of new-protein arginine and total, acid-extractable arginine (14).

enzymes requires approximately 1 hour. Third, feedback inhibition of ornithine synthesis is immediate and complete. This was established by finding an immediate cessation of entry of ^{14}C-glutamate into arginine and its precursors after addition of arginine (13). Fourth, the intracellular arginine pool increases for about 1.5 hr (10). Much of the arginine which enters actually goes into the vesicles, but the even more rapid uptake from the medium favors an immediately higher steady-state concentration in the cytosol. By measurement of the specific radioactivity of new proteins in suitable labelling experiments, we have found that the cytosolic concentration rises from less than 0.2 mM (in minimal medium) to about 15 mM when arginine is entering the cell (14). It is the new cytosolic steady-state concentration that appears to explain the immediacy of the other responses referred to above.

We thus attribute the immediate and adaptive onset of catabolic conditions to two main factors: the presence of substantial arginase and ornithine transaminase in the cells before arginine is added, and the differential rate of uptake between the plasma and vesicular membranes. As we shall discuss further below, entry of arginine into the vesicles in these conditions leads to an almost immediate discharge of over 90% of the vesicular ornithine to the cytosol. This, with a possible blockade to further entry of ornithine, leads to conditions favoring catabolism of this ornithine, as well as of the ornithine arising from the arginase reaction. The major point to be made is that the vesicular membranes serve a major regulatory role in controlling metabolism.

C. Response to Withdrawal of Arginine

A last indication of the role of the vesicular membranes in control is seen upon the withdrawal of arginine from cells growing in arginine-containing medium. Upon the exhaustion of arginine, such cultures cease catabolism (as measured by urea synthesis) within a few minutes, despite the presence of induced levels of arginase and a huge intracellular arginine pool (10). It is clear that most of the arginine is in the vesicles, and that the cytosolic arginine concentration is quickly reduced below the threshhold required by arginase. Yet the arginine in the vesicles emerges at a rate sufficient to satisfy the needs of protein synthesis, as determined by the continued growth of an arginine auxotroph (10). Thus vesicular membranes, even in this extreme condition, regulate the cytosolic concentration of arginine between the threshhold of arginase (ca. 0.2 mM) and the needs of arginyl-tRNA synthetase ($Km = 2 \times 10^{-5}M$).

III. ORNITHINE

A. Anabolic Conditions

In cells grown in minimal medium, ornithine is distributed in three pools: vesicles, cytosol, and mitochondria, the last location being the place where ornithine is made. Labeling studies (3,6) show the cytosol to have about 1% of the ornithine, yielding a concentration of about 0.2 mM if cytosolic water is 80% of cell water. The mitochondria also have about 1% of the ornithine, yielding a nominal concentration of about 1.0 mM if 13% of cell water is mitochondrial. We presume the other 98% of ornithine is the large vesicular pool. The disposition of ornithine is determined by its rate of synthesis and consumption, and the fluxes across mitochondrial and vesicular membranes. The latter have been

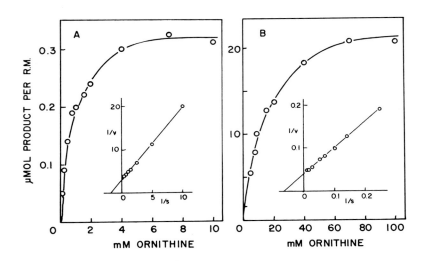

FIGURE 3. Substrate saturation curves for (A) ornithine
decarboxylase and (B) ornithine transaminase. Lineweaver-
Burk plots of the data are shown as insets. Ornithine decarboxylase was assayed in crude, desalted extracts at pH 6.5 by
the method of Morris et al. (15); ornithine transaminase was
assayed in crude, desalted extracts at pH 7.4 by the method
of Davis and Mora (16).

independently measured in our labelling studies in vivo (6,7).
     Our primary interest here is in the cytosolic enzymes
which use ornithine. The first is ornithine decarboxylase,
which yields the polyamine precursor putrescine. The saturation curve for this enzyme (Fig. 3A) is Michaelian, with a K_m
of about 0.5 mM in standard assay conditions. The enzyme
would not be saturated at the cytosolic ornithine concentration we have inferred above if the K_m in vivo is 0.5 mM.
This, as we shall see below, raises the question of how the
rate of putrescine synthesis responds to a large increase in
the cytosolic concentration of ornithine in catabolic
conditions.
     The second cytosolic enzyme of interest is ornithine
transaminase. We have regularly found that in minimal medium,
cells catabolize about 5-10% of the ornithine produced by the
cell (3,6). This is in marked contrast to the case of arginine in the same conditions: no arginine is catabolized, as
noted above. The saturation curve of ornithine transaminase
in vitro, is Michaelian, with a Km of about 15 mM (Fig. 3B).
Even at concentrations between 0.25 and 1.0 mM, there is no

sign of sigmoid kinetics. While we do not know the actual
intracellular conditions in which it operates, a Michaelian
enzyme would permit a finite rate of catabolism even at low
cytosolic ornithine concentrations. The catabolic drain on
cytosolic ornithine in cells grown in arginine-free medium is
probably not wasteful. This is because all the ornithine
which is catabolized by such cells is actually converted to
proline (3), thus sparing the independent biosynthetic pathway for proline. Catabolism of ornithine to glutamate only
happens when ornithine is present at high levels (9) in the
cytosol.

B. Catabolic Conditions

We now consider how the distribution and flow of ornithine
changes in response to addition of arginine. With regard to
biosynthesis of arginine, we have shown above that ornithine
immediately stops being made in the mitochondria. This presumably reflects feedback inhibition at the level of the
acetylglutamate synthase and kinase steps. All ornithine
which appears in the cytosol thereafter comes from the
vesicles or from the arginase reaction (7). However, a
serious economic problem remains: CPSase A is completely
insensitive to feedback inhibition of any kind. This has
been established not only with the purified enzyme (9), but
also by in vivo tests (6,9). While the enzyme is repressible,
repression takes over eight hours. Because no other enzyme
is repressed, the possible recycling of ornithine is a phenomenon the cells deal with in another way. Our labelling
studies show, in fact, that upon arginine administration,
citrulline synthesis is immediately reduced to about 20% of
the rate characteristic of cells grown in arginine-free
medium (6,7). The rate is reduced ultimately to zero over
the next eight hours (three doublings of dry weight) as
repression of CPSase-A becomes complete (6). There is no
evidence that ornithine transcarbamylase is inhibited by
arginine. We have therefore speculated (7), that cytosolic
arginine prevents the entry of cytosolic ornithine into the
mitochondria. Thus we see, if this hypothesis is correct,
that the mitochondrial membranes serve a regulatory role in
minimizing anabolic flux shortly after "catabolic" conditions
are established.

The net effect of arginine addition on ornithine flow,
then, is as follows. First, almost all the ornithine of the
vesicles is discharged into the cytosol, and further uptake
by the vesicles is blocked. Second, ornithine biosynthesis
ceases. Third, ornithine entry into the mitochondria is
greatly reduced. Over 80% of the ornithine in the cytosol is

TABLE II.   Rates of Enzyme Reactions In Vivo After
Addition of 1 mM Arginine[a]

Enzyme[b]	Interval analyzed		
	Prior to arginine addition	0-60 minutes after argi- nine addition	Steady- state in arginine
OTCase	0.86	0.17	0
ODCase	0.09	0.13	0.11
OTAase	0.13	0.61	1.07
Arginase	0	0.96	1.30

[a]Units: nmoles per min. per mg. dry weight.
[b]Abbreviations: OTCase, ornithine transcarbamylase; ODCase, ornithine decarboxylase; OTAase, ornithine transaminase.

immediately diverted into the ornithine transaminase and ornithine decarboxylase reactions (Table II).   The other 20% is initially "cycled" via ornithine transcarbamylase in the mitochondria (6).   Thus the transaminase, responding to the sudden increase in the cytosolic ornithine concentration, becomes the major consumer of ornithine.   As time goes on, the arginase reaction becomes the only continuing source of ornithine, and consumption by the mitochondria stops.   The rate of the ornithine decarboxylase reaction rises only slightly, using catabolic rather than anabolic ornithine as a substrate.   (This finding is not compatible with the raw in vitro enzyme data shown in Figure 3A because the enzyme is well below substrate saturation before catabolic conditions are imposed.)   As time goes on, the entire catabolic system is enhanced by further induction of the catabolic enzymes, and much of the ornithine carbon finds its way to glutamate in addition to proline.

V.   CONCLUSIONS

The system we have described above displays a profound interplay between kinetic and spatial factors in regulating flux and distribution of metabolite pools.   The kinetic features are familiar: the substrate-velocity relations of enzymes, feedback inhibition of ornithine biosynthesis, the repression of one enzyme, CPSase A, and the induction of two catabolic enzymes, arginase and ornithine transaminase.

The "spatial" regulatory mechanisms are less familiar, and can be accounted for by transport across the plasma-membrane, and the membranes of the vesicles and mitochondria. These mechanisms are of course ultimately kinetic. However, they endow the cell with three major benefits: (a) adaptive regulation of cytosolic arginine and ornithine concentrations; (b) storage of large pools of these compounds without catabolism or disturbance of anabolic regulatory mechanisms; and (c) possible use of the mitochondrial membrane as the equivalent of a feedback-inhibition mechanism. It is very likely that all eucaryotic cells possess similar capabilities. Therefore, compartmentation must increasingly be integrated into our view of biochemical regulation.

REFERENCES

1. Srb, A. M., and Horowitz, N. H., J. Biol. Chem. 154: 129 (1944).
2. Weiss, R. L., and Davis, R. H., J. Biol. Chem. 248: 5403 (1973).
3. Karlin, J. N., Bowman, B. J., and Davis, R. H., J. Biol. Chem. 251: 3948 (1976).
4. Weiss, R. L., J. Biol. Chem. 248: 5409 (1973).
5. Subramanian, K. N., Weiss, R. L., and Davis, R. H., J. Bacteriol. 115: 284 (1973).
6. Bowman, B. J., and Davis, R. H., J. Bacteriol. 130: 274 (1977).
7. Bowman, B. J., and Davis, R. H., J. Bacteriol. 130: 285 (1977).
8. Davis, R. H., Lawless, M. B., and Port, L. A., J. Bacteriol. 102: 299 (1970).
9. Davis, R. H., Unpublished experiments.
10. Weiss, R. L., and Davis, R. H., J. Bacteriol. 129: 866 (1977).
11. Mora, J., Salceda, R., and Sanchez, S., J. Bacteriol. 110: 870 (1972).
12. Weiss, R. L., and Anterasian, G. P., J. Biol. Chem. 252: 6974 (1977).
13. Weiss, R. L., Lee, C. A., and Goodman, I., unpublished experiments.
14. Weiss, R. L., J. Bacteriol. 126: 1173 (1976).
15. Morris, D. R., Wu, W. H., Applebaum, D., and Koffron, K. Ann. N. Y. Acad. Sci. 171: 968 (1970).
16. Davis, R. H., and Mora, J., J. Bacteriol. 96: 383 (1968).

DISCUSSION

A. BOLLON: Can you get modulation of the compartmented systems by using arginine auxotrophs and varying concentrations of exogenous arginine or arginine analogues?

R. DAVIS: One of the modulations we can see is the growth of a partial mutant on minimal medium. This leads to no impairment of growth, but to a great reduction in the cellular pool of arginine. That is one such modulation; growth even at low levels of arginine availability. It seems to be directed in favor of protein synthesis rather than storage. I think perhaps Dick Weiss can answer the question more fully because he has done exactly the experiment you suggest.

R. WEISS: Well, you can't modify the uptake rates in quite the manner in which you suggested. What we have done is to use a mutant in which amino acid uptake is limited to a general amino acid permease system. We have used competitive inhibitors of the uptake system and looked at the effect of arginine uptake rates on the steady state level of arginine and on the rates of biosynthesis and of degradation. No matter how slowly arginine is taken up it appears to prevent further biosynthesis completely. In addition, the rate of degradation appears to be proportional to the rate of uptake in the absence of enzyme induction. Ultimately the rate of enzyme induction is also directly proportional to the rate of uptake across the plasma membrane. So all the regulatory and degradative responses appear to be directly related to the rate of transport across the plasma membrane.

J. WILLIAMSON: In the arginine-rich system is there any possibility that ammonia is rate limiting for carbamyl phosphate synthesis?

R. DAVIS: Yes, in conditions of arginine excess. These are conditions of ammonia production from arginine and from urea. I don't think there is any ammonia limitation necessarily. Do you mean the ammonia transport into the mitochondria?

J. WILLIAMSON: Well, free ammonia can make carbamyl phosphate. You don't get that from arginine.

R. DAVIS: No, but you get it from urea which is degraded to ammonia.

J. WILLIAMSON: Oh, I didn't realize that Neurospora contained urease.

R. DAVIS: Yes, in fact we have to interpose a mutant to block that reaction to do most of our measurements.

J. BLUM: Have any experiments been done on the isolated vesicles to investigate their transport characteristics?

R. DAVIS: That is a very good question and that is why we are trying to study it. We have isolated vesicles and found a number of amino acids in them. The basic amino acids are in high concentration. They are a distinct organelle but they have not been made to take up amino acids, even by exchange, at this point.

M. E. JONES: The loss of ornithine from the vesicles, when you have arginine in the medium, suggests that there is a limited capacity to the vesicles. Have your metabolic studies given you any idea of what that capacity is?

R. DAVIS: We haven't done the total "ninhydrin positive" capacity of the vesicle, but we do know that after adding arginine to cells there is achieved a limit of about 300 nanomoles of arginine per milligram dry weight internally, which is about ten-fold the figure for growth on minimal media. That seems to be a limit imposed by the capacity of the vesicles for arginine, and this is about the maximal capacity even for ninhydrin positive material. The implication is that when arginine is added to the vesicle it displaces everything else and becomes the main occupant. Thus there does seem to be a capacity, but we don't know what determines it.

C. deDUVE: One of the important properties of lysosomes which I will talk about tomorrow (this volume, pg 371), is their ability to concentrate weak bases by proton trapping. I wonder whether your vesicles might not be similar to vacuoles or other plant organelles related to lysosomes and whether they might also rely on an internal acidity to concentrate the basic amino acids.

R. DAVIS: I really neglected to say that I feel that these vesicles are very much like the yeast and plant vacuoles (which may have different roles in different types of organisms). In Neurospora in particular, we are entertaining the possibility of vesicular polyphosphates (polyanions) which bind these basic amino acids internally.

F. LIPMANN: There is frequently a connection between the two pathways that use carbamyl phosphate, one leading to uridylic

acid and the other to arginine. Have you ever paid attention
to that?

R. DAVIS: I have paid considerable attention to that in the
past. It appears that there are two enzymes of carbamyl
phosphate synthesis in Neurospora. One of them is localized
in the nucleolus (the pyrimidine specific enzyme) and the
one for the arginine pathway is localized in the mitochondria.
The pathways are completely independent in such a way that
if you block one of them by mutation, the carbamyl phosphate
of the other pathway does not supplement the deficient one.
Thus they are wholly independent metabolic systems. That is
why we feel that this story about arginine is not confused
by demands of the pyrimidine pathway for carbamyl phosphate.

J. DeMOSS: I would like to ask you the question which you
asked Dr. Moses. Neurospora has been shown to grow in a
very heterogeneous fashion with protein synthesis occurring
mainly in the growing tip and the older part of the mycelium
is highly vacuolated. Is it possible that the apparent separation of the so-called vesicle pool from the metabolic
pool is due to the fact that it is sequestered in vacuoles
in the older parts of the mycelium?

R. DAVIS: That is a problem that concerned us quite a bit.
I am not sure I can reconstruct the argument clearly for you,
but starting with labelled orthinine as an added precursor
we get the derived arginine compartmented just as if arginine were added directly. Thus the anabolic reactions
serving protein synthesis are in direct proximity to the
storage vesicles.

THE REGULATION OF <u>DE NOVO</u> PYRIMIDINE BIOSYNTHESIS
BY CELLULAR PHOSPHORIBOSYL PYROPHOSPHATE LEVELS
IN CULTURED EHRLICH ASCITES CELLS[1]

Jane-Jane Chen[2]
Mary Ellen Jones

Department of Biochemistry
School of Medicine
University of Southern California
Los Angeles, California

INTRODUCTION

Phosphoribosyl 1-pyrophosphate (PRPP)[3] is the common substrate for the biosynthesis of purine, pyrimidine and nicotinamide nucleotides. The effect of the level of cellular
PRPP on purine biosynthesis has been studied quite extensively (1-6) because patients with Lesch-Nyhan syndrome lack
hypoxanthine-guanine phosphoribosyltransferase which utilizes
PRPP. The over-production of uric acid in these patients has
been attributed to the higher levels of cellular PRPP observed in their erythrocytes and fibroblasts (1-6). It would
appear from these studies that cellular concentration of PRPP
might normally be rate-limiting for purine biosynthesis.
Recently, however, Hershfield and Seegmiller have obtained

---

[1] Supported in part by NIH Grant HD 06538 and NSF Grant
PCM 75-05490 and the Calif. Foundation for Biochem. Research.
[2] This work was performed in partial fulfillment of the
requirement for the Ph. D. degree at the University of
Southern California.
[3] Abbreviations used are: PRPP, 5-phosphoribosyl 1-
pyrophosphate; CPSase II, carbamyl phosphate synthetase;
ATCase, aspartate transcarbamylase; DHOase, dihydroorotase;
OPRTase, orotate phosphoribosyltransferase; OMPdecase,
orotidine-5'-monophosphate decarboxylase; glu-NH_2, glutamine; CAP, carbamyl phosphate; CAA, carbamyl aspartate;
DHO, dihydroorotate; OA, orotic acid; OMP, orotidine-5'-
monophosphate; UMP, uridine-5'-monophosphate; EDTA,
ethylene diamine tetraacetate.

Copyright © 1978 by Academic Press, Inc.
All right of reproduction in any form reserved.
ISBN 0-12-660550-5

a mutant deficient in hypoxanthine-guanine phosphoribosyltransferase from human lymphoblast in which the increased
intracellular concentration of PRPP does not increase the
rate of de novo purine biosynthesis (7).

De novo pyrimidine biosynthesis could be regulated by
the level of PRPP; however, much less work has been done on
this pathway in vivo. Fausto (8) has shown that the PRPP
level in the regenerating liver was about three times higher
than that in the normal liver. From this he suggests that
PRPP might be a rate-limiting factor for pyrimidine biosynthesis. Ferris and Clark (9) also showed that the rapid
incorporation of $[^{14}C]OA^3$ into both DNA and RNA after partial
hepatectomy was inhibited in a dose-dependent fashion by
previous injection of nicotinamide. There are two potential
regulatory sites at which de novo pyrimidine biosynthesis
(Fig. 1) could be regulated by the cellular PRPP levels.

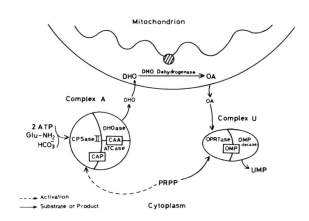

FIGURE 1. Two potential regulatory sites of de novo
biosynthesis of pyrimidine that may be regulated by
cellular PRPP levels.

The first regulatory site is at CPSase II[3], the first enzyme
of the de novo pyrimidine biosynthetic pathway. PRPP stimulates CPSase II activity by increasing the affinity of the
enzyme for the substrates, $MgATP^{-2}$ and free Mg^{+2} (10,11).
The other site is at the fifth step of the pathway where
PRPP is one of the substrates for OPRTase[3] (12). PRPP and
Mg^{+2} stabilize OPRTase and OMPdecase[3] activities when a
solution of Complex U is diluted (13) and promote the conversion of both enzymes to a more active form (Traut and
Jones, unpublished results).

The present work investigates how de novo pyrimidine bio-synthesis responds to changes in cellular PRPP as a result of the addition of adenine or guanine to Ehrlich ascites cells growing in culture by measuring the levels of intermediates and products of the pathway. These studies allow one to suggest which of the two enzyme sites is the primary site of regulation in vivo.

MATERIALS AND METHODS

Materials

$[^{14}C]NaHCO_3$ (46.1 mCi/mmole), $[4-^{14}C]orotic$ acid (46.86 mCi/mmole) and $[7-^{14}C](carboxyl)-orotic$ acid (39.6 mCi/mmole) were provided by New England Nuclear. Glucose, sodium PRPP, glutamine, adenine, alkaline phosphatase type III (E. coli, activity = 27.5 μmoles product/min/mg at 25° C, pH 8.0) and yeast OPRTase and OMPdecase (activity = 400 nmoles of product/h/mg at 25° C, pH 8.0) were purchased from Sigma Chemical Company. Bio-Gel P-2 (200-400 mesh) was provided by Bio-Rad Laboratories. Fetal calf serum and Eagle's minimal essential medium in Earle's salt (powder form) were provided by Grand Island Biological Company.

Cell Culture

Ehrlich ascites cells were grown in Eagle's minimal essential medium with Earle's salts supplemented with 5% fetal calf serum (heat denatured at 56° C for 30 min), 1 mg glucose/ml and 2 mM glutamine (14). Cells were grown in suspension in the presence of 95% air and 5% CO_2. Antibiotics were not used. The doubling time for these cells under the conditions used was about 16 h. Cells were routinely screened for mycoplasma by scanning electron microscopy (15) incorporation of $[^3H]uracil$ and $[^3H]uridine$ into RNA (16), and culturing in nutrient broth and on agar plates. All tests for mycoplasma were negative.

Incorporation of $[^{14}C]NaHCO_3$ and $[4-^{14}C]OA$ into Cells

Cells in the log or stationary phase were used for the studies on incorporation of $[^{14}C]NaHCO_3$ and $[4-^{14}C]OA$ into cellular metabolites. Adenine and guanine were used to decrease the cellular levels of PRPP. Thirty min after the

addition of adenine (160 μM) or guanine (0.03 mg/ml added as
solid), either [^{14}C]NaHCO$_3$ (100 μCi) or]4-^{14}C]OA (220 μCi)
was added to 50 or 100 ml of a cell suspension and the incubation was continued for another 30 or 40 min. At the end of
the incubation, the cells were pelleted by centrifugation at
3,000 X g for 5 min. The cells were resuspended in water and
then acidified with sufficient 70% HClO$_4$ to yield a final
concentration of 1 N HClO$_4$. This acid denatured mixture was
then kept on ice for 30 min, after which it was centrifuged
at 7,000 X g for 10 min. The acid-soluble fraction was then
boiled at 100° C for 1 h, adsorbed onto charcoal, then washed
3 times with 10 ml aliquots of H$_2$O, and the intermediates
were eluted with a mixture of ammonium hydroxide:ethanol:H$_2$O
(1:2:2) as described by Kusama and Roberts (17). The eluate
was evaporated nearly to dryness and then resuspended in a
small volume of water. The acid-insoluble pellets were resuspended in 8% tricloroacetic acid, boiled for 15 min, and
then centrifuged at 7,000 X g for 10 min. The supernatants
(0.5 ml) were mixed with 5 ml of the Madson's scintillation
cocktail (18) and counted in a Beckman 100C scintillation
counter in order to measure the incorporation of radioactivity into nucleic acids.

Assay of the Cellular Content of PRPP

Extraction of cellular PRPP was done by using a modification of the method described by Hershka et al. (19). A 5 ml
cell suspension (0.5 - 1.5 X 10^6 cells/ml) was transferred to
a test tube and centrifuged immediately at 4° C. Cell pellets were then resuspended in 1 ml of 1 mM sodium phosphate
buffer (pH 7.4) containing 1 mM EDTA[3]. This suspension was
placed in a boiling water bath for 30 sec and then cooled in
an ice bath. The denatured proteins were removed by centrifugation at 7,000 X g for 10 min. The supernatant was then
assayed for PRPP by a method similar to that of May and
Krooth (20). Complete enzymatic conversion of PRPP to UMP[3]
and [^{14}C]CO$_2$ was accomplished by adding [7-^{14}C]OA, MgCl$_2$ and
a yeast preparation containing OPRTase and OMPdecase in excess. The final assay solution contained Tris buffer, 40 mM
(pH 8.0); β-mercaptoethanol, 1 mM; MgCl$_2$, 2 mM; OA, 72 mM
(4 mCi/mmole); yeast OPRTase and OMPdecase (activity =
3 nmoles UMP/min at 37° C); and 0.82 ml of cell extract in
a final volume of 1 ml. The reaction was started by addition
of yeast OPRTase and OMPdecase and then incubated for 15 min
at 37° C to allow complete conversion of PRPP to UMP. The
[^{14}C]CO$_2$ produced was trapped and counted as described by
Prabhakararao and Jones (21). Since yeast OPRTase and

OMPdecase are inhibited by various nucleotides (22), controls
containing known amounts of PRPP were also included in the
assay mixture under every set of conditions. Knowing the
amount of standard PRPP converted to UMP in the absence of
the Ehrlich ascites cell extract and in the presence of cell
extract, as well as the amount of PRPP in the cell extract
alone, we were able to calculate the efficiency of the assay
in the presence of cell extract. The amount of cellular PRPP
can thereby be corrected according to the efficiency obtained
for the standard PRPP with the given cell extract.

Analysis of the Intermediates and Products
of the de novo Biosynthesis of Pyrimidine

Bio-Gel P-2 columns have been useful in separating
nucleotides, nucleosides and free bases (23). We have used
a Bio-Gel P-2 column to separate the intermediates and products of pyrimidine biosynthesis. Bio-Gel P-2 was swollen in
10 mM potassium phosphate buffer (pH 8.9). After degassing,
a column (0.7 cm X 82 cm) was packed and equilibrated in the
same buffer at a flow rate of 10 ml/h with a Buchler poly-
staltic pump. The cell extract (150 µl) was mixed with 100
nmoles of each non-radioactive standard, UMP, orotidine,
uridine, OA and uracil to a final volume of 200 µl, then
applied to the column. The column was eluted with 10 mM
potassium phosphate (pH 8.9) and fractions of 0.55 ml were
collected. The elution of the unlabeled standards was monitored spectrophotometrically with a Zeiss PM 6 spectrophotometer at 280 nm for OA and 260 for the other standards.
After reading the absorbance, each fraction was mixed with
5 ml of Madson's scintillation cocktail and the radioactivity
was then measured in a Beckman 100C scintillation counter.

Identification of UMP

The UMP fraction from the column can contain an unknown
radioactive anion. Therefore, one must confirm whether all
of the radioactivity in this peak is UMP. To do so, a portion of the samples was treated with alkaline phosphatase
before application to the Bio-Gel column and the amount of
material which moved as uridine after alkaline phosphatase
treatment was determined. Samples eluted from charcoal were
treated with alkaline phosphatase (activity = 1.54 µmoles/min
at 37° C (pH 8.0)) at 37° C for 1 h in the presence of Tris-
Cl (50 mM, pH 8.0) and UMP (1.14 mM). The reaction was
stopped by adding $HClO_4$ to a final concentration of 0.3 N

and then neutralizing with KOH and KHCO$_3$ to pH 8.9.   The
KClO$_4$ precipitated was removed by centrifugation.   The supernatant was applied to the Bio-Gel P-2 column with unlabeled
orotidine and OA as markers.

RESULTS

The Depletion of Cellular PRPP

Adenine is the most effective reagent known for reducing
cellular PRPP (24).   Cellular PRPP is decreased when cells
are centrifuged and resuspended in the same medium at a
higher cell density (7; Chen and Jones, unpublished results).
As a result, we have added adenine directly to cultures of
Ehrlich ascites cells without so perturbing the cells.   The
effect of various concentrations of adenine on cellular PRPP
levels under this condition is shown in Fig. 2.   As the concentration of adenine increased, the level of cellular PRPP
decreased.   When the concentration of adenine was 50 µM or
higher, there was a low steady-state concentration of PRPP
that could not be depleted further by adding more adenine.
This is in agreement with the results of Henderson and Khoo
(24) with Ehrlich ascites cells grown in the mouse, and the
results of Bagnara and Finch (25) with Escherichia coli
cells.

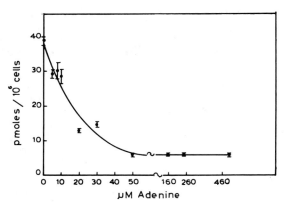

FIGURE 2.   Depletion of cellular PRPP levels by addition
of adenine.   Adenine (5 mM) was added to an Ehrlich ascites
culture with a density of 1.4 X 10^6 cells/ml to obtain the
final concentration indicated and maintained at 37° C for 30
min.   Cell extracts were assayed for PRPP as described in
Methods.

The time course for the depletion of cellular PRPP levels is shown in Fig. 3. The level of cellular PRPP decreased very rapidly after the addition of 170 μM adenine and some-what slower with 20 μM adenine. In addition, a different steady-state concentration of cellular PRPP was reached and maintained after 30 min with each of the above concentra-tions of adenine. This may be due to the different rates of the conversion of adenine to AMP by adenine phosphoribosyl-transferase or the different rate of adenine uptake into cells at the two concentrations of adenine.

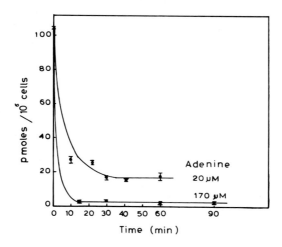

Time (min)

FIGURE 3. Time course for the depletion of cellular PRPP levels after the addition of adenine. Adenine (5 mM) was added to an Ehrlich ascites culture with a density of 1.2 X 10^6 cells to reach the final concentration indicated. Cell extracts were prepared and assayed for PRPP as de-scribed in Methods.

Effect of the Decreased Cellular PRPP Levels
on the Incorporation of [^{14}C]NaHCO$_3$ into Intermediates
and Products of de novo Pyrimidine Biosynthesis

As mentioned in the introduction, in vitro studies with enzyme preparations have shown that there are two potential sites in the de novo pyrimidine biosynthesis that could be regulated by cellular levels of PRPP, namely, as an activa-tor of CPSase II or as a substrate for the OPRTase reaction (Fig. 1). The question we asked is whether or not pyri-midine biosynthesis in intact growing cells is sensitive to changes of cellular PRPP levels and, if so, which of these enzymes is more strongly regulated by PRPP. If OPRTase is more sensitive than CPSase II, then the accumulation of OA[4] should be observed when cells are labeled with [^{14}C]NaHCO$_3$ at certain low PRPP levels. On the other hand, if CPSase II is equally, or more, sensitive than OPRTase, then none of the intermediates should accumulate, but UMP synthesis would be reduced. Under this condition, one should only see the inhibition of the incorporation of [^{14}C]NaHCO$_3$ into UMP and nucleic acid. The results of experiments designed to answer this question are presented in Table I and Fig. 4. The typical elution profile of the acid-soluble fraction of cells labeled with [^{14}C]NaHCO$_3$ is shown in Fig. 4A. The pattern of elution did not change with the addition of either adenine or guanine to the culture medium. None of the intermediates (CAA[3], DHO[3], OMP[3], OA), and especially OA, was observed to accumulate in any case (Fig. 4A and Table I). When alkaline

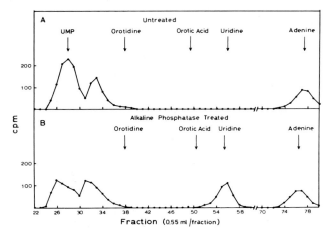

FIGURE 4. Elution profile of the acid-soluble fraction of cells labeled with [^{14}C]NaHCO$_3$ from a Bio-Gel P-2 column. Ehrlich ascites cell culture (50 ml) with a density of 1.0 X 10^6 cells/ml was used for labeling at 37° C for 30 min. The cell extract was prepared and applied onto the column as described in Methods. (A) Profile of an extract that was not treated with alkaline phosphatase. (B) Profile of an extract treated with alkaline phosphatase as described in Methods.

---

[4]If OA accumulated to certain levels, the accumulation of CAA[3] and/or DHO[3] may also occur as a result of the inhibition of DHOase and/or DHO dehydrogenase. On elution from a Bio-Gel P-2 column, the peaks of CAA-hydantoin, orotidine and DHO were in three consecutive fractions.

TABLE I. Effect of the Decreased Levels of Cellular PRPP on the Incorporation of the $[^{14}C]NaHCO_3$ into UMP and Nucleic Acids

	PRPP[a] (pmoles/10^6 cells)	UMP (%) (apparent)[b]	UMP (%) (identified)[c]	Nucleic acids (%)
Exp. 1				
Control	88.9	100	100	100
Guanine	42.3	94.9	104	97.3
Exp. 2				
Control	235	100	100	-
Adenine	19.6[e]	53.0	53.3	-
Exp. 3				
Control	22.8	100	100	-
Adenine	2.0[e]	77.9	50.0	-
Exp. 4				
Control	25.0	100	100	-
Adenine	2.0[e]	97.0	49.5	-
Exp. 5				
Control	8.0	100	100	-
Adenine	2.0[e]	49.4	10.0	-
Exp. 6				
Control	72.6	100	100	100
Adenine[d]	15.4	67.0	70.5	58.4
Adenine	2.0[e]	45.1	54.5	59.5

There was no accumulation of CAA, DHO, OA or OMP in any of these experiments.

[a]The levels of cellular PRPP varied in the control samples above because the cells used were at different states of growth.

[b]Radioactivity that co-migrated with unlabeled UMP prior to alkaline phosphatase treatment.

[c]Radioactivity that co-migrated with unlabeled uridine after alkaline phosphatase treatment.

[d]In this experiment adenine was 20 μM rather than 160 μM.

[e]These values are near or at the limit of detection. In experiment 2, the number of cells assayed was lower than in the other experiments.

phosphatase was used to verify the identity of the radioactivity which co-migrated with carrier UMP, a new radioactive peak that co-migrated with carrier uridine was observed as expected (Fig. 4B). However, there was a significant amount of radioactivity that remained in the initial
position, even though the added carrier UMP was completely
converted to uridine. At present we do not know the chemical
nature of the alkaline phosphatase resistant materials which
remain in the initial position; it would seem that the unknown is not a nucleotide nor a monophosphate ester. We also
know that the unknowns are not oligonucleotides because snake
venom phosphodiesterase together with alkaline phosphatase
does not shift the position of these materials. When cells
containing various PRPP concentrations (235 to 2 pmoles/10^6
cells or lower) were labeled with [^{14}C]NaHCO$_3$, there was inhibition of the incorporation of [^{14}C]NaHCO$_3$ into UMP
(Table I). However, in no case did we see the accumulation
of OA; therefore, it is most likely that CPSase II is more
sensitive to lowered PRPP levels than OPRTase in vivo. However, since the rate of the OPRTase reaction is dependent on
CPSase II for the production of OA from bicarbonate, it is
still possible that CPSase II and OPRTase are equally sensitive in vivo to cellular PRPP.

Effect of Decreased Cellular PRPP Levels
on the Incorporation of [4-^{14}C]OA into Pyrimidines

As mentioned above, the OPRTase reaction in vivo is dependent on the rate of OA production by the first four enzymes of this pathway; therefore, it is difficult to tell
whether or not OPRTase is tightly regulated by cellular PRPP
from studies using [^{14}C]NaHCO$_3$ as the radioactive substrate.
To try to observe directly the effect of PRPP on OPRTase,
[4-^{14}C]OA was used to label pyrimidine metabolites of the
Ehrlich ascites cells. The results of these experiments are
shown in Table II. Either adenine or guanine was used to
decrease the cellular PRPP levels. When cellular PRPP levels
were decreased from 85 μM to 42 μM (experiment 1), there was
no difference in the conversion of [4-^{14}C]OA to [^{14}C]UMP or
in the incorporation of radioactivity into nucleic acids.
When cellular PRPP levels were depleted further, from 44 μM
to 2 μM or from 35 μM to 1.6 μM (Table II), there was still
no inhibition of the synthesis of [^{14}C]UMP. Incorporation of
radioactivity into nucleic acid showed either no inhibition
(experiment 2) or a slight inhibition (experiment 3). From
the results of Table II, it might seem apparent that OPRTase
is relatively insensitive to changes in cellular PRPP levels.

TABLE II. Effect of the Decreased Levels of Cellular PRPP
on the Incorporation of [4-^{14}C]OA
into UMP and Nucleic Acids

	PRPP (pmoles/10^6 cells)	UMP[a] (%)	Nucleic acids[b] (%)
Exp. 1			
Control	84.8	100	100
Guanine	42.2	92.3	91.5
Exp. 2			
Control	44.0	100	100
Adenine	2.0	101	99.1
Exp. 3[c]			
Control	35.0	100	100
Adenine	1.6	99.7	77.7

[a]For Exp. 1, 100% = 1.07 nmoles; for Exp. 2, 100% = 1.01 nmoles; for Exp. 3, 100% = 0.72 nmoles.

[b]For Exp. 1, 100% = 0.50 nmoles; for Exp. 2, 100% = 0.28 nmoles; for Exp. 3, 100% = 0.13 nmoles.

[c]Cells were prelabeled with [4-^{14}C]OA for 30 min before the addition of adenine.

Since growing cells were used for labeling in all these ex-periments, the rate of uptake of [4-^{14}C]OA into cells becomes a major concern for the interpretation of these results. If the rate of uptake of OA is so slow as to be rate-limiting, then we cannot draw any definite conclusion about the effect of PRPP on OPRTase by this approach. For this reason, the rate of cellular uptake of OA was determined at several time points by rapid filtration of the cells incubated with [4-^{14}C]OA through a layer of oil (dibutyl phthalate, density = 1.043). The results are shown in Fig. 5. The rate of up-take of [4-^{14}C]OA was 0.096 nmoles/10 min/10^7 cells when 50 μM OA was present in the incubation medium. The rate of the conversion of [^{14}C]OA to UMP and nucleic acid (Table II) was 0.039 nmoles/10 min/10^7 cells. Thus, the rate of uptake of OA is of the same magnitude as the rate of the conversion of OA to UMP. When the activities of OPRTase in whole cells and homogenates were compared, the activity of the homogenate (under optimal conditions) was about two hundred times higher than that of whole cells (10 nmoles/10 min/10^7 cells[5] vs. 0.039 nmoles/10 min/10^7 cells). Therefore, the rate of uptake of OA into cells would seem to be so rate-limiting that we cannot interpret the results in Table II as indicating that OPRTase is insensitive to changes in cellular PRPP. To resolve this question, other approaches will have to be used. Currently we are trying to develop a method that can overcome the problem of slow OA transport.

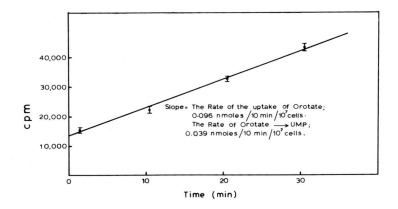

FIGURE 5. Time course of the uptake of $[4\text{-}^{14}C]OA$ into Ehrlich ascites cultured cells. Ehrlich ascites cells, 200 ml, with a density of 1.0 X 10^6 cells/ml were pelleted and resuspended in 10 ml of the same medium. $[4\text{-}^{14}C]OA$ (57.4 mCi/mmole) was added to the cell suspension to obtain a final concentration of 50 μM and incubated at 37° C. At the end of each time period, 0.5 ml of cell suspension was transferred to a Brinkmann centrifuge tube which contained 0.5 ml of dibutyl phthalate and then centrifuged in a Brinkmann 3200 centrifuge for 30 sec. After carefully removing the supernatant and oil, the cell pellets were resuspended in 0.5 ml of water, mixed with 5 ml of Madson's scintillation cocktail, then counted as described in Methods.

---

[5]This activity of OPRTase is about 5-fold that reported by Shoaf and Jones (26). This increase of activity may be due to the addition of dithiothreitol to both extraction and assay media.

DISCUSSION

Our results show that CPSase II is an enzyme responsible
for inhibition of de novo pyrimidine biosynthesis in growing
whole cells when cellular PRPP is decreased by the addition
of adenine. This inhibition was observed only when cellular
PRPP levels were 20 pmoles/10^6 cells or lower. These results
are consistent with those of Nuki et al. (27), who found that
the rates of de novo pyrimidine biosynthesis were similar in
both control lymphoblasts and lymphoblasts which contain
higher PRPP levels as a result of the deficiency in hypoxanthine-guanine phosphoribosyltransferase.

The apparent K_m of PRPP for OPRTase from Ehrlich ascites
cells is about 16 μM (13). The apparent concentration of
PRPP for half-maximal activation of CPSase II from Yoshida
ascites hepatoma cells is about 5 μM (10,11). From these
in vitro data it would seem that OPRTase, rather than CPSase
II, should respond first as the PRPP concentration is lowered. However, our growing whole cell experiments show just
the opposite result.

All our experiments were short, i. e., 30-40 min, compared to the cell generation time of 16 h, therefore our results should not be complicated by long-term effects. The
levels of the intermediates of the de novo pyrimidine pathway
are very low under normal conditions (28,29). The low levels
of the intermediates make the short-term labeling valid since
the isotope will not be diluted by an existing pool. When
adenine was added to the cell culture medium, it was rapidly
taken up by the cells and converted mainly to ATP, while ADP
and AMP and adenine were present in very small amounts (30).
ATP is a very weak inhibitor of OPRTase (31); therefore, the
elevation of cellular ATP by the addition of adenine into
cell culture should not cause inhibition of OPRTase. The
results shown in Tables I and II agree with this argument.
CPSase II is known to be subject to feed-back inhibition by
UTP (10,32). UTP decreases the affinity of CPSase II for
MgATP^{-2}, while PRPP increases the affinity of CPSase II for
MgATP^{-2} (10). After addition of adenine to a culture of
E. coli, Bagnara and Finch observed decreased levels of UTP
and CTP (25). As shown in Table I, the total uridine nucleotides decreased. Therefore, the addition of adenine might
decrease the feed-back inhibition of CPSase II by UTP, but
certainly not inhibit CPSase II activity. Since ATP is required for CPSase II reaction, the increased levels of
cellular ATP resulting from the addition of adenine would
also tend to increase the activity of CPSase II. Therefore,
the inhibition shown in Table I after the addition of

adenine can probably be attributed to the decreased levels of cellular PRPP.

Our experiments and the reasoning above show that the kinetic values determined in vitro did not correctly predict the site at which de novo biosynthesis of UMP from bicarbonate would be regulated when the intracellular PRPP is lowered by adenine addition. This contradiction between the results of our experiments with growing intact cells and kinetic experiments performed in vitro by other investigators may be due to a preferential use of cellular PRPP by OPRTase. However, direct support for this postulate has not yet been obtained.

In E. coli, the addition of adenine to the culture medium was shown to cause the inhibition of the incorporation of $[^{14}C]OA$ into nucleic acid (33). PRPP has also been shown to activate CPSase from Salmonella typhimurium (34), an organism closely related to E. coli. The effect of the depletion of PRPP on the CPSase II and OPRTase reactions in E. coli has been investigated by R. I. Christopherson and L. R. Finch (personal communication). They observed an accumulation of OA after the addition of adenine to the culture. Therefore, the enzyme most sensitive to a lowered cellular PRPP concentration seems to be CPSase II in the Ehrlich ascites cell, while it is OPRTase in E. coli.

ACKNOWLEDGMENTS

The established Ehrlich ascites cell line was a kind gift from Dr. Carl A. Hirsch, for which the authors are most grateful. We are also grateful for the expert technical assistance of Ms. Mary O. Lei. Travel support for Jane-Jane Chen from the USC Graduate School is greatly appreciated.

References

1. Rosenbloom, F. M., Henderson, J. F., Caldwell, I. C., Kelley, W. N., and Seegmiller, J. E., J. Biol. Chem. 243:1166 (1968).
2. Wood, A. W., Becker, M. A., and Seegmiller, J. E., Biochem. Genet. 9:261 (1973).
3. Lever, J. E., Nuki, G., and Seegmiller, J. E., Proc. Natl. Acad. Sci. U.S.A. 71:2679 (1974).
4. Zoref, E., de Vries, A., and Sperling, D., J. Clin. Invest. 56:1093 (1975).
5. Becker, M. A., J. Clin. Invest. 57:308 (1976).

6. Becker, M. A., Biochim. Biophys. Acta 435:132 (1976).
7. Hershfield, M. S., and Seegmiller, J. E., J. Biol. Chem. 252:6002 (1977).
8. Fausto, N., Biochim. Biophys. Acta 182:62 (1969).
9. Ferris, G. M., and Clark, J. B., Biochem. J. 128:869 (1972).
10. Tatibana, M., and Shigesada, K., J. Biochem. (Tokyo) 72:549 (1972).
11. Mori, M., and Tatibana, M., Biochem. Biophys. Res. Commun. 67:287 (1975).
12. Lieberman, I., Kornberg, A., and Simms, E. S., J. Biol. Chem. 215:403 (1955).
13. Kavipurapu, P. R., and Jones, M. E., J. Biol. Chem. 251:5589 (1976).
14. Live, R. T., and Kaminskas, E., J. Biol. Chem. 250:1786 (1975).
15. Brown, S., Teplitz, M., and Revel, J-P., Proc. Natl. Acad. Sci. U.S.A. 71:464 (1974).
16. Schneider, E. L., Stanbridge, E. J., and Epstein, C. J., Exp. Cell Res. 84:311 (1974).
17. Kusama, K., and Roberts, E., Biochemistry 2:573 (1963).
18. Pande, S. V., Anal. Biochem. 74:25 (1976).
19. Hershko, A., Razin, A., and Mayer, J., Biochim. Biophys. Acta 184:64 (1969).
20. May, S. R., and Krooth, A. S., Anal. Biochem. 75:329 (1976).
21. Prabhakararao, K., and Jones, M. E., Anal. Biochem. 69:451 (1975).
22. Umezu, K., Amaya, T., Yoshimoto, A., and Tomita, K., J. Biochem. (Tokyo) 70:249 (1971).
23. Khym, J. Y., Anal. Biochem. 58:638 (1974).
24. Henderson, J. F., and Khoo, M.K.Y., J. Biol. Chem. 240:2358 (1965).
25. Bagnara, A. S., and Finch, L. R., Eur. J. Biochem. 41:421 (1974).
26. Shoaf, W. T., and Jones, M. E., Biochemistry 12:4039 (1973).
27. Nuki, G., Astrin, K., Brenton, D., Cruikshank, M., Lever, J., and Seegmiller, J. E., Adv. Exp. Med. Biol. 76B:326 (1977).
28. Hager, S. E., and Jones, M. E., J. Biol. Chem. 240:4556 (1965).
29. Hitchings, G. H., Adv. Enz. Reg. 12:121 (1973).
30. Hawkins, R. A., Berlin, R. D., Biochim. Biophys. Acta 173:324 (1969).
31. Traut, T. W., and Jones, M. E., Biochem. Pharm. 26:2291 (1977).

32. Pausch, J., Wilkening, J., Nowack, J., and Decker, K., Eur. J. Biochem. 53:349 (1975).
33. Hosono, R., and Kuno, S., J. Biochem. (Tokyo) 75:215 (1974).
34. Abdelal, A.T.H., and Ingraham, J. L., J. Biol. Chem. 250:4410 (1975).

DISCUSSION

B. CHANCE: Might I say, if you have problems with the rates of diffusion, which apparently you do, ascites cells work over a pretty wide range of temperatures. They don't do everything, but they do a lot and maybe you might be lucky at some different temperatures. What temperature did you use?

M. E. JONES: 37°.

R. DAVIS: I would like to ask you, Mary Ellen, whether, despite the fact you didn't see label accumulating in the intermediates, you did measurements of intermediate pools that might be there before hand in your cells.

M. E. JONES: Not really. Right Jane?

J. CHEN: We did not measure pools of intermediates because the pool size of these intermediates is low under normal conditions. Values reported by Hitchings, G. H., for orotate and OMP from rat liver are 0.4 and 0.07 nmoles/g of wet tissue. The value for dihydroorotate reported by Decker et al. is less than 15 nmoles/g of wet tissue. Since the first three enzymes for the pyrimidine biosynthetic pathway are present as an enzyme complex, the levels of carbamyl phosphate and carbamyl aspartate would be anticipated to be rather low in the cells, as in the case of OMP. If we assume Σ UMP is 1 mM in cells (Pausch, J. G. et al., Eur. J. Biochem. 76, 157 (1977) and Jackson, R. C. et al., Life Science 19, 15-31 (1976) and that all the CPM incorporated into UMP from [^{14}C]-NaHCO$_3$ is equal to Σ UMP, we can calculate the upper limit of our ability to detect the four stable intermediates. It should be a cellular concentration of about 30 μM, with the assumption that 10^9 cells equals 1 ml. The real sensitivity would be lower than 30 μM because the labeling time is short (30 min compared to doubling time of 16 hr). When azauridine is added to the cell culture the accumulation of orotate can be detected (Chen and Jones, unpublished results). Therefore, if OPRTase reaction is limited by low levels of PRPP we should expect to see the accumulation of orotate.

COMPARTMENTATION OF GLUCOSE METABOLISM IN LIVER

Joseph Katz
Robert Rognstad

Department of Biochemistry
Cedars-Sinai Medical Center
Los Angeles, California

I. INTRODUCTION

The anabolic and catabolic functions of liver are the most diverse of any organ. According to needs liver takes up glucose, or converts it to various products, or glucose and glycogen may be formed from pyruvate but the carbohydrate also serves as precursor for acetyl CoA and lipid. The question before us is whether anabolic and catabolic functions are carried on in the same or different cells or compartments (1). Liver tissue is composed from several kinds of cells, but one cell type, the parenchyma constitutes close to 90% of the tissue mass. Methods to isolate parenchyma cells in good yield have been developed and these preparations are now extensively used. These hepatocytes carry out gluconeogenesis, glycolysis, pyruvate oxidation, and many other functions at rates similar to those in vivo. It is commonly held that these cells are metabolically homogenous, but this view has been challenged.

A large body of experiments with ^{14}C labeled substrates have established a coupling between gluconeogenesis and oxidation. Oxalacetate is a common intermediate for gluconeogenesis and for the Krebs cycle, a precursor of PEP and citrate. However as shown below, it has been impossible to fit quantitative isotopic data with a simple model consisting of a single pool of oxalacetate, but on the other hand solid evidence for multiple pools of oxalacetate and citrate is still unavailable.

Copyright © 1978 by Academic Press, Inc.
All right of reproduction in any form reserved.
ISBN 0-12-660550-5

A second problem discussed here is compartmentation of the reactions between glucose and pyruvate. Most of the intermediate steps are reversible, but there are 3 irreversible sequences, between glucose and glucose 6-P, fructose 6-P and fructose 1,6-diP, and PEP and pyruvate where the opposite reactions are catalyzed by separate enzymes. It has been recently established, that during gluconeogenesis the glycolytic enzymes, glucokinase, phosphofructokinase and pyruvate kinase are still active and thus gluconeogenesis and glycolysis proceed simultaneously. This causes ATP breakdown without any corresponding metabolic change. The occurrence of such so-called futile cycles in liver has been reviewed (2). Most investigators believe that the opposing reactions proceed in the same cell but recently, Jungermann and coworkers have provided evidence for metabolic heterogeneity of liver parenchyma, with some cells being gluconeogenic and others glycolytic. Their evidence and ideas have been summarized in a recent review (3) and will be discussed below.

A. Gluconeogenesis and the Krebs Cycle

It has long been known that ^{14}C from CO_2, acetate or fatty acid is incorporated into glucose. The incorporation of these compounds, which are not substrates for gluconeogenesis were accounted by the "crossover" between gluconeogenesis and the Krebs cycle at the oxalacetate level. The isotope distribution in glucose formed from specifically labeled acetate or pyruvate firmly established this coupling. However when several isotopes were used simultaneously, serious discrepancies become apparent. An example for such experiments with isolated hepatocytes by Mullhofer and coworkers (4) is shown in Table 1.

They incubated rat hepatocytes in a bicarbonate buffer with lactate and octanoate, with ^{14}C either in lactate, CO_2 or octanoate, and they isolated and degraded carboxylic acids and glucose (Table 1). The data obtained from the different labeled compounds were inconsistent. The specific activities of malate and citrate from HCO_3 and 1-^{14}C octanoate were much higher than expected from the results with lactate. The specific activity of the acetyl moiety should be twice or more than that of the OAA moiety of citrate.

The specific activity of the acetoacetate was nearly 3 times that of the acetyl unit of citrate. Glutz and Walter (5) also compared the specific activities of acetoacetate and citrate formed by liver mitochondria from 1-^{14}C palmitate and 2-^{14}C pyruvate and found the specific activity ratio higher

TABLE I. Relative Specific Activities of Intermediates
in Hepatocytes

Cells from fasted rats incubated for 30 minutes with 10 mM lactate and 1 mM octanoate in 95% O_2 -
5% CO_2. (After Mullhofer et al., Eur. J. Bioch. 75,
331, 1977.)

Label	$1-^{14}C$ Lactate	$H^{14}CO_3$	$1-^{14}C$ Octanoate
Intermediates:			
HCO_3	-	1.00	-
Lactate	1.00	0	-
(2-C) Citrate	0	0	1.00
(4-C) Citrate	0.60	1.09	0.85
Malate	0.52	0.86	1.09
Glucose	0.57	0.84	0.91
Acetoacetate	-	-	5.4

or lower respectively than theoretical. These experiments
support the proposal of Fritz (6) of two separate mitochondrial pools of acetyl CoA, one derived from fatty acids
and used preferentially for ketone body formation and one
derived from pyruvate, used preferentially for citrate
synthesis.

Another example for inconsistency in isotopic data is
shown in Table 2 from unpublished experiments by Grunnet in
our lab. Hepatocytes were incubated with lactate as substrate
in the presence of trace amounts of $1-^{14}C$ and $2-^{14}C$ propionate
and the ^{14}C yields in glucose and CO_2 determined and the glucose isolated and degraded. From metabolic carbon balance and
manometric determination of O_2 uptake, it is possible to calculate directly the oxidation via the Krebs cycle. The Krebs
cycle flux was also calculated from the isotopic data, based
on a conventional model, with a single precursor pool of OAA
for PEP and citrate. Propionate is a rather convenient tracer
for such experiments, yielding simple expressions for such
calculations. As shown in Table 2, the relative fluxes of OAA
to PEP compared to that of citrate as calculated from the
ratio of yields in ^{14}C labeled CO_4 and glucose was higher,
especially from $1-^{14}C$ propionate, than the flux obtained from
the O_2 uptake. On the other hand the flux ratio calculated
from the C-4/C-5 ^{14}C ratio in glucose from $2-^{14}C$ propionate
was less than that obtained by non-isotopic methods. Similar

discrepancies were obtained with labeled lactate. The discrepancy could not be adequately accounted for by futile
cycling between PEP and pyruvate. The findings suggest that
there is a system in which propionate and the acetyl CoA from
pyruvate are oxidized predominantly to CO_2 and water with
little, or even without any gluconeogenesis, and another system where the outflow from OAA to PEP is much higher than
that to citrate.

There is now compelling evidence for multiple acetyl CoA
pools in liver. There are (see above), apparently two mitochondrial pools derived from pyruvate and fatty acids respectively. Another acetyl CoA pool which can be derived from
acetate is extramitochondrial, and serves preferentially as
precursor for fatty acid and cholesterol synthesis as shown by
Dietschy and McGarry (7). Recent experiments indicate the
possibility of another peroxisomal pool of acetyl CoA.
Lazarow and DeDuve (8) have recently shown that fatty acids
oxidation occurs in these organelles, and in clofibrate
treated animals an important site of fatty acid oxidation may
be peroxisomal.

It remains to be determined, how many pools there are and
how they interact and whether they occur in the same organelle, or that there are different types of mitochondria, or
that there are different cell types. Moreover with isolated
hepatocytes, the possibility must be considered that there are
damaged cells, which may have lost the capacity for gluconeogenesis but still can oxidize citrate.

The existence of separate acetyl CoA pools suggests also
the existence of two citrate pools. It is impossible to fit
isotopic data to simple models with a single acetyl CoA and
single citrate pool. In Tetrahemena, Raugi et al. (9) was
successful in fitting isotopic data to a model with 3 acetyl
CoA pools. The application of complex models with multiple
pool to liver metabolism is a difficult but important task for
the future.

B. Isotopic Evidence for Multiple Pools
of Phosphate Esters

There are a considerable number of studies in which, after
administration of a labeled compound, specific activities of
glycolytic intermediates were determined. Large differences
in the specific activities of phosphate esters, such as
glucose 6-P, fructose 6-P, PEP and phosphoglyceric acid were
observed, and such results were taken to indicate the existence of multiple pools of glycolytic intermediates. Most of
this work has been done with muscle tissue and is not

TABLE II. Krebs Cycle Flux in Rat Hepatocytes,
Calculated by Several Methods

Hepatocytes from fasted rats were
incubated with 10 mM lactate, or with lactate
plus either 10 mM NH_4Cl or 1 mM oleate (with 1%
albumin). 1-14C or 2-14C propionate were added
in trace amounts. The yields of ^{14}C in glucose
and CO_2 were determined and glucose from 2-14C
propionate was isolated and degraded. (Grunnet
and Katz, unpublished.)

Additions		-	NH_4Cl	Oleate
Glucose formed μmoles/g/min		60	76	95
		Ratios of ^{14}C Yields		
CO_2/glucose from 1-14C propionate	$= R_1$	0.33	0.32	0.35
CO_2/glucose from 2-14C propionate	$= R_2$	5.1	4.8	8.8
C-4/C-5 of glucose from 2-14C propionate	$= R_3$	0.16	0.13	0.12
		Ratio of Flux (OAA to Citrate)/(OAA to PEP)		
Calculated from O_2 uptake and analysis		0.58	0.51	0.51
From R_1		1.01	1.06	0.93
From R_2		0.65	0.68	0.40
From R_3		0.47	0.35	0.32

Equation for calculations of the ratio (OAA to PEP)/(OAA
to citrate) = e/g.

The equations are:

For R_1: $e/g = \dfrac{1-R_1}{2-R_1}$; For R_2: $= \dfrac{4g^2+5ge}{e(2e+g)}$; For R_3: $e/g = \dfrac{2R_3}{1-2R_3}$.

Since g, the rate of PEP formation is twice that of the
formation of glucose, the flux of OAA to citrate, e, can
be calculated.

Joseph Katz and Robert Rognstad

considered here. It has been extensively although somewhat
uncritically, reviewed by Ottoway and Mowbray (1). In liver
there are only a few such studies. Threlfall and Heath (10)
injected rats intravenously with U-^{14}C fructose and followed
the change in specific activities of UDP glucose, glucose 6-P
and glycerol 3-P. The specific activity of UDPG was always
greater than that of glucose 6-P. Threlfall and Heath suggested that there are 2 kinds of hepatocytes, gluconeogenic
and glycolytic. However they did not obtain an adequate fit
to the data with a 2 pool model. The system in vivo is of
great complexity and the amount of experimental data required
to analyze such a system are a great deal more than obtained
by them. Moreover their analysis is encumbered by an awkward
mathematical technique.

Das et al. (11) injected ^{14}C glucose intravenously into
rats and determined the specific activity of glucose 1-P, glucose 6-P and UDPG. Two minutes after injection the ratio of
specific activity of G1P/UDPG was 7, decreasing to 3 at 30
minutes. The specific activity of glucose 6-P was much less
than that of UDPG. Veneziale (12, 13) reported a marked difference in the specific activities of PEP and phosphoglyceric
acid from livers perfused with ^{14}C pyruvate or ^{14}CO$_2$.

The existence of a single compartment does not necessarily
imply equal specific activity of closely related intermediates. Equal specific activities will be attained in a
closed system at equilibrium. Even with flow from a single
substrate, when there are branch points and alternate pathways, unequal specific activities may be consistent with a
single compartment. Also so-called equilibrium reactions,
catalyzed by enzymes whose activity in vitro assay is
extremely high, may be much slower in the cell. For example,
the activity of triose-P isomerase in vitro is some 2 orders
of magnitude greater than that of irreversible reactions such
as phosphofructokinase or PEP carboxykinase. Still it has
been repeatedly observed that the triose phosphates are not
completely equilibrated, as shown by the unequal incorporation
of labeled glycerol or pyruvate in the top or bottom carbons
of glucose.

From an experimental point of view it seems to us that a
good deal of the data on specific activities of phosphate
esters are questionable. There is a lack of consistency and
reproducibility and so far none of the results in muscle (14,
15) or liver have been confirmed. Some as the widely quoted
claims of Veneziale (12, 13) could not be duplicated (15).
The determination of the specific activities of intermediates
present at low concentration requires rigorous methods of
purification. From our experience with the isolation of phosphate esters from hepatocytes (17) sole reliance on

chromatographic methods is inadequate, and specific enzymatic procedures as used by Mullhofer (4, 16) are essential to isolate pure glycolytic intermediates.

C. Metabolic Zonation of the Liver

According to currently prevalent concepts, the functional unit of liver structure is considered to be the lobule. It is not a clearly defined morphological unit but a structure determined by hepatic blood supply. It is delineated at the periphery by the terminal afferent portal and arterial vessels, arranged about a central efferent terminal hepatic vein. A diagram of a lobule according to Rappaport (18) is shown in Figure 1. The lobule is made of irregular sheets of parenchyma cells, one cell thick, which forms an anastomising three-dimensional network that extends radially from the afferent to the efferent central vessels. The space between the parenchyma sheets constitute the liver sinusoids. (Endothelial and Kupffer cells, which line the sinusoids are neglected here for simplification.) Portal and arterial blood enters and mixes in the sinusoids at one end and exits into the terminal hepatic venule at the efferent end. The cells along the sinusoid take up and secrete material, and there is a gradient of oxygen, CO_2, of substrate and of products in the sinusoid blood. There are many observations on morphological and histochemical heterogeneity of the cells in the liver lobule reviewed by Rappaport (18). He has proposed a division into 3 zones, a periportal one close to the afferent portal arterial terminal vessels, a perivenous or perilobular in the center around the hepatic venule, and an intermediate zone. In normal liver the distinction between zones is faint, but it is markedly enhanced in some pathological conditions or by drugs, for example, phenobarbital injection (19).

There are a number of studies, based on cell morphology and histochemical enzyme assays, that suggest metabolic zonation in the lobule. (See review in 18.) The cells in the periportal zone were said to be mainly oxidative with a high Krebs cycle, and those in the periportal mainly biosynthetic. However an examination of the literature reveals conflicting observations and in our opinion the experimental support for such classification is weak. Nolte and Pette (20) investigated by histochemical and microspectrographic methods the distribution of some 15 enzymes. Differences in enzyme activities was observed only for glutamic dehydrogenase, isocitric dehydrogenase and succinic dehydrogenase. The activity of succinic dehydrogenase in the periportal zone was 1.6 times that in the perivenous. The inverse distribution was found

for TPNH linked isocitrate dehydrogenase. In thyroid treated
rats there was no difference in activity between the zones.
We think this hardly establishes a zonation of oxidative
metabolism.

   We present here in some detail the extensive recent work
by the Freiburg group in the localization of the enzymes of
glycolysis and gluconeogenesis. Sasse et al. (22) using
histochemical techniques reported a marked glycogen zonation
in glycogen and glucose 6-Pase. In fed rats glycogen was uniformly distributed throughout the lobule, but on fasting the
glycogen was first lost in the periportal zone. (Figure 2A
and B.) The activity of G6Pase in Figure 3 is much greater in
the periportal than in the perivenous zone. Wansen et al.
(19) found however a nearly even distribution of G6Pase in the
liver lobule of normal rats.

   Histochemical techniques are only qualitative, and to
obtain quantitative data N. Katz and coworkers (23, 24) have
used microdissection techniques, as developed by Lowry. A
segment consisting of 100-200 cells, weighing about 0.5 micrograms, was dissected out from periportal and perivenous zones
of frozen and lyophilized sections and the activities of
G6Pase, glucokinase and FDPase were assayed. Guder and
Schmidt has used similar microtechniques for the assay of
pyruvate kinase and PEP carboxykinase (25). These data are
summarized in Table 3.

   In cells of fed rats the periportal/perivenous (PP/PV)
activity ratio of glucose 6-Pase and FDPase was 2:1, whereas
the ratio for glucokinase was about 1:2. Fasting increased
the activity of G6Pase in both periportal and perivenous
cells, but had little effect on the activity of FDPase and
glucokinase (Table 3). The difference between the zones was
decreased in fasting. The distribution of PEP carboxykinase
and pyruvate kinase exhibited the same reciprocal pattern as
with the hexose ester enzymes. The PP/PV activity ratio for
PEP carboxykinase was about 3, whereas the inverse ratio was
found for pyruvate kinase (Table 3). It should be noted that
the activities of PEP carboxykinase shown by Guder are much
less than found by others (26).

   Metabolic zonation for glucose metabolism has been shown
for kidney tubule cells (27, 28). The activity of PEP
carboxykinase in the cells of the proximal tubules was some 10
times higher than in that of the distal end. The activity
ratio was reversed for hexokinase and phosphofructokinase, and
the activity of pyruvate kinase in the loop of Henle and the
convoluted distal end was some 30 times that in proximal convoluted tubule. Thus glucose synthesis seems to occur solely
in the proximal tubule cells, and glycolysis in the loop of
Henle and in the distal cells. In liver distinction between

TABLE III. Activity of Some Gluconeogenic and Glycolytic Enzymes in Periportal (PP) and Perivenous (PV) Zones of Livers of Fed and Fasted Rats

(After N. Katz et al. and Guder and Schmidt.)

Enzyme	FED			FASTED		
	Periportal	Perivenous	PP/PV Ratio	Periportal	Perivenous	PP/PV Ratio
	μmoles/min/g*			μmoles/min/g*		
G6Pase	15±5	6.7±2.5	2.3(1.4-3.4)	31±13	18±5.3	1.7(1.2-2.3)
FDPase	24±7	13±4	1.9(1.6-3.3)	27±9	18±4	1.5(1.4-1.6)
Glucokinase	7.2±2.6	14±3	0.51(0.35-0.81)	8.3±1.8	14±4	0.60(0.48-0.75)
PEP Carboxykinase	0.72	0.25	2.9	1.5	0.91	1.7
Pyruvate Kinase	280	640	0.45	270	360	0.80

*Gram dry weight.

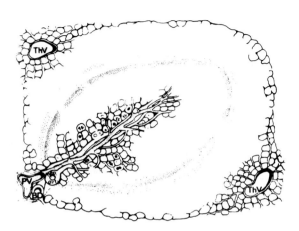

FIGURE 1. Diagramatic Cross Section of a Liver Lobule
PV, portal vein, BD, bile duct, THV terminal hepatic vein.
The triangular portal vein, the bile duct and hepatic artery
constitute the so-called triad. Blood flow in the portal vein
and hepatic artery in this diagram is perpendicular to the
plane of the paper. A terminal portal venule and terminal
arteriole are shown to branch from the triad, and extend
approximately in the plane of the paper. Sheets of parenchyma
cells separated by sinusoids, extend between the portal-
arterial and hepatic vessels. Mixed portal-arterial blood
flows through the sinusoids draining into the hepatic vein.
The distance between PV and THV is of the order of 0.5 mm.
Shading indicates the border of the periportal zone. (From
Rappoport (18).)

the zones is much less pronounced than in kidney. Also their
relative size is variable. The perivenous zone in rat liver
is enlarged upon fasting (19) and upon barbital treatment.
     Jungermann and coworkers have proposed that liver paren-
chyma cells fall into 2 functional classes, gluconeogenic and
glycolytic cells (3). The first group produces glucose and
the second takes it up. They also propose that fatty acid
oxidation and ketogenesis is localized in the periportal gluconeogenic cells, and lipogenesis in the glycolytic cells.
Other processes may also be predominant or restricted to one
cell type. The regulation of circulating glucose levels and
shifts from hepatic glucose production to uptake represent
a balance of the output and uptake of the periportal and

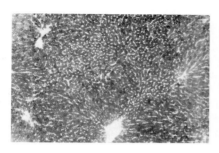 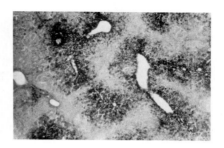

A   B

FIGURE 2. Sections of Liver Stained for Glycogen.
Rat fed ad libitum. A, 8 a.m. the whole parenchyma is filled
uniformly with glycogen. B, 4 p.m. glycogen prominent only
in the perivenous zone. (From Sasse et al. 22.)

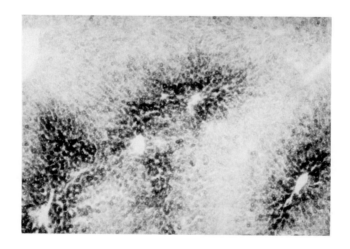

FIGURE 3. Liver Section Stained for G6Pase Reaction
The enzyme activity is prominent only in the periportal zone.
(From Sasse et al. 22.)

perivenous cells. The net direction and flux will be determined by the activities of the cells and the relative size of
the zones. Since considerable amounts of gluconeogenic and
glycolytic enzymes occur in all zones, they believe that
futile cycles occur in each cell type, with a net flux in
opposite directions. Superimposed upon the futile cycles
occurring in each cell at the levels of glucose 6-P, fructose
6-P, and PEP ("small" futile cycles) there is another "large"
futile cycle due to the opposed flux in the two zones.

Our own studies with tritiated sugars or on the randomization of glucose (2) clearly establish the occurrence of
intracellular futile cycling. If the metabolism in each cell
type were unidirectional, there would be no difference in
isotope utilization between ^{14}C and tritium labeled glucose
nor randomization of carbon from position 1 to position 6 in
glucose.

Jungermann et al. (3) suggest that a metabolic system composed of "small" and "large" futile cycles is advantageous
for metabolic regulation in that it provides added sensitivity
in response to hormonal and dietary stimuli. Whether this is
true or not, the existence of cell types in liver with distinct metabolic functions would require, if established, a
revision of current ideas in the regulation of liver
metabolism. The experiments seem to establish heterogeneity
in the enzyme makeup of liver cells, but in our opinion the
division of the cells into gluconeogenic and glycolytic cells
offers considerable problems.

The concept of "gluconeogenic" and "glycolytic" cells is
consistent with the prevailing idea that uptake of glucose by
liver has a major role in regulation of blood glucose levels
with the glucose being converted to glycogen and fatty acids
(exported as lipo proteins). Recent work indicates however
that at least in rodents, glucose uptake by liver is rather
limited except under nonphysiological glucose loads. Studies
with perfused liver (29) and hepatocytes (30) show that after
refeeding fasted rats, the precursors of liver glycogen are
gluconeogenic substrates, and glycogen synthesis is a "gluconeogenic" process. Net synthesis of glycogen from glucose
occurs only at concentrations above 40 mM (30). It has also
been shown with hepatocytes (31) and in vivo (32), that glucose is a rather poor substrate for hepatic fatty acid synthesis in rodents. The preferred substrate for fatty acid
synthesis in liver of fasted-refed rats appears to be glycogen
and lactate (31). Thus the substrate for glycolysis in liver
is glycogen rather than glucose. This suggests that at some
stage the same cell is "gluconeogenic" accumulating glycogen,
becoming at a later stage "glycolytic" and lipogenic.

Great care has to be exercised to deduce rates of flux in intact cells or tissues from rates of in vitro assays. To cite one example the assayed rate of active phosphorylase exceeds greatly that of glycogen synthase even under conditions of rapid glycogen deposition. A difference in assayable activity by a factor of 2 or 3 may not reflect the rates in the intact cell. To establish definitely metabolic zonation in liver, measurement of activities of key enzymes of pathways specific to liver, such as urea synthesis, drug detoxification, or bile acid production, are required. A combination of several procedures, such as histochemical staining, microphotometry in conjunction with the use of fluorescent antibodies, as well as microdissection, should permit definitive conclusions on the localization of enzymes and metabolic zonation in the liver lobule.

To sum up compartmentation in liver is still an unsolved issue. There is evidence for its occurrence, but it is not definitive at this time. The histochemical and microdissection studies described here are of great interest and no doubt will stimulate advances in methods for the study of metabolic zonation.

ACKNOWLEDGMENT

This paper would be impossible without the cooperation of Drs. D. Sasse and K. Jungermann, who kindly provided manuscripts in press, and the microphotographs for Figures 2 and 3.

REFERENCES

1. Ottoway, J. H., and Mowbray, J., Curr. Topics on Cell. Regu. 12:107 (1977).
2. Katz, J., and Rognstad, R, Curr. Topics in Cell. Regu. 10:237 (1976).
3. Jungermann, K., Katz, N., Teutsch, H. and Sasse, D, in "Alcohol + Aldehyde Metabolizing Systems", Academic Press, New York, 1978 (In Press).
4. Mullhofer, G., Muller, C., Stetten, I. V. and Gruber, E., Eur. J. Biochem. 75:331 (1977).
5. Glutz, V. G. and Walter, P., Eur. J. Bioch. 60:147 (1975).

6.   Fritz, I. B., in "Cellular Compartmentalization and Control of Fatty Acid Metabolism" (F. C. Grun, ed.) p. 39. Academic Press, New York, 1968.

7.   Dietschy, J. M. and McGarry, J. D., J. Biol. Chem. 249: 52 (1974).

8.   Lazarow, P. B. and DeDuve, C., Proc. Nat. Acad. Sci. 73: 2043 (1976).

9.   Raugi, G. J., Liang, T., and Blum, J. J., J. Biol. Chem. 248:8064 (1973).

10. Threlfall, C. J. and Heath, D. F., Bioch. J. 110:303 (1968).

11. Das, I., Sie, H.G., and Fishman, W. H., Arch. Bioch. Biophys. 144:715 (1971).

12. Veneziale, C. M., Gabrielli, F., and Lardy, H. A., Biochemistry. 9:3900 (1970).

13. Veneziale, C. M., Biochemistry. 10:2793 (1971).

14. Marcus, O., and Kalant, N., Canad. J. Bioch. 55:31 (1974).

15. Das, I., and Chain, E. B., Bioch. J. 154:765 (1976).

16. Mullhofer, G., Schwab, A., Muller, C., Stetten, C. V., and Gruber, E., Eur. J. Bioch. 75:319 (1977).

17. Katz, J., Wals, P. A., and Rognstad, R., J. Biol. Chem. In Press (1978).

18. Rappaport, A. M., in "Diseases of the Liver" (4th Edition), (L.S. Schiff, ed.) p. 1, Lippincott Press, Philadelphia, Pennsylvania, 1975.

19. Wanson, J. C., Drochmans, P., May, C., Penasse, W., and Popowski, A., J. Cell. Biol. 66:23 (1975).

20. Nolte, J., and Pette, D., Jour. Histo. Cytochem. 20:567 (1972).

21. Dasse, D., Histochemie 20:237 (1975).

22. Sasse, D., Katz, N., and Jungermann, K., FEBS Letters 57:83 (1975).

23. Katz, N., Teutsch, H. F., Sasse, D., and Jungermann, K., FEBS Letters 76:226 (1977).

24. Katz, N., Teutsch, H. F., Jungermann, K., and Sasse, D., FEBS Letters 83:272 (1977).

25. Guder, W. W., and Schmidt, U., Zeit. f. Physiol. Chemie. 257:1793 (1976).

26. Soling, H. D., and Kleinecke, J., in "Gluconeogenesis, its Regulation in Mammalian Spec ies" (R.W. Hansen and M.A. Mehlman, eds.), p. 369. J. Wiley, New York, 1976.

27. Guder, W. W., and Schmidt, U., Proc. 6th Int. Congress of Nephrology, (Karger, Basel) 1976.

28. Schmidt, U., Murosvami, I., and DuBach, U. L., FEBS Letters 53:26 (1975).

29. Hems, D. A., Whitton, P. D., and Taylor, F. A., Bioch. J. 129:529 (1977).
30. Katz, J., Golden, S., and Wals, P. A., Proc. Nat. Acad. Sci., USA. 73:3433 (1976).
31. Clark, D. G., Rognstad, R., and Katz, J., J. Biol. Chem. 249:2028 (1974).
32. Hems, D. A., Rath, E. A., and Vervirden, T. R., Bioch. J. 150:167 (1975).

DISCUSSION

R. WELCH: I have a comment for Dr. Katz regarding the role of organization of glycolysis in liver cells. Hubocher, Mayer and Hansen (Bioenergetics, 2, 115, 1971) presented a somewhat theoretical argument that, based upon the known concentrations of glycolytic enzymes in liver parenchymal cells, the enzymes must be localized either in a complex or in some membraneous type of compartment. They were concerned primarily with transient times. I think they were a little distraught at the emphasis being placed on the lack of a transit time argument for cells like yeast, where the concentrations of some glycolytic enzymes are as high as 10^{-4} to 10^{-5}M. These authors showed for large cells, like the liver parenchymal cells, diffusion (or transit times) would play a role.

J. KATZ: I have not read that paper and my personal feeling is having read all I could find about compartmentation of glycolysis in the liver cell, that there is really no convincing evidence for compartmentation. I do not put much stress on the theoretical arguments. I can't understand them. I doubt that they are convincing and we have to have better evidence than that. I think to establish compartmentation you have really to show that the experimental data fit such a model. The approach must be like that of Dr. Blum's who has found a nice fit for his data with a single glycolytic compartment. It is not enough to have messy data that you can't interpret and claim that there is compartmentation. If you assume compartments it is up to you to show that the data fits a two compartmental system, and no one so far has come even close to it.

R. WELCH: May I give a retort?

B. CHANCE: What do you have left?

R. WELCH: Well, people have argued for years that the organization of glycolysis would not be important even in a cell
like a bacterium, but we now see convincing evidence which
suggests it is, indeed a complex (cf paper by Welch and
DeMoss. This volume, pg 323). Are we to suppose that larger
eukaryotic cells are less "sophisticated", or less "logical",
than the prokaryotic cells in this respect? I think not. In
fact, accumulating evidence indicates that glycolysis is
spatially organized in a variety of cell types [(e.g., Welch,
G. R., Prog. Biophys. Mol. Biol. <u>32</u>, 103 1977)].

B. CHANCE: Franz Matschinsky presented our data on redox
scanning of the liver in two dimensions. Figure 1 shows a
three dimensional result that outlines volumes that are more
oxidized than the background. These are regions of the order,
as you might expect, of millimeters that have the same redox
state. Therefore, it seems possible to gouge out the parts of
the same redox state and make the appropriate assays.

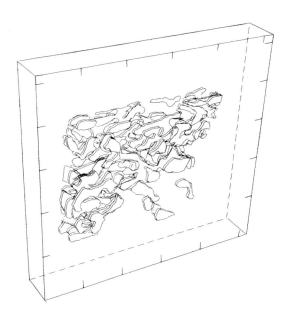

Figure 1. A 3D representation of redox states in perfused
liver (6 x 6 x 0.6 mm^3). The area within the contours represent F_p/PN ratios of oxidized states of mitochondria (Expts.
with B. Quistorff and J. Haselgrove).

J. KATZ: Well people do it, Dr. Matschinsky did it and the Freiburg group did it. The Freiburg group shows that there is no doubt that the cells are heterogeneous. That means the assayed enzyme activity is not uniform across the lobule. What it means in terms of metabolic rates I am not sure.

B. CHANCE: They may be rather small changes.

J. KATZ: Yes.

INTERRELATIONS BETWEEN FATTY ACID SYNTHESIS,
FATTY ACID OXIDATION AND KETOGENESIS IN LIVER [1]

J. Denis McGarry
Daniel W. Foster

Department of Internal Medicine and Biochemistry
University of Texas Health Science Center at Dallas
Dallas, Texas

I. INTRODUCTION

In seeking to explain the biochemical basis for the so-
called "carbohydrate sparing" of hepatic fatty acid oxidation,
recent studies from this laboratory have uncovered a potentially novel control mechanism. If correct, the model prom-
ises to shed new light not only on the problem of ketogenesis
and its regulation but on the much broader issue of the hormonal control of interactions between hepatic carbohydrate and
lipid metabolism. The present paper will summarize these new
findings.

A. Background

The notion that carbohydrate in some manner suppresses hepatic fatty acid oxidation and ketone body production has been
intermittently expressed by many investigators since the turn
of the century (1-8). However, the underlying mechanism has
remained an enigma. Our interest in this phenomenon stemmed
from the finding of a reciprocal relationship between the
glycogen content and ketogenic capacity of rat liver. In the
fed state the liver exhibited high glycogen levels and a limited ability to produce acetoacetic and β-hydroxybutyric acids
when perfused with long-chain fatty acids; conversely, livers

[1]Supported by NIH grant AM18573.

Copyright © 1978 by Academic Press, Inc.
All right of reproduction in any form reserved.
ISBN 0-12-660550-5

from fasted, diabetic or acutely glucagon-treated animals were
largely depleted of glycogen and displayed high rates of ketogenesis when perfused with oleate (9,10). In contrast to the
situation with intact livers, liver homogenates, supplemented
with the appropriate cofactors (ATP, CoASH and carnitine), oxidized oleic acid to ketone bodies at high and equal rates,
irrespective of the nutritional or hormonal status of the
donor animals. Moreover, we could detect no difference in
apparent Km values for the fatty acid substrate or for any of
the cofactors involved in the initiation of fatty acid oxidation by homogenates from normal and ketotic livers (11). Since
we had previously postulated that primary control over hepatic
fatty acid oxidation is exerted at the first step in the pathway, the carnitine palmitoyltransferase (CPT) reaction (12),
our bias was that some component of carbohydrate metabolism,
which normally serves to suppress this reaction in the fed
state, might have been diluted to non-inhibitory levels by
disruption of the tissue, thus accounting for the high rates
of fatty acid oxidation seen in homogenates. One might logi-
cally have sought the putative inhibitor in the sequence of
intermediates between glycogen and pyruvate, or perhaps in the
pentose phosphate pathway or the Krebs cycle. However, an exhaustive search among the metabolites involved in these sequences failed to reveal a component capable of significantly
inhibiting fatty acid oxidation in homogenate preparations(13).

B. Role of Malonyl-CoA in the Regulation
of Hepatic Fatty Acid Oxidation

At this point we began to examine the problem from a different prespective, and asked whether a clue to the control of
hepatic fatty acid oxidation might be found in a consideration
of the opposing system of fatty acid biosynthesis. It was,
after all, well established that under circumstances where the
ability of the liver to oxidize fatty acids is low (carbohy-
drate-fed state) the capacity for fat synthesis is high; when
rates of fatty acid oxidation and ketogenesis are high fatty
acid synthesis is low. Thus, the possibility existed that the
elusive "carbohydrate factor" responsible for "turning off"
fatty acid oxidation might reside not in the glycogen → pyruvate pathway, but in the more distal sequence of reactions
leading from acetyl-CoA to long-chain fatty acids. Since hepatic levels of malonyl-CoA, the first committed intermediate
in the conversion of glucose into fat, had been shown by others
to fluctuate in parallel with the activity of the fatty acid
biosynthetic sequence (14,15) it was attractive to suppose
that this compound might play a role in controlling the activity of the fatty acid oxidative pathway. Table 1 shows the

TABLE I. Effect of Malonyl-CoA on the Oxidation of
[1-^{14}C]-oleate by a Rat Liver Homogenate [a]

Additions	nmol[1-^{14}C]-oleate → product·12 min^{-1}	
	CO_2	Ketone bodies
None	0.92	94.0
D-Octanoylcarnitine(1mM)	0.53	42.0
Malonyl-CoA (0.5 mM)	0.16	1.8

[a] 0.5 ml of a 5% (w/v) liver homogenate from a fed rat was
incubated with 0.1 mM albumin-bound [1-^{14}C]-oleate in the
presence of optimal quantities of ATP, CoASH and carnitine
(final volume, 2.5 ml). At the indicated time, reactions
were terminated with perchloric acid and the incorporation
of ^{14}C into CO_2 and ketone bodies (acetoacetate + β-hydroxybutyrate) was determined. (See ref 13 for further experimental details).

first experiment in which this hypothesis was tested. D-Octa-
noylcarnitine, a known inhibitor of the CPT reaction (16),
caused a 55% inhibition of oleate oxidation at a concentration
of 1mM, but malonyl-CoA was almost totally inhibitory when
used at half this concentration. Furthermore, the effect was
completely reversible and specific for the malonyl ester of
CoASH (11,13).

C. Site of Malonyl-CoA Inhibition
of Fatty Acid Oxidation

Table 2 shows that the inhibitory effect of malonyl-CoA on
the oxidation of oleate was also seen when palmitate or palmitoyl-CoA served as the ketogenic substrate. All three compounds require both CPT I and CPT II for oxidation (Fig 1). In
contrast, the oxidation of octanoic acid, and of palmitoylcarnitine was totally resistant to malonyl-CoA inhibition. Octanoate requires neither CPT I nor CPT II for oxidation while
palmitoylcarnitine utilizes only CPT II. It thus appeared
that the site of the malonyl-CoA effect was at the level of
CPT I. To establish this point more definitively it was necessary to examine the effect of malonyl-CoA directly on transferase activity. For this purpose a mitochondrial fraction
from rat liver was prepared in hypotonic medium (0.01M potassium phosphate buffer) on the assumption that the resulting

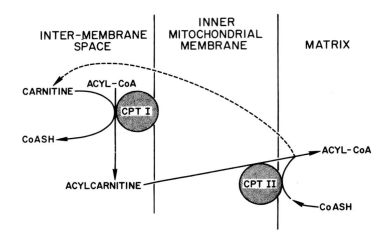

FIGURE 1. Current concepts on the roles of carnitine palmitoyltransferase I (CPT 1) and carnitine palmitoyltransferase
II (CPT II) in the translocation of long-chain fatty acids
across the inner mitochondrial membrane. The model has evolved from studies reported in refs 17-22.

TABLE II.   Effect of Malonyl-CoA on the Oxidation
            of Various Fatty Acid Substrates by Rat
            Liver Mitochondrial Fraction [a]

Substrate	% inhibition of oxidation by malonyl-CoA
Oleate	98
Palmitate	96
Palmitoyl-CoA	94
Octanoate	0
Palmitoylcarnitine	1

[a]Albumin-bound [1-14C]-labeled substrates (40 µM), together
with the necessary cofactors, were incubated with a mitochondrial fraction from rat liver in the absence or presence
of 20 µM malonyl-CoA. Rates of fatty acid oxidation were
measured as described in Table 1. See ref 23 for further
experimental details.

TABLE III. Radioisotopic Assays Employed for the
Measurement of Carnitine Palmitoyltransferase Activity [a]

Assay	Reaction components at zero time			
I	Palmitoyl-carnitine	CoASH $\rightleftharpoons$	Palmitoyl-CoA	[^{14}C]-Carnitine
II	-	- $\rightleftharpoons$	Palmitoyl-CoA	[^{14}C]-Carnitine
III	[^{14}C]-Palmitoyl-carnitine	CoASH $\rightleftharpoons$	-	-

[a]After addition of mitochondrial membranes the rate of formation (assays I and II) or loss (assay III) of labeled palmitoylcarnitine was followed. See ref 23 for full experimental details.

vesicles would be largely devoid of matrix components (23) and
more suitable for transferase assays than the intact organelles. Carnitine palmitoyltransferase activity was measured
using the radioisotopic methods depicted in Table III.
    The curve shown in Figure 2 represents a typical response
of mitochondrial CPT activity to increasing concentrations of
malonyl-CoA. Two points are noteworthy. First, under the
assay conditions employed, maximal inhibition (generally 40-
60%, depending upon the batch of mitochondria) was invariably
achieved at a malonyl-CoA concentration of about 20 μM. The
fact that half the total activity escaped inhibition suggested
that only one of the two transferases was susceptible to the
inhibitor. Second, it appeared that a concentration of only
1.5 μM malonyl-CoA was sufficient to produce a 50% suppression
of the inhibitor-sensitive enzyme. Since the same concentrations of malonyl-CoA producing half-maximal and complete inhibition of the suppressible CPT activity (1.5 μM and 20 μM)
produced a 50% and 100% inhibition, respectively, of palmitate
oxidation by intact mitochondria (23), it seemed clear that
the malonyl-CoA-sensitive enzyme was indeed CPT I.
    Why was CPT II insensitive to malonyl-CoA inhibition? At
least three possibilities existed. First, it was conceivable
that because of the impermeability of the inner mitochondrial

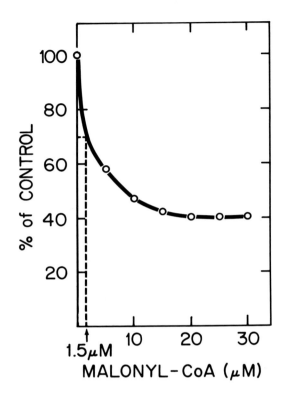

FIGURE 2.   Effect of malonyl-CoA concentration on CPT activity of mitochondrial membranes from rat liver.   Enzyme activity was measured using the isotope exchange assay (assay I) depicted in Table III and described fully in ref 23.   The broken line represents the concentration of malonyl-CoA required for 50% suppression of the malonyl-CoA-sensitive enzyme.

membrane to CoASH esters malonyl-CoA simply could not gain access to the presumed location of CPT II (Fig 1).   Second, a buried location of CPT II within the inner membrane might have precluded its inhibition by malonyl-CoA even if both sides of the membrane were exposed to the CoASH ester.   Third, it was possible that CPT I and CPT II are intrinsically different with regard to their sensitivity to malonyl-CoA, as has been suggested for other properties of the two enzymes (21,22). The first of these alternatives could be eliminated by the finding that even after sonication of mitochondria in the presence of malonyl-CoA, a procedure which should result in exposure of

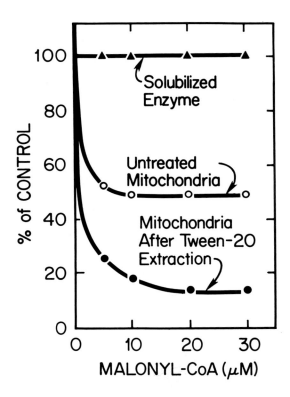

FIGURE 3. Effect of malonyl-CoA on solubilized and membrane-bound CPT activity. Mitochondrial membranes were treated with the detergent, Tween-20, which resulted in the solubilization of approximately one half of the original enzyme activity. Aliquots of the untreated membranes, the residual membranes and the Tween-20 extract (after exhaustive dialysis against detergent-free buffer) were then assayed for CPT activity in the presence of the indicated concentration of malonyl-CoA using assay I depicted in Table III. See ref 23 for full details.

both aspects of the inner membrane to the bulk phase solution, only one half of the total CPT activity could be suppressed (23). To distinguish between the remaining alternatives we made use of the detergent, Tween-20, which had previously been employed by others as a tool in the solubilization of CPT I (24). Two important points emerged from these studies. First,

the enzyme that was solubilized by the detergent proved to be
totally insensitive to malonyl-CoA (Fig 3) and second, the enzyme that remained associated with the membrane fraction displayed far greater sensitivity to malonyl-CoA than that pres-
sent in the untreated preparation. In light of previous
studies (20) we feel that a reasonable interpretation of these
findings is as follows. The detergent-releasable enzyme is
CPT I. However, its sensitivity to malonyl-CoA requires that
CPT I be present in its natural environment on the mitochondrial membrane. Analogous observations were made by Fritz and
co-workers regarding the inhibition of mitochondrial CPT by
(D)-acylcarnitines (24,25). CPT II is normally insensitive
to malonyl-CoA by virtue of its deeper location within the
inner membrane, but becomes sensitive to the inhibitor if the
membrane is damaged, as for example after treatment with
Tween-20. We recognize, of course, that alternative explanations for these data are possible and that a complete understanding of the present findings must await more detailed
knowledge regarding the anatomical relationship between CPT I
and CPT II on the inner mitochondrial membrane. An important
issue yet to be resolved is whether the two enzymes are identical but positioned differently within the membrane or whether,
in addition, they constitute distinct protein entities. While
the studies outlined above do not discriminate between these
alternatives the different responses to malonyl-CoA could be
helpful in future studies of the two enzymes.

D. Mechanism of the Malonyl-CoA Inhibition of Mitochondrial Carnitine Palmitoyltransferase

While an unequivocal answer cannot yet be given to the
question of how malonyl-CoA inhibits the CPT I reaction a number of observations point to a competitive type of interaction
between the inhibitor and the acyl-CoA substrate. For example, when the rate of oxidation of oleate by a mitochondrial
fraction from rat liver was made dependent upon added CoASH
(ATP and carnitine present in excess) the kinetics of malonyl-
CoA inhibition were typical of a competitive inhibitor with a
K_i in the region of 2 μM (11). Second, when the CPT activity
of mitochondrial membranes was measured using all three isotopic assays depicted in Table III, only the activity monitored by assays I and II was suppressible by malonyl-CoA
(Fig 4). It should be noted that, unlike assay III, both
assays I and II are dependent upon the interaction of palmitoyl-CoA and carnitine. Finally, when assay II was run with
varying levels of palmitoyl-CoA in the presence of fixed concentrations of malonyl-CoA the data shown in Figure 5 were

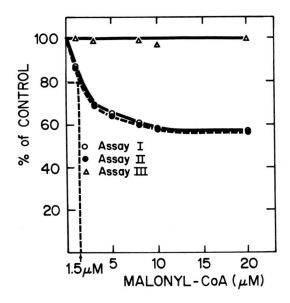

FIGURE 4. Effect of increasing concentrations of malonyl-CoA on CPT activity of mitochondrial membranes as measured using the three assays depicted in Table III. The vertical broken line shows the concentration of malonyl-CoA required to inhibit the malonyl-CoA-sensitive enzyme by 50%. See ref 23 for full details.

obtained. The loss of malonyl-CoA sensitivity with increasing palmitoyl-CoA concentration is clearly evident. Whereas the control incubations yielded typical rectangular hyperbolic kinetics, those containing malonyl-CoA exhibited distinct sigmoidicity at low substrate concentrations. As a result, when the data are expressed in Lineweaver-Burk form (Fig 6) the control points lie on a straight line but those obtained in the presence of malonyl-CoA deviate markedly from linearity at low palmitoyl-CoA concentrations. Nevertheless, extrapolation of the curves through the ordinate and abscissa again suggests that malonyl-CoA acted as a competitive inhibitor with a calculated K_i of approximately 2 μM.

Obviously, it is impossible to draw firm conclusions from the preliminary kinetic studies outlined above. The fact that only the membrane-bound enzyme appeared to be inhibitable by

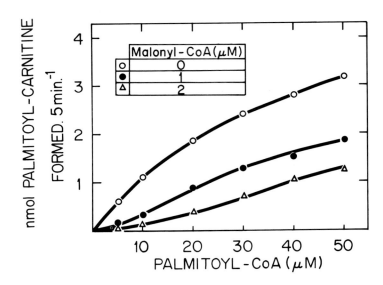

FIGURE 5. Effect of malonyl-CoA on mitochondrial CPT activity in the presence of varying concentrations of palmitoyl-CoA. CPT activity was measured using assay II depicted in Table III. Each data point refers to the suppressible fraction of CPT, i.e., the difference between total enzyme activity and that expressed in the presence of 20 µM malonyl-CoA. The concentration of albumin in the reaction mixtures was kept constant at 2%. See ref 23 for full details.

malonyl-CoA in itself suggests that the interaction does not conform to classical concepts of the mechanism of action of enzyme inhibitors. Also unclear is whether the data of Figs 5 and 6 reflect an allosteric type of interaction between acyl-CoA, malonyl-CoA and the CPT I - membrane complex.

The question remains as to whether the inhibitory effect of malonyl-CoA on mitochondrial CPT activity described above has physiological relevance for the control of hepatic fatty acid oxidation in normal and ketotic states. Suggestive evidence that it does comes from measurements of hepatic malonyl-CoA levels in fed and fasted rats. Using a new radioisotopic procedure for the assay of malonyl-CoA we have found values of approximately 10-15 and 2-4 nmol per g wet wt in livers from meal-fed and fasted rats, respectively. While these numbers are somewhat lower than those reported by Cook et al (15), the directional changes are the same in both studies. It is not possible to extrapolate directly from units of total tissue

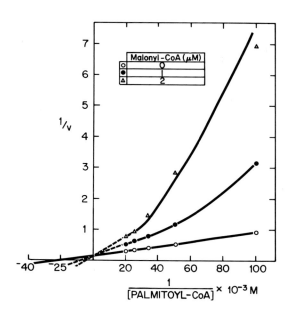

FIGURE 6. Lineweave-Burk plot of the data from Figure 5.

content to units of activity for a particular metabolite within a subcellular compartment. Nevertheless it seems reasonable to suppose that the liver content of malonyl-CoA, expressed in nmol per g wet wt, approximates the micromolar concentration of this intermediate in the vicinity of mitochondrial carnitine palmitoyltransferase. With this proviso, it
may be concluded that in vivo the hepatic malonyl-CoA level
fluctuates through a concentration range consistent with its
demonstrated ability to modulate the flow of fatty acid carbon
through the β-oxidation pathway in vitro.

E. Hormonal Considerations

If the above postulate is correct the question arises as to
how the reduction of hepatic malonyl-CoA levels is accomplished by elevated glucagon levels (with or without insulin
deficiency) (10). One possibility, favored by Cook et al (15),
is that glucagon causes inhibition of acetyl-CoA carboxylase,
the enzyme responsible for the formation of malonyl-CoA.
While this is an attractive thesis, a mechanism to explain the
link between glucagon binding to the liver and the resultant

inhibition of the carboxylase has not been established. Another possibility would be that glucagon, in addition to causing the discharge of hepatic glycogen stores as free glucose, causes blockade of the glycolytic sequence through a cyclic AMP-mediated inhibition of key enzymes (26,27). The resultant fall in pyruvate generation would be expected to produce a secondary reduction in malonyl-CoA concentration such that the rate of fatty acid synthesis would decrease, with concomitant derepression of fatty acid oxidation. The latter mechanism would be consistent with the observations of Watkins et al (28) who found that glucagon caused a marked fall in the citrate content of isolated chicken hepatocytes at a time when the incorporation of ^3H_2O into fatty acids was severely depressed. The same authors showed that addition of pyruvate to the cells restored both the citrate concentration and fatty acid synthesis to normal levels, even in the presence of glucagon. It should be noted, however, that in contrast to the findings of Watkins et al with chicken hepatocytes (28), those of Cook et al (15) revealed no fall in the citrate content of rat liver 15 min after injection of fed animals with glucagon, despite the fact that hepatic malonyl-CoA levels fell precipitously over this short time interval. Furthermore, incubation of hepatocytes from fed rats with dibutyryl cyclic AMP was found to result in a profound reduction of lactate and pyruvate release coupled with concomitant depression of fatty acid synthesis at a time when the citrate content of the cells actually increased (29). It is evident, therefore, that further studies are needed to clarify the mechanism whereby glucagon reduces the concentration of malonyl-CoA in liver.

Finally, while this paper has concentrated on the role of malonyl-CoA in the regulation of hepatic fatty acid oxidation the point should not be overlooked that elevation of the circulating [glucagon]:[insulin] ratio has another important effect that is central to the issue, i.e., it also brings about an increase in liver carnitine content (30). Since carnitine serves as a substrate for the CPT I reaction an increase in its concentration, coupled with removal of the inhibitor, malonyl-CoA, constitutes a doubly effective mechanism for the accelerated ketone body production characteristic of insulin deficient states.

SUMMARY

Evidence is presented that the inhibitory effect of malonyl-CoA on mitochondrial fatty acid oxidation is exerted at the level of carnitine palmitoyltransferase I, which is presumed to be present on the outer aspect of the inner mitochondrial membrane. Carnitine palmitoyltransferase II, is normally insensitive to malonyl-CoA, probably because of its buried location within the inner membrane. Inhibition of carnitine palmitoyltransferase I by malonyl-CoA requires that the enzyme be associated with the membrane. While the inhibitory mechanism has not been established, malonyl-CoA appears to act competitively towards acyl-CoA with an apparent K_i in the region of 2 μM. The exquisite sensitivity of carnitine palmitoyltransferase I, the first step in fatty acid oxidation, to malonyl-CoA, the first committed intermediate in the conversion of glucose into fat, indicates that malonyl-CoA represents an important element in the so-called "carbohydrate sparing" of hepatic fatty acid oxidation and ketogenesis. Its strategic location in the intermediary metabolism of glucose suggests that malonyl-CoA plays a central role in the overall coordination of fat synthesis and degradation in liver.

REFERENCES

1. Embden, G., and Kalberlah, F., Beitr. Z. Chem. Physiol. u. Path. 8:121 (1906).
2. Embden, G., and Wirth, J., Biochem. Z. 27:1 (1910).
3. Blixenkrone-Møller, N., Z. Physiol. Chem. 252:117 (1938).
4. Mirsky, I. A., J. Am. Med. Assoc. 118:690 (1942).
5. Weinhouse, S., Millington, R. H., and Friedman, B., J. Biol. Chem. 181:489 (1949).
6. Lossow, W. J., and Chaikoff, I. L., Arch. Biochem. Biophys. 57:23 (1954).
7. Lossow, W. J., Brown, G. W., Jr., and Chaikoff, I. L., J. Biol. Chem. 220:839 (1956).
8. McGarry, J. D., and Foster, D. W., Arch. Intern. Med. 137:495 (1977).
9. McGarry, J. D., Meier, J. M., and Foster, D. W., J. Biol. Chem. 248:270 (1973).
10. McGarry, J. D., Wright, P. H., and Foster, D. W., J. Clin. Invest. 55:1202 (1975).
11. McGarry, J. D., Mannaerts, G. P., and Foster, D. W. Submitted for publication.
12. McGarry, J. D., and Foster, D. W., J. Biol. Chem. 246:6247 (1971).
13. McGarry, J. D., Mannaerts, G. P., and Foster, D. W., J. Clin. Invest. 60:265 (1977).
14. Guynn, R. W., Veloso, D., and Veech, R. L., J. Biol. Chem. 247:7325 (1972).
15. Cook, G. A., Nielsen, R. C., Hawkins, R. A., Mehlman, M. A., Lakshmanan, M. R., and Veech, R. L., J. Biol. Chem. 252:4421 (1977).

16. McGarry, J. D., and Foster, D. W., Diabetes 23:485 (1974).
17. Fritz, I. B., Advances in Lipid Research 1:285 (1963).
18. Yates, D. W., and Garland, P. B., Biochem. J. 119:547 (1970).
19. West, D. W., Chase, J. F. A., and Tubbs, P. K., Biochem. Biophys. Res. Comm. 42:912 (1971).
20. Hoppel, C. L., and Tomec, R. J., J. Biol. Chem. 247:832 (1972).
21. Kopec, B., and Fritz, I. B., J. Biol. Chem. 248:4069 (1973).
22. Brosnan, J. T., Kopec, B., and Fritz, I. B., J. Biol. Chem. 248:4075 (1973).
23. McGarry, J. D., Leatherman, G. F., and Foster, D. W., J. Biol. Chem. (1978). In press.
24. Kopec, B., and Fritz, I. B., Can. J. Biochem. 49:941 (1971).
25. Fritz, I. B., and Marquis, N. R., Proc. Natl. Acad. Sci., U.S.A. 54:1226 (1965).
26. Pilkis, S. J., Riou, J. P., and Claus, T. H., J. Biol. Chem. 251:7841 (1976).
27. Feliu, J. E., Hue, L., and Hers, H. G., Proc. Natl. Acad. Sci., U.S.A. 73:2762 (1976).
28. Watkins, P. A., Tarlow, D. M., and Lane, M. D., Proc. Natl. Acad. Sci., U.S.A. 74:1497 (1977).
29. Harris, R. A., Arch. Biochem. Biophys. 169:168 (1975).
30. McGarry, J. D., Robles-Valdes, C., and Foster, D. W., Proc. Natl. Acad. Sci., U.S.A. 72:4385 (1975).

DISCUSSION

J. WOOD: Denis, I was wondering, since you saw no effect of malonyl CoA on the detergent solubilized enzyme, does the detergent itself limit the access of malonyl Co-A to the enzyme? Have you tried to release the external enzyme with digitonin? Does malonyl-CoA have an effect on this activity?

D. MCGARRY: As to your first question, we too were concerned about the possibility that the detergent prevented inhibition of the solubilized enzyme by malonyl-CoA. We feel that this is unlikely to be the case for the following reasons. First, the data I showed were obtained after extensive dialysis of the solubilized enzyme. However, we recognize that this does not necessarily mean that the detergent had been removed from the enzyme protein. Second, we have been able to effect a partial solubilization of the enzyme without the use of detergents and again have found a major reduction in its inhibitability by malonyl-CoA. We have not studied the effect of digitonin on the system.

J. LOWENSTEIN: In solubilizing the enzyme you may be removing a regulatory subunit.

D. MCGARRY: While that is possible, experiments in which mixtures of the solubilized enzyme and residual mitochondrial membranes were tested for malonyl-CoA sensitivity yielded additive results. In other words, if a regulatory sub-unit had remained associated with the membranes, its function did not seem to be expressed in the mixing experiments. Obviously the relationship of the outer enzyme (CPT I) with the inner mitochondrial membrane is complex, and exactly how malonyl-CoA exerts its inhibitory effect is not known at this time.

J. ONTKO: That is very nice, Denis. You may have an important contribution. I have a comment. Regarding the glucagon effect, have you observed any effect of cylic AMP on the malonyl-CoA concentration?

D. MCGARRY: We have not yet made the malonyl-CoA measurements. One of the problems here is that this is a very difficult measurement to make spectrophotometrically. While Dr. Veech has developed a spectrophotometric method we are working on an alternative assay which I think will increase the sensitivity.

J. ONTKO: Does Dr. Veech have data bearing on that point? Does cyclic AMP effect the malonyl-CoA concentration?

R. VEECH: Yes. It lowers the concentration of malonyl-CoA.

J. ONTKO: With regard to cellular heterogeneity within the liver lobule, ketogenesis and gluconeogenesis may occur predominantly in certain cells whereas glycolytic and fatty acid synthetic activity (and thereby malonyl CoA generation) may be concentrated in other cells. This possibility remains open.

D. MCGARRY: That is quite possible, Joe.

V. JOSHI: Does malonyl-CoA act as a substrate for CPT-I?

D. MCGARRY: I think we can say the following on this point. First, in our hands malonyl-CoA does not act as a substrate for commercial preparations of carnitine acetyltransferase. Second, if one adds malonyl-CoA to rat liver mitochondria, one detects a potent malonyl-CoA deacylase activity. If, in addition, we add carnitine we do not see an increased rate of release of coenzyme A. This is suggestive evidence that malonyl-CoA does not act as a substrate for mitochondrial carnitine acyltransferase.

C. deDUVE: As I am sure you know, Paul Lazarow has found in our laboratory that much of hepatic β-oxidation is carried out by peroxisomes. What evidence do you have that the system you are studying is mitochondrial? Could the partial inhibition you observe with malonyl-CoA reflect the fact that only the mitochondrial or the peroxisomal system is inhibited.

D. MCGARRY: We prepare mitochondria by conventional techniques and to what extent they may be contaminated by peroxisomes we cannot say. I would add the following, however. In crude liver homogenates from clofibrate-treated rats (which are presumably greatly enriched with peroxisomes) malonyl-CoA is still profoundly inhibitory to the overall oxidation of fatty acids. This would suggest that if the carnitine acyltransferase system is common to mitochondria and peroxisomes both systems are inhibited by malonyl-CoA.

C. deDUVE: Then it remains to be seen whether the mitochondrial system is inhibited. May I suggest that you refer to your preparation as a mitochondrial fraction rather than mitochondria. These are two different things.

D. MCGARRY: I agree.

H. MORGAN: Can the effect of glucagon be reversed by pyruvate?

D. MCGARRY: We have examined this question in isolated hepatocytes and the answer appears to be yes. In other words, addition of carnitine and glucagon to hepatocytes from fed rats markedly stimulates the oxidation of oleic acid. However, the addition of lactate and pyruvate prevents the stimulation. One interpretation would be that glucagon suppresses carbon flow from glucose to pyruvate and therefore prevents the formation of malonyl-CoA. Consistent with this notion is the fact that glucagon completely blocks lactate output by these cells. Addition of lactate or pyruvate, however, might be expected to raise the malonyl-CoA concentration back to a level sufficient to inhibit fatty acid oxidation. We are presently examining this possibility.

MULTIENZYMIC SYSTEMS

A GLUCOSE BINDING-TRANSPORT FACTOR ISOLATED FROM NORMAL
AND MALIGNANTLY TRANSFORMED CHICKEN FIBROBLASTS

Fritz Lipmann[1]
Sung G. Lee[2]

The Rockefeller University
New York, New York

INTRODUCTION

At the beginning of his biochemical career, F.L. worked
for some time on the excess aerobic glycolysis in chicken
fibroblasts (1, 2), and compared it with the increase in glycolysis that occurs on malignant transformation (3). In the
latter case, a quite dramatic increase also occurs in the uptake of glucose (4). Although this increased uptake has been
extensively studied, it has been done almost exclusively by
measuring physico-chemical parameters. Having had some experience recently in a bacterial system with the induction of
amino acid binding proteins as the initial stage of uptake (5),
we undertook to look for a glucose binding protein in order to
compare it, quantitatively and qualitatively, before and after
transformation of chick fibroblasts by Rous sarcoma virus
(RSV).

RSV is a RNA virus of small size, 6×10^6 daltons, consisting of presumably identical halves with molecular weights
of 3×10^6 daltons. In Figure 1, each half is shown to contain four genes for messages of: 1) a group-specific antigen;
2) a reverse transcriptase, which transcribes the RNA virus
into DNA for insertion into the chick nuclear DNA and therefrom
back into numerous RNA messages, thus producing new virus; 3)

---

[1] Supported by NIH grant GM-13972.
[2] Supported by NSF grant PCM75-21165

Copyright © 1978 by Academic Press, Inc.
All right of reproduction in any form reserved.
ISBN 0-12-660550-5

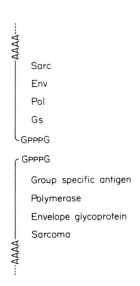

FIGURE 1.   The genome of Rous sarcoma virus.

a specific surface glycoprotein;   and 4) the sarc gene containing the message for transformation, the expression of which in
protein language is so far unknown.   Furthermore, each 3 x 10^6
dalton moiety of the RSV genome is associated with a trypto-
phan-tRNA (7).   In the temperature-sensitive strain T68 of
Kawai and Hanafusa (8) which we used in our experiments, the
expression of sarcoma gene is suppressed at 41° without influencing virus replication;   however, at 36° it is expressed,
causing transformation.

Figure 2 shows normal fibroblasts, which are elongated,
relatively slender cells.   For comparison, Figure 3 shows in-
fected cells grown at the nonpermissive temperature of 41°
that, at this stage, are quite analogous to normal ones.   In
Figure 4, however, one sees the same cells after 20-24 hours
at 37°, now fully transformed into typical sarcoma cells,
squarely compact or rounded, and very different from normal
fibroblasts.

ISOLATION OF THE GLUCOSE BINDING FACTOR

The method used (9) is the same as the one we had applied
in experiments on tyrocidine synthesis for localizing amino

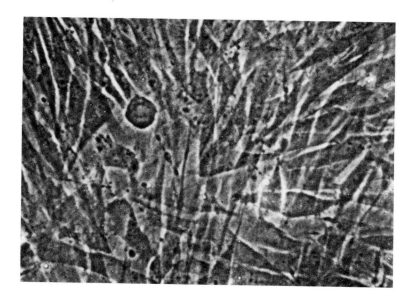

FIGURE 2. Normal cells.

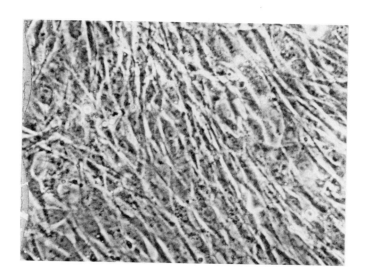

FIGURE 3. RSV-TS68 at 41°, nonpermissive.

Fritz Lipmann and Sung G. Lee

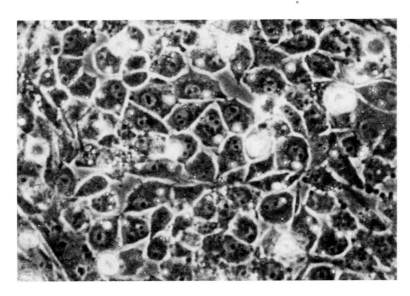

FIGURE 4. RSV-TS68 at 37°, transformed

acid binding proteins (5); it consists of charging Sephadex
G-200 with a uniform base level of the radioactive compound to
be studied, i.e., in this case glucose. When the protein
reaches the charged glucose, radioactivity peaks appear above
the base line. Several such are shown in Figure 5, from which
their molecular weights can be roughly estimated. The first
and highest peak is in the exclusion volume, molecular weight
larger than 400,000; the second peak, or rather a shoulder,
is in the rebound region, molecular weight <u>ca</u>. 200,000; and a
third peak has a molecular weight of about 100,000. This
means that the protein easily aggregates; if chromatographed
at pH 5, disaggregation is more pronounced. Since our fractions were impure, we did not attempt to determine the true
subunit molecular weight. However, recent work (unpublished)
on purification, to be mentioned at the end, indicates a molecular weight of 70,000-80,000.

Three fractions are collected as described in the legend
of Figure 6. These fractions from normal and transformed cells
are compared in Table I. It appears first that the total of
the glucose binding fraction is 2.3 times higher in transformed
than in normal cells. Furthermore, its distribution among the
fractions is highest in the supernatant from normal cells, but
this is reversed after transformation when the highest activity
appears in the membrane fraction, extracted with Triton X-100

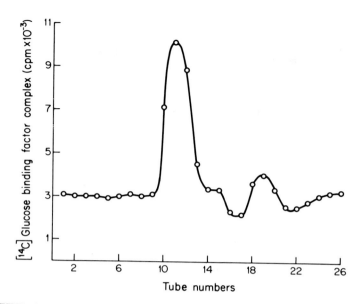

FIGURE 5. Separation of D-glucose binding activity by Sephadex G-200 chromatography (6). The glucose binding activity was determined by the method of Hummel and Dreyer (9). The glucose binding factor applied to the column was from the membrane-Triton X-100 fraction.

without losing its activity. This discrepancy is more pronounced in Figure 6 where the low membrane and high supernatant of the normal cells can be seen on the left, and the much higher membrane concentration in the transformed cells on the right. Recent experiments have shown that if fast-growing normal cells are used instead of cells that have stopped growing, i.e., that have become confluent as in the experiments of Table I and Figure 6, then the abundant appearance of the binding factor in the wash fluid goes down and more of the glucose binding activity is found in the membrane fraction. This means that the tumor cell, not unexpectedly, resembles more the fast-growing normal cell, although the cells in the tumor preparation, still exceeding it, have become confluent. However, these confluent cells do not stop growing but, rather, tend to pile on each other because they are not contact-inhibited.

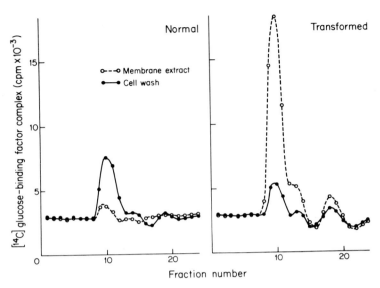

FIGURE 6. Distribution of glucose binding factor in cell wash and in membrane-bound form in normal and RSV-transformed chicken embryo fibroblasts. After thoroughly draining the culture medium, the confluent culture of normal cells (120 dishes, 100-mm diameter), or the RSV-transformed cell culture (52 dishes), was incubated for 20 min at 37° with 2 ml/dish of wash solution (10 mM triethanolamine buffer, pH 7.6, 1 mM EDTA, 100 mM NaCl). Sheets of cells that peeled off the dishes were collected together with the wash solution and pelleted by centrifugation for 5 min at 2,000 rpm. The supernatant (cell wash) was lyophilized and the resulting material was dissolved in 10 ml of water and chromatographed on a Sephadex G-200 column equilibrated with 50 mM NaCl, 5 mM phosphate buffer, pH 7, and 0.005 μCi $\underline{/}^{14}C\underline{/}$glucose (250 mCi/mmole). The cell pellets were suspended in 30 ml of wash solution and homogenized with a Dounce homogenizer. The homogenate was centrifuged for 5 min at 2,000 rpm to remove cell debris and nuclei, and the resulting supernatant was centrifuged for 20 min at 30,000 x g. The membrane-containing 30,000 x g pellets were suspended in 10 ml of 10 mM triethanolamine buffer containing 0.2% Triton X-100 and 1 mM EDTA, and the suspension was sonicated for 20 seconds at step 5 with a Branson sonifier. The sonicated material was then centrifuged for 20 min at 30,000 x g and the resulting supernatant (membrane extract) was chromatographed as above.

TABLE I. Distribution of $[^{14}C]$Glucose Binding
Activity in Various Fractions

Fractions	Normal cells[a]		Transformed cells[b]	
	cpm x 10^{-3}	% of total	cpm x 10^{-3}	% of total
Cell washing	41.9	66.9	17.9	13.1
Postmembrane supernatant	10.1	16.1	24.1	17.5
Membrane extract	10.6	16.9	95.0	68.4
Total	62.6	100.0	137.0	100.0

The three glucose binding fractions, prepared as described
(6), were applied to Sephadex G-200 columns equilibrated with
5 mM phosphate buffer (pH 6.0), containing 100 mM NaCl and
$[^{14}C]$glucose (0.01 μCi/mol), and the columns were eluted with
the same radioactive solution. The Sephadex chromatography
yielded three glucose binding peaks for each of the three
fractions. The combined radioactivity of these three peaks is
shown in the table.

[a] Cells amounting to 296 mg of protein (208 dishes) were used.
Average value of their $[^{3}H]$2-deoxyglucose uptake was 91,000
cpm/mg of cell protein when determined as described (6).

[b] Cells amounting to 278 mg of protein (102 dishes) were used.
Average value of their $[^{3}H]$2-deoxyglucose uptake was 316,000
cpm/mg of cell protein.

STIMULATION OF GLUCOSE UPTAKE BY BINDING FACTOR

We turn now to experiments that show this binding factor
to have a function in glucose uptake. To test this effect,
quiescent cells were obtained by growing them for 6 to 7 days
without renewing the serum. In Table II it can be seen that
the addition of 1 μg/ml of glucose binding factor already
triples the rate of uptake. Aliquots were used in runs of 15
min with deoxyglucose, which is not metabolized further after
phosphorylation but with regard to uptake, behaves in short-
term experiments analogously to glucose. On addition of 3 μg/
ml, the uptake increases about sevenfold which amounts to
almost maximal stimulation. A double reciprocal plot in Figure
7 of rates of uptake by serum-starved cells against that by
factor-complemented cells, shows that the V_{max} in the latter
cells (lower curve) is much higher than in the starved cells,
but the K_m remains the same as seen by the meeting of the

TABLE II. Promotion of $\sqrt{3}H\sqrt{7}$2-Deoxyglucose Uptake
of Quiescent Cells by Glucose Binding Factor

Glucose binding factor (μg in 6 ml medium)	$\sqrt{3}H\sqrt{7}$2-Deoxyglucose uptake/dish (cpm)
0	5,500
6	15,400
12	26,200
18	35,800
30	39,500

The glucose binding fraction was from membrane extracts
of transformed cells purified by Sephadex G-200 chromatography.
Varying amounts of glucose binding factor in 3 ml of glucose-
free Hanks' medium were added to the quiescent secondary culture dishes, and the dishes were preincubated for 30 min at
37°. They then received 3 μCi of $\sqrt{3}H\sqrt{7}$2-deoxyglucose in 3 ml
of glucose-free Hanks' medium, making a total of 6 ml, and
were incubated for 15 min at 37°. $\sqrt{3}H\sqrt{7}$2-Deoxyglucose uptake
was determined as described (6).

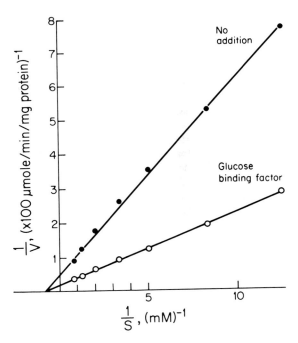

FIGURE 7. Kinetics of $\sqrt{3}H\sqrt{7}$2-deoxyglucose uptake in the
presence or absence of glucose binding factor. The confluent
culture of normal cells grown in 100-mm diameter dishes was

washed with three 12-ml portions of Hanks' solution. The culture dishes were preincubated for 30 min at 37° with either 3 ml of Hanks' solution alone or 3 ml of Hanks' solution containing 22 µg of glucose binding factor from Sephadex G-200 chromatography (see Fig. 6). At the end of the preincubation, varying concentrations of $/^3H/$2-deoxyglucose in 0.5 ml of Hanks' solution were added to the culture dishes to a final concentration of 0.08-1.2 mM, and the dishes were incubated for 10 min at 37°. The $/^3H/$2-deoxyglucose uptake was determined as described (6).

curves at the lower left of the Figure. After addition of the factor, development of the increase goes through an induction period of about 30 min, then approaches maximum as shown in Figure 8. Accordingly, in all the experiments of Table II, these cells were first preincubated with factor for 30 min in the absence of $/^3H/$2-deoxyglucose before measuring its uptake. The cause of this delay has not been explored.

COMPARISON OF GLUCOSE BINDING FACTOR WITH OTHER SUBSTANCES THAT INCREASE UPTAKE

In Figure 9, serum action on glucose uptake with serum-depleted cultures is compared with factor action. The time points in all curves refer to samples taken for 15-min determination of $/^3H/$2-deoxyglucose uptake during the incubation period. Other than the omission of serum or its replacement with the factor, the incubation medium here was a secondary culture medium containing Scherer's solution and tryptose phosphate broth. When measured after 1 hr, the stimulation is similar for factor and serum. On further incubation with factor, stimulation falls off and reaches a plateau at about half the peak uptake. In contrast, the serum uptake curve rises further, beginning to fall off after the third hour and then continuing rather rapidly to fall to a plateau. On the other hand, if serum is incubated together with the glucose binding factor, the curve of uptake rises more rapidly and the differential between the sample containing serum and glucose binding factor reaches a level approximately 1.5 times that of serum after 3 hr, and then plateaus instead of falling off. In other words, the combined effect of the two compounds is cumulative.

In another similar experiment (Figure 10), the effect of our factor is compared with insulin and serum; the former is also known to increase glucose uptake by chicken fibroblasts.

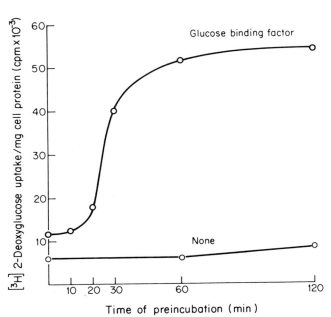

FIGURE 8.   Kinetics of the activation of $[^3H]$2-deoxygluc-
ose uptake by glucose binding factor.   Quiescent 7-day old
secondary culture dishes were supplied with 82 μg of glucose
binding factor (obtained from the cell washing fraction and
purified by Sephadex G-200) in 3 ml of glucose-free Hanks'
medium, and the dishes were incubated at 37° for varying
periods.   At the end of each period, the culture dishes received 3 μCi of $[^3H]$2-deoxyglucose in 3 ml of glucose-free
Hanks' medium and were then incubated for 15 min.   At the end
of the incubation, $[^3H]$2-deoxyglucose uptake was determined as
described (6).

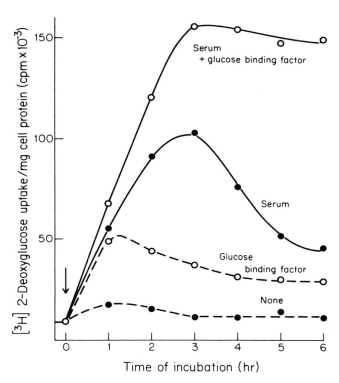

FIGURE 9. Activation of $[^3H]$2-deoxyglucose uptake by serum and glucose binding factor (6). The quiescent secondary culture was divided into four groups. At the time indicated by an arrow, the culture dishes were supplied with fresh secondary medium containing serum-free medium, serum-free medium supplemented with 52 μg of glucose binding factor, 5% serum, or 5% serum + 52 μg of glucose binding factor. The culture dishes were incubated at 37° in a humidified CO_2 chamber for varying lengths of time. At the end of each incubation, $[^3H]$-2-deoxyglucose uptake was determined by dissolving the cells after twice washing them with saline in 0.1 NaOH.

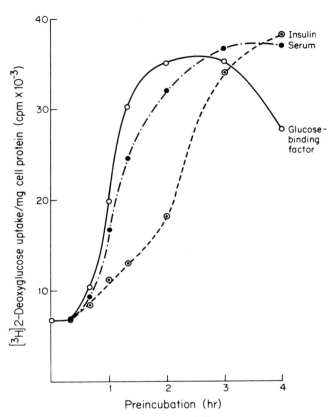

FIGURE 10.   Stimulation of $\overline{/^3H/}$2-deoxyglucose uptake of
serum starved cells by serum, insulin, or glucose binding factor.   The subconfluent culture of normal cells was grown in
serum-free Scherer's culture medium for 36 hr.   The medium was
decanted and the dishes were washed with three 12-ml portions
of Hanks' salt solution and then preincubated at 37° for varying lengths of time with 3 ml of Hanks' salt solution containing 5% serum, 9 μg of insulin, or 26 μg of glucose binding factor.   At the end of the preincubation, 2.5 μCi of $\overline{/^3H/}$2-deoxy-
glucose (10 mCi/μmole) in 0.5 ml of Hanks' salt solution was
added to each dish and the dishes were incubated for an additional 15 min. $\overline{/^3H/}$2-Deoxyglucose uptake was determined as
described (6).

The pre-treatment of cells in this case was to reduce the glucose uptake, after initial incubation with serum, by replacing
the fluid with serum-free medium. To stimulate glucose uptake

the cell samples were then incubated with serum, insulin, or the factor in Hanks' salt solution. In this set-up, the rise in glucose uptake is highest with the binding factor but falls off after incubation for 3 hr, while the serum curve rises more slowly to reach a plateau at 4 hr; with insulin, the uptake rises in a sigmoid curve, also reaching a plateau after 4 hr that is similar to the one formed by the serum. However, in contrast to the binding factor effect, these two curves do not fall off. What interests us most in this type of experiment is that, in the initial period before it falls off, the glucose binding factor effect is equivalent to or even better than the serum or insulin effects.

We would now like to introduce an important observation that shows that, in contrast to serum and insulin, the binding factor does not affect cell division. Table III shows that serum and insulin addition increased eightfold the incorporation of $[^3H]$thymidine over the control, while addition of the glucose binding factor left it unchanged. This difference shows that the factor effect is not due to any contamination by stimulators present in serum or by traces of insulin.

TABLE III. Mitogenic Activity of the Factors
Stimulating Glucose Uptake

Factors	$[^3H]$Thymidine incorporation into DNA/mg protein (cpm)	$[^3H]$2-Deoxyglucose uptake/mg cell protein (cpm)
None	48,000	14,400
Glucose binding factor (11 μg/ml)	47,300	88,900
Insulin (3 μg/ml)	400,200	95,400
Serum (5%)	394,300	104,600

Subconfluent normal cells were brought into G_0 phase by growing them in a serum-free culture medium for 16 hr, at which time serum, insulin, or the factor was added to the culture medium and the cells were grown for 8 hr. The culture medium was then removed and the cell samples were incubated for 1 hr at 37° with $[^3H]$thymidine (5 μCi) in 4 ml of Hanks' salt solution. The radioactive solution was then decanted, cell samples were washed with Hanks' salt solution and dissolved in 0.1 N NaOH. The labeled DNA was precipitated with trichloroacetic acid, collected on a Millipore filter, and the radioactivity was determined. The uptake of $[^3H]$2-deoxyglucose was determined as described (6).

The identity of the factor that binds glucose and stimulates uptake of deoxyglucose is affirmed by competing experiments using $[^3H]$2-deoxyglucose together with cold monosaccharides in high concentrations. It may be seen in Tables IV and V that the inhibition by D-glucose and D-glucosamine is strong in both the binding and uptake experiments; in contrast, L-glucose, fructose, and galactose have little or no effect. There is one feature, tested in the competitive experiment for binding of Table IV, that reflects on the very firm binding of the glucose: the competing monosaccharide has to be added at the same time as the $[^3H]$2-deoxyglucose. If the labeled glucose is added first and then followed later by the competing monosaccharide, no inhibition is observed. Apparently, once the glucose has anchored itself to the binding factor, its displacement is not possible under these conditions. This is also shown by the fact that protein denaturation by trichloroacetic acid or by heating does not release the glucose, which is only released on heating with normal hydrochloric acid. In

TABLE IV. Inhibition of $[^3H]$2-Deoxyglucose Binding by Various Sugars

Sugars	$[^3H]$2-Deoxyglucose bound (cpm)	Control (%)
None	3,020	100
D-Mannose	1,770	58.5
D-Glucose	1,030	34.2
D-Galactose	2,480	82.2
L-Glucose	2,720	90.0
D-Glucosamine	1,240	41.0

The cell wash fraction containing glucose binding factor was prepared from confluent normal cells as described in the legend to Fig. 6, and chromatographed on a Sephadex G-200 column equilibrated with 5 mM phosphate buffer, pH 6.5, containing 50 mM NaCl. The column was eluted with the same solution and the material eluting at the void volume was used as the source of binding factor. To measure the effect of monosaccharides on the binding of $[^3H]$2-deoxyglucose to the factor, about 80 μg of the factor in 3 ml of 5 mM phosphate buffer containing 50 mM NaCl was incubated for 30 min at $37°$ with 0.05 mM $[^3H]$2-deoxyglucose (0.5 μCi) alone, or with the mixture of $[^3H]$2-deoxyglucose and 0.5 mM of monosaccharides. The factor was then collected on a HAMK Millipore filter, the filter was washed with five 10-ml portions of the same buffered salt solution, and its radioactivity was determined.

TABLE V. Inhibition of $[^3H]$2-Deoxyglucose
Uptake by Various Sugars

| Sugars | $[^3H]$2-Deoxyglucose uptake (cpm) | |
	Without binding factor	With binding factor
None	12,830	35,060
L-Glucose	13,320	35,850
D-Glucose	6,470	17,200
D-Fructose	12,010	35,720
D-Galactose	12,510	35,400
D-Mannose	5,420	16,950
D-Glucosamine	7,120	18,250

Confluent normal cell culture dishes were incubated for
15 min at 37° with 0.05 mM $[^3H]$2-deoxyglucose (3 µCi) alone,
or with the mixture of $[^3H]$2-deoxyglucose and monosaccharides
in 3 ml of Hanks' salt solution, and $[^3H]$2-deoxyglucose uptake was determined as described (6).

Table V, in an analogous experiment on glucose uptake, the
effect of the factor is affected in a similar manner by a
spectrum of monosaccharides. This confirms the binding factor
as being part of the glucose transport system.

PURIFICATION

The purification of the binding factor has caused difficulties. We have only recently been able to obtain what seems
to be a rather highly purified preparation and have achieved
this by affinity chromatography. There, the binding factor
charged with glucose binds very tightly. It is adsorbed onto
immobilized concnavalin A and released by using methyl gluco-
side in the presence of Triton X-100. In this manner, about
half the binding factor is released in a rather highly purified form. Since sodium dodecyl sulfate electrophoresis gave
a fairly homogeneous spot corresponding to a molecular weight
between 70,000 and 80,000, we assume that this may represent
the true molecular weight of the glucose binding factor.

REFERENCES

1. Lipmann, F., Biochem. Z. <u>26</u>: 157 (1933).
2. Lipmann, F., in "Symposium on Respiratory Enzymes", p. 48. University of Wisconsin Press, Madison (1942).
3. Warburg, O., "Stoffwechsel der Tumoren". Springer, Berlin (1926).
4. Hatanaka, M., Biochim. Biophys. Acta (Reviews on Cancer) <u>355</u>: 77 (1974).
5. Lipmann, F., and Lee, S. G., J. Cell. Physiol. <u>89</u>: 523 (1976).
6. Lee, S. G., and Lipmann, F., Proc. Nat. Acad. Sci. USA <u>74</u>: 163 (1977).
7. Haseltine, W. A., Maxam, A. M., and Gilbert, W., Proc. Nat. Acad. Sci. USA <u>74</u>: 989 (1977).
8. Kawai, S., and Hanafusa, H., Virology <u>46</u>: 470 (1971).
9. Hummel, J. P., and Dreyer, W. J., Biochim. Biophys. Acta <u>63</u>: 530 (1962).

DISCUSSION

S. BESSMAN: Is the glucose bound to the carrier a substrate for hexokinase?

F. LIPMANN: So far we haven't tested it but we hope we will. We were more concerned with the purification and spent a great deal of time trying to purify the carrier with the glucose on it, but it would be wonderful if the hexokinase might react with it and remove the glucose.

B. CHANCE: Is this protein present in ascites and other types of cell lines?

F. LIPMANN: We haven't tried, but I guess there should be something similar there. It should be rather wide spread in tumors in which a large amount of glucose must be transported.

P. SRERE: Is there an increase in the utilization of glucose when you do the temperature shift?

F. LIPMANN: Oh, yes that comes pretty early. In about five hours you get an increase before full transformation occurs. Dr. Hanaka has mentioned these experiments in his review article (Biochem. Biophys. Acta Rev. on Cancer, <u>355</u>, p81,

Fig. 8). Puromycin will suppress transformation from the
temperature shift in both ways. Thus, interestingly enough,
you need protein synthesis for transformation. If you go
back to high temperature you can reverse in about 12 hours
and get again the untransformed cells, and puromycin inhibits
this process too, as mentioned.

S. BESSMAN: May I ask one more question. This is something
that is also mysterious. Are these cells grown in the presence of glucose?

F. LIPMANN: Well, yes.

S. BESSMAN: Why isn't the protein saturated with glucose,
because you have shown that the binding is apparently irreversible?

F. LIPMANN: You see, we run an aliquot first through the
column where it picks up glucose to identify the protein. But
for the experiment, uncharged carrier protein is used.

S. BESSMAN: What I meant was that since cells are grown in a
medium already containing glucose, why didn't they pick up
the glucose in the medium? This would make it difficult to
find it by binding glucose since it binds glucose so tightly.

F. LIPMANN: To measure uptake from one of a number of parallel incubated culture dishes (10 cm dia.) containing glucose in the medium, the medium is decanted and the culture
washed twice with glucose-free medium. Labeled deoxyglucose
containing glucose-free medium is then added and the mixture
is incubated for 15 min at 37°. The radioactive solution is
decanted, again washed twice, and the cell sheet dissolved
in 5 ml of 0.1 M NaOH; 0.5 ml is measured for radioactivity.
The carrier-linked deoxyglucose enters the cell, as has been
checked by using limited amounts of labeled deoxyglucose.

R. WELCH: I have a question regarding the nature of this
transport protein. Is it that the large increase you see
in the amount is due to a new protein, or is it the same
protein? That is to say, is the cell in the transformed
state making more of the same transport protein or is this
possibly another isozyme, say a fetal isozyme?

F. LIPMANN: I would say from all we have seen, the chromatogram of the protein looks just the same. The concentration
effect that we measure in the uptake experiment shows that

it is probably more of the same. Of course, I can't guarantee that it's the same protein.

M. JONES: Do you have any idea why more of it remains membrane bound in the transformed cells?

F. LIPMANN: It has something to do with the rate of growth because fast growing tissue culture has more membrane-bound material. It may actually be related to the fact that a fast growing tissue culture takes up more glucose. Yet there is always an increase when you transform the cells. We have thought of the possibility that it's different, but I doubt it from all we have seen. It looks more as if it is the same. How the transformation achieves it is really interesting to explore. The fact that the temperature-sensitive strain depends on protein synthesis to transform it makes it quite clear. What I have not emphasized is that at the nonpermissive temperature it makes lots of virus. Other people have found that generally temperature sensitivity means temperature sensitivity of the protein. The protein may be made but it seems to be temperature-inactivated. On the other hand, a temperature-sensitive strain has been described that is the opposite - it is cold sensitive.

S. BESSMAN: Do you have to use a special medium to generate this protein? Do you grow your sarcoma cells in a particular medium or just standard medium and you just add your virus.

F. LIPMANN: It is standard medium. It is very agreeable to have this situation because then you start out with a completely normal cell, add the virus and wait for 36 hrs. Then you switch from high (41°) to low (36°) temperature and you get a completely transformed sample.

S. BESSMAN: It sounds like the hemoglobin A1C where the glucose binds and then undergoes an Amadori rearrangement and you can't get it off.

F. LIPMANN: Yes, I have heard about that. I wasn't aware of the fact that the glucose binds covalently and that in diabetics the glucose is a very bad devil.

R. DAVIS: You have used 2-deoxyglucose for your assays of the binding protein and found it is hard to get off the protein afterwards. Do some of the other things that compete with deoxyglucose binding bind as tightly and as irreversibly to the isolated protein?

<u>F. LIPMANN</u>: We have not tried that. That is a good question. We actually should saturate the protein once with a competitive monosaccharide and then add the deoxyglucose. I guess you would find that we wouldn't get it on. We haven't done any reverse experiments.

FATTY ACID SYNTHETASE OF YEAST AND 6-METHYLSALICY-
LATE SYNTHETASE OF PENICILLIUM PATULUM - TWO MULTI-
ENZYME COMPLEXES

F. Lynen, H. Engeser, J. Friedrich, W. Schindlbeck,
R. Seyffert, and F. Wieland

Max-Planck-Institut für Biochemie, Martinsried,FRG

The biosynthesis of fatty acids from acetyl CoA
is achieved by the action of acetyl CoA carboxylase
and the multienzyme complex fatty acid synthetase.
We have studied the latter enzyme of yeast. From
ruptured yeast cells we isolated a protein fraction
which synthesizes a mixture of palmityl and stearyl
CoA according to the following equation (n=7 or 8):

$$\text{Acetyl CoA} + n \text{ malonyl CoA} + 2 \text{ } n \text{ NADPH} + 2n \text{ H}^+$$

$$\longrightarrow CH_3(CH_2CH_2)_n \text{ CO-CoA} + n \text{ CO}_2 + n \text{ CoA}$$

$$+ 2n \text{ NADP}^+ + n \text{ H}_2O$$

The purified fatty acid synthetase proved to be
homogeneous by electrophoresis and ultracentrifugation and could be crystallized from ammonium sulfate
solution (1). Its molecular weight was estimated
to be 2.3 million.
    The transformation of malonyl CoA into fatty
acids is achieved through intermediates which are
covalently bound to two types of sulfhydryl groups
of the multienzyme complex which we denoted as
"central" ($-S_cH$) and "peripheral" (-SpH) and which
belong either to 4'-phosphopantetheine, the functional group of the acyl carrier protein (ACP) component, or to cysteine in the active center of the
condensing enzyme.
    The synthetic process, as summarized in Figure 1
is initiated by the transfer of an acetyl residue
from acetyl CoA to the "peripheral" SH-group via the
"central" SH-group. After the following transfer of
a malonyl residue from malonyl CoA to the "central"
SH-group, condensation occurs between the two
enzyme-bound acyl groups, resulting in the formation
of acetoacetate with the concomitant liberation of

Copyright © 1978 by Academic Press, Inc.
All right of reproduction in any form reserved.
ISBN 0-12-660550-5

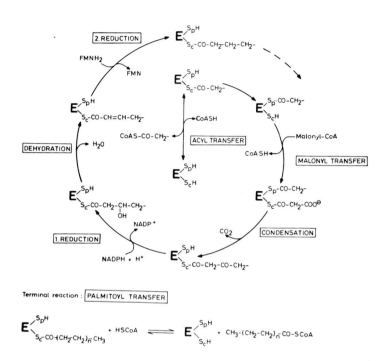

FIGURE 1.   Reaction scheme of fatty acid biosynthesis

CO_2. The stepwise conversion of the ß-keto acid into
the saturated acid is accomplished with acids bound
to the "central" SH-group.   At the stage of the
saturated acid, the butyryl group finally is transferred to the "peripheral" SH-group, thus liberating
the "central" group for introduction of the next
malonyl residue.   The reaction sequence is then repeated until long-chain saturated fatty acids with
16 or 18 carbon atoms are formed, which in the terminal step are transferred from the "central" SH-
group to coenzyme A with the formation of palmityl
or stearyl CoA and the regenerated enzyme.

The multienzyme complex may be visualized as a strict compartmentation of a metabolic multistep reaction sequence in the smallest possible space. According to this concept the multienzyme complexes represent intracellular factories in which the building blocks are assembled piece by piece and only the finished product is released from the complex. With this picture in mind it is tempting to draw an analogy between the yeast fatty acid synthetase and the mitochondrion. The function of the mitochondrial membrane, serving as a selective barrier which guarantees the availability of certain metabolites and the exclusion of others in the fatty acid synthetase, is taken over by the acyl transferase enzyme components which deliver acetyl and malonyl fragments to the complex and release the long chain fatty acids from it. In fatty acid synthesis the transferases play the critical role in compartmentalization.

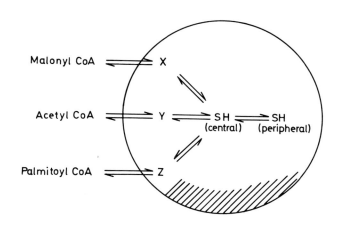

FIGURE 2.   Schematic representation of the functions of acyl transferases in fatty acid synthetase

$SH_{central}$: ACP component

$SH_{peripheral}$: Functional group of the condensing enzyme

X, Y, and Z : Active sites of acyl transferases

It was found that the active sites of all transferases labelled X, Y, and Z in Figure 2, are represented by the OH-groups of serine residues. However,
even more interestingly, it was found by genetic
analysis in Schweizer's laboratory (2), and also by
binding-studies as well as by protein chemical analysis of the binding-sites performed by Engeser (3)
in our laboratory, that one and the same transferase
component enzyme is responsible for the transfer of
malonate and that of palmitate. As a result the
incorporation of malonate into fatty acids is
blocked as long as the long chain fatty acids are
not released from the complex. That may be of great
regulatory significance.

In order to explain the double specificity of
this acyl transferase we may assume that there exist
three binding sites in the active center of this
enzymic domain. The first interacts with the thiolester grouping, which would be present in all acyl
thiolester intermediates of the synthetic process.
The additional binding sites leading to the specificity of the enzyme are assumed to be represented
by a positively charged group of the enzyme which
can interact with the negatively charged carboxylate
anion of malonyl thiolesters and an hydrophobic
area of the enzyme more distant from the first binding site which comes into play if the number of carbon atoms in the acyl residue exceeds thirteen. As
Sumper and Oesterhelt (4) in our laboratory have
calculated from their experiments the binding energy
for this site increases by 0.9 Kcal for each $-CH_2-$
group in the acyl residue exceeding thirteen.

With respect to the architecture of the multienzyme complex, Schweizer (2) in 1973 showed with
genetic methods that all partial activities are
coded for by only two gene loci, designated as fas 1
and fas 2, each coding for one single multifunctional polypeptide chain. By genetic analysis the
distribution of most of the partial reactions on the
gene products of fas 1, named polypeptide chain ß,
and fas 2, named chain α, could be found (Figure 3).
The gene product for fas 2, α, carries the condensing enzyme activity, the first reductase as well as
the integrated acyl carrier protein. On ß are located malonyl/palmitoyl-transferase, acetyl transferase, dehydratase and the second reductase. By SDS-
gel-electrophoresis the two subunits were analytically separated and their molecular weights were

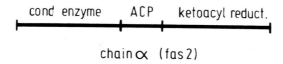

chain α (fas 2)

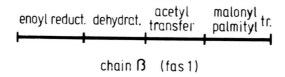

chain ß (fas 1)

FIGURE 3.   Localization of the component
enzymes on the polypeptides α and ß

TABLE I.   Composition of yeast fatty acid
synthetase

Yeast Fatty Acid Synthetase

	Mol. Weight
Native Enzyme ($\alpha_6 \beta_6$)	2.3×10^6
Chain α	185 000
Chain ß	180 000

estimated to be about 185 000 and 180 000 (Table I).
For the experiments to be discussed in the following, it should be mentioned that Kresze et al. (6)
were able to confirm by protein chemical methods
that the condensing enzyme activity is located on
chain α.   It was known from previous studies of
Oesterhelt and Hagen in our laboratory that iodo-
acetamide is a specific reagent for the "peripheral"
SH-group, which represents the active site of the
condensing enzyme.   Fatty acid synthetase was specifically labelled with ^{14}C-iodoacetamide and analyzed
by SDS-gel electrophoresis.   Radioactivity was found
only in the α chain.

Fatty acid synthetase can be reversibly dissociated by the freezing and thawing procedure of Sumper (7). In this procedure the solution of the multienzyme complex in the presence of 1 M lithium chloride is repeatedly frozen and thawed. This leads to the loss of enzymic activity concomitant to the disaggregation of the complex to the separated polypeptide chains. But our attempts to separate the two subunits prepared in this way were without success.

The separation became only possible when Felix Wieland (8) tried to modify the complex chemically, hoping to change the chemical properties of one chain more than those of the other one. Acylation of the ε-amino-group of lysine by treatment with cyclic dicarbonic anhydrides like citraconic anhydride and dimethylmaleic anhydride under mild conditions led to a total loss of the overall activity. On disk-gel-electrophoresis a resolution into two proteins could be observed.

The preparative isolation of the two subunits became possible on Martin and Ames sucrose density gradients. Centrifugation for 45 hours at 230 000xg led to the appearance of two protein peaks (Figure 4), of which the slower sedimenting protein contained all radioactivity and therefore represented α. The faster one showed high activity in acetyl transferase which was not observed in α but was present in ß (see Figure 3).

Table II summarizes the distribution of the partial enzymic activities in both fractions: acetyltransferase, dehydratase, malonyl-transferase and enoyl reductase were found in peak I protein (ß), whereas the condensing enzyme is located in peak II protein (α) as shown by its radioactivity, due to the labelling with the ^{14}C-carboxamidomethyl group.

Using dimethylmaleic anhydride in order to dissociate the complex is advantageous, because the ε-amino-lysyl-dimethylmaleic amide formed is much easier to hydrolyse under mild acidic conditions than the products of other cyclic dicarbonic anhydrides. Its half life at pH 3.5 and 20° C was found to be about 2 minutes. Therefore it could be expected that the dissociation of the complex by treatment with dimethylmaleic anhydride could be reversed. The reconstitution was finally achieved by removal of dimethylmaleic acid by incubation at pH 4.6 in the presence of ammonium sulfate at 0° C (10 hrs).

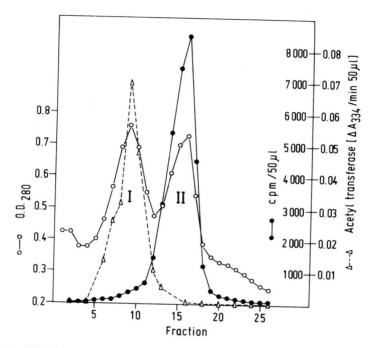

FIGURE 4.   Separation of chain α and ß
            after treatment of fatty acid synthe-
            tase with dimethylmaleic anhydride
            (DMMA).

Centrifugation for 42 hrs at 230 000 xg in a
linear density gradient (10-20 percent sucrose)
5-6 mg purified and ^{14}C-iodoacetamide treated
enzyme per ml of 0.3 M potassium phosphate,
pH 7.5, containing 10 mM 2-mercapto-ethanol
were brought to 10 mM DMMA and incubated for 30
minutes at 0° C.   The sample was then chromatographed over a Sephadex G-50 column in 20 mM
Tris-HCl, pH 7.5, 1 mM dithiothreitol and
loaded on sucrose density gradients containing
the same buffer.

TABLE II.   Distribution of the component enzyme
            activities on the two protein frac-
            tions from Figure 4

peak I protein	peak II protein	Activity
+	–	Acetyl transfer
+	–	Malonyl transfer
–	–	β-Ketoacylreduction
–	+	Condensation (Radioactivity)
+	–	Dehydratation
+	–	Enoylreduction

Though the reactivated protein exhibits only about
50 % of the original activity, it sedimented like
untreated fatty acid synthetase in the analytical
ultracentrifuge.   In addition the protein behaves
like the untreated complex in the Maurer disc-gel
electrophoresis system.   From this we may conclude
that, at least under appropriate conditions, the
complex state of the enzyme is favoured over the
subunit state and over possible intermediate sub-
complexes which we were not able to find with this
method.
     The isolated α and ß polypeptides were used by
Wieland to immunize rabbits and in this way he obtained specific antibodies, which, in collaboration
with Dr. Elmar Siess, he used to obtain some insight
into the architecture of the multienzyme complex.
Native fatty acid synthetase was incubated with non-
precipitating amounts of each immunoglobulin fraction.   Such incubations were centrifuged in sucrose
density gradients with the results shown in Figure 5.
Fatty acid synthetase treated with control immunoglobulin from non-immunized rabbits shows only one

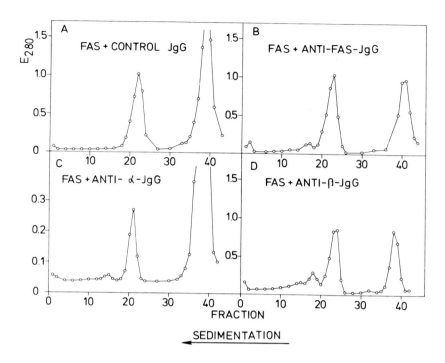

FIGURE 5. Sucrose density gradient centrifugation of fatty acid synthetase in
presence of non-precipitating
amounts of antibodies

peak corresponding to native fatty acid synthetase.
Incubation with anti-α immunoglobulin led to the
appearance of small amounts of a faster sedimenting
protein peak before fatty acid synthetase and so
did also the incubation with anti-ß immunoglobulin
and fatty acid synthetase immunoglobulin. This
faster sedimenting material was expected to be immunoglobulin crosslinked fatty acid synthetase dimers
or oligomers.
      Figure 6a, an electronmicrograph of untreated
fatty acid synthetase, shows a random distribution
of the individual complex molecules over the whole
area. In Figure 6b, protein from the faster sedimenting peak of the specific immunoglobulin fatty
acid synthetase interaction is shown. As expected
they are no longer randomly distributed but fatty

acid synthetase molecules are predominantly arranged
in dimeric and oligomeric groups. Anti-α immunoglobulin crosslinked and anti-ß immunoglobulin crosslinked material now was investigated at higher
magnification, and Figure 6c gives a representative
survey of anti-ß crosslinked fatty acid synthetase.

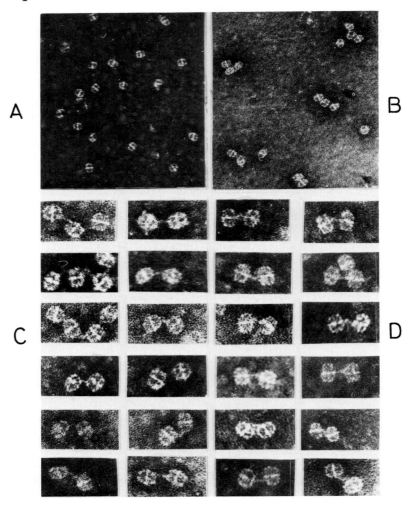

FIGURE 6.   Electronmicrographs of fatty acid
            synthetase

Alone (a) or after interaction with anti-FAS
antibodies (b), anti-ß antibodies (c) and
anti-α antibodies (d)

For interpretation it must be added, that only those structures were taken into account, which possessed a visible immunoglobulin as a link between the synthetase molecules. Many other dimeric and oligomeric structures without visible antibody were present but were not evaluated. We don't know why antibody bridges were not always visible and why in some of the dimers the molecules were closely attached. It may be that parts of the antibodies are able to penetrate into the hollow body of the enzyme and bind internally. In our pictures of evaluated structures we are able to localize a preferable region for anti-ß antibody binding on fatty acid synthetase. This region is spanned in the central part between equator and poles of the enzyme structure. Figure 6d gives a survey of typical anti-α antibody crosslinked complexes. The region of complexation by anti-α immunoglobulin seems to be concentrated at the equator of the enzyme structure.

This information was used to extend a three dimensional model for the yeast fatty acid synthetase complex in our laboratory in the past year. A comparison of the molecular weights of the subunits with the molecular weight of the complex as already mentioned suggests that each subunit is present six times in the complex (see Table I). Further evidence for this stoichiometry results from the presence of 5.5 to 6 FMN molecules (1) and between 5 and 6 phosphopantetheine molecules (9) per one molecule of fatty acid synthetase complex. Small angle X-ray scattering analysis of the complex made with Pilz and Kratky (10), as well as the results of three dimensional electronmicroscopy performed by Hoppe and his colleagues (11), supported the assumption that the enzyme is a hollow body, separated into two halves by a center wall, having a 3/2 symmetry.

To combine these data with the analytical results mentioned above, we assumed in Figure 7 that the complex is built from six protomers, each consisting of one A and one B subunit, which are connected in the form of the letter v. Combination of these six protomers in such a manner that all of the polypeptides of one type are arranged in hexagonal order forming a single plane. The binding of these polypeptide chains is achieved by the interaction of identical binding sites, i.e. in our model the gray sites bind to the gray sites and the black

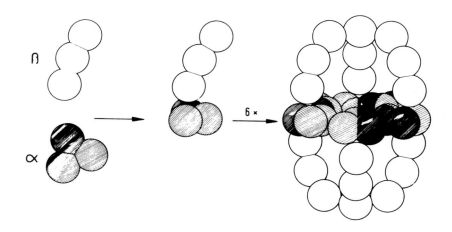

FIGURE 7.   Three dimensional model of yeast
            fatty acid synthetase

sites to the black sites.   The result is a hexagonal basic disc resembling the central wall of the
complex, from which three polypeptide chains of the
other type protrude upward and three subunits protrude downwards.   Those chains protruding upwards
are displaced by 60 degrees from those protruding
downwards. This model has a shape similar to the
shape of the complex seen in electronmicrophoto-
graphs and (see Figure 6a) is compatible with the
proposed symmetry.   Twisting three times around the
long axis and twice around the short axis results in
a identical, hollow rotation ellipsoid.
    From our electronmicroscopic studies with spe-
cific antibodies, we would like to propose that the
central wall consists of six α-subunits, separating
the complex into two halves, each of which is built
from three ß-subunits.

Let me now turn to a discussion of recent results with the 6-methylsalicylate synthetase of <u>Penicillium</u> <u>patulum</u>. We were interested in this multienzyme complex because it uses the same substrates as fatty acid synthetase, namely: acetyl CoA as primer, malonyl CoA, and NADPH. But instead of straight chain fatty acids, it synthesizes the benzene derivative 6-methylsalicylic acid (6-MSA) according to the following equation:

$$\text{Acetyl CoA} + 3 \text{ malonyl CoA} + \text{NADPH} + \text{H}^+ \longrightarrow$$

$$+ \ 4 \text{ CoA} + 3 \text{ CO}_2 + \text{NADP}^+ + \text{H}_2\text{O}$$

Friedrich (12) in our laboratory recently developed a new purification procedure which leads to a homogeneous protein. This is summarized in Table III.

TABLE III. Purification of 6-MSA-synthetase from <u>Penicillium</u> <u>patulum</u>

PURIFICATION OF 6-MSA-SYNTHETASE FROM PENICILLIUM PATULUM

Step	Volume (ML)	Total Activity (mU)	Protein (mg)	Specific Activity (mU/mg)	Recovery (%)
1. Centrifuged extract	3 000	54 400	38 900	1.4	100
2. Polyethylene-glycol-6000-precipitation (3 - 10 % w/v)	410	42 950	6 400	6.7	79
3. Polyethylene-glycol-6000-precipitation (4 - 9 % w/v)	75	66 110	2 900	22.7	121
4. 22 - 37 % Ammonium-sulfate fractionation	52	56 060	1 940	28.8	103
5. Hydroxyapatite concentrated eluate	24	35 880	356	101	66
6. Centrifugation in a discontinuous sucrose gradient	10	28 730	177	162	53

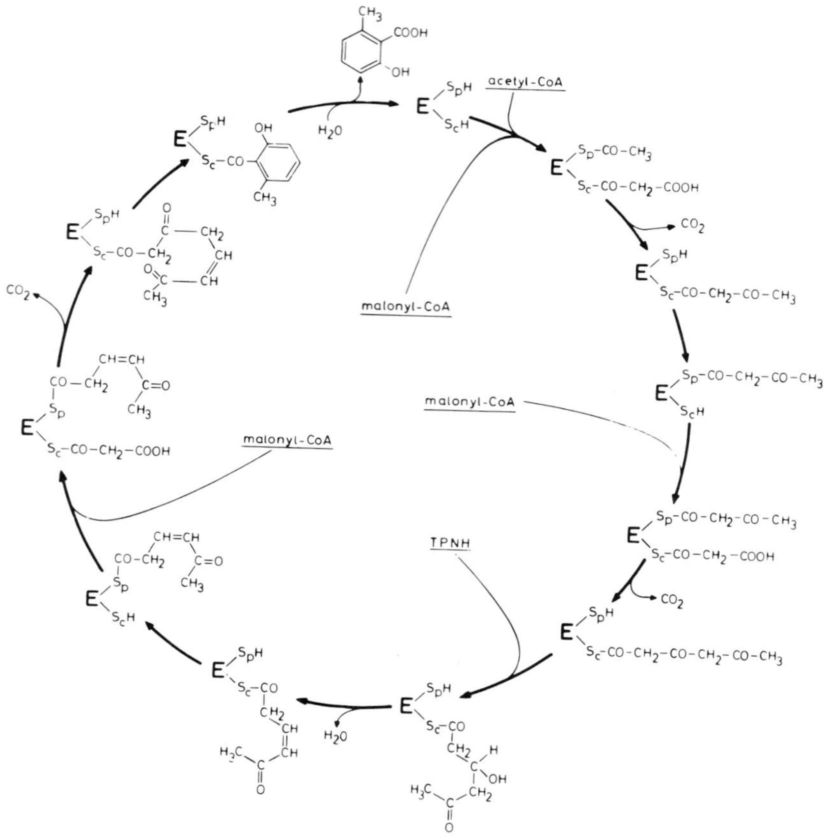

FIGURE 8.   Reaction scheme of 6-methylsalicylic
acid biosynthesis

The enzyme catalyzes the synthetsis of 6-MSA in
the following way (Figure 8). It contains two types
of SH-groups, analogous to fatty acid synthetase,
which we again called "central" and "peripheral" and
which belong to 4'-phosphopantetheine (13) bound at
a serine residue of the multienzyme complex and to a
cysteine residue in the active centre of the condensing enzyme component. The synthesis of 6-MSA proceeds in a manner rather analogous to fatty acid
synthesis: First transfer of acetyl and malonyl residues to the active SH-groups, then condensation of
sulfur-bound acetate and malonate to form acetoacetate. Whereas in fatty acid synthesis acetoacetate
is reduced, in 6-MSA synthesis it condenses once
more with malonate to form triacetic acid before re-

duction occurs. After dehydration, which probably leads to the formation of 5-keto-cis-3-hexenoic acid, the condensation with the third malonyl-unit follows and the product then cyclizes by an aldol condensation to form 6-MSA bound to the enzyme. In the final step the product is released from the enzyme complex by hydrolysis.

TABLE IV. Comparison of 6-MSA-synthetase and fatty acid synthetase

Partial reactions of	
6-MSA synthetase	fatty acid synthetase
1. acetyl transfer	1. acetyl transfer
2. malonyl transfer	2. malonyl transfer
3. condensation $C_2 \rightarrow C_4 \rightarrow C_6$	3. condensation $C_2 \rightarrow C_4$
4. β-keto acyl reduction	4. β-keto acyl reduction
5. dehydration $[\beta, \gamma \rightarrow cis]$?	5. dehydration $[\alpha, \beta \rightarrow trans]$
	6. enoyl acyl reduction
3.' condensation $C_6 \rightarrow C_8$	repetition of 2. to 6.
6. condensation (aldol type) $\rightarrow$ aromatic ring	
7. hydrolysis	7. palmitoyl transfer to CoA-SH (stearoyl transfer)

Table IV (in the left column) summarizes the reactions just mentioned and compares them with the partial reactions of fatty acid synthesis (in the right column).

In order to demonstrate many of the reactions listed here we applied two methods:

1. The enzyme complex was used in stoichiometric amounts and the transfer of the acyl groups from ^{14}C-acetyl- or ^{14}C-malonyl-CoA to the carrier sites of the complex was measured directly. In this way Schindlbeck (14) could demonstrate that acetate and malonate were not only bound to

SH-groups on the enzyme but also to OH-groups.
We assume that the latter groups represent the
active sites of acetyl and malonyl transferase
respectively and belong to peptide bound serine
residues as in the case of fatty acid synthetase.
Friedrich (12) continued these studies and obtained experimental evidence showing that in
6-MSA synthetase the acyl transferases for acetate and malonate are identical, or in other
words, the same catalytic domain transfers acetate and malonate.

2. The second method took advantage of the fact
that some of the enzymic functions of 6-MSA
synthetase, like those of fatty acid synthetase,
can also act on substrate models. For comparative studies Seyffert (15) used either triacetic
acid ethyl ester (I) or S-acetoacetyl-N-acetyl
cysteamine (II) as substrate models.

$$CH_3-\overset{\overset{\displaystyle O}{\|}}{C}-CH_2-\overset{\overset{\displaystyle O}{\|}}{C}-CH_2-\overset{\overset{\displaystyle O}{\|}}{C}-OC_2H_5$$

I (TAE)

$$CH_3-\overset{\overset{\displaystyle O}{\|}}{C}-CH_2-\overset{\overset{\displaystyle O}{\|}}{C}-SCH_2CH_2NH-COCH_3$$

II (AAC)

In the experiment shown in Figure 9, various
protein fractions obtained by sucrose gradient centrifugation during our enzyme purification procedure
were assayed with both substrate models: acetoace-
tyl-N-acetyl cysteamine (AAC) and triacetic acid
ethyl ester (TAE). It was found that the heaviest
protein fraction, representing fatty acid synthetase,
very actively catalyzes the reduction of AAC, whereas the middle fraction, representing 6-MSA synthetase, is inactive in that respect. On the other
hand this fraction can catalyze the reduction of
TAE. Fatty acid synthetase can also reduce TAE but
only at a slow rate. The observations of Seyffert
in our laboratory indicate that the specificity of
the reducing enzyme, to some extent, determines
which product is formed by the particular multienzyme complex. In both processes, fatty acid synthe-

sis and 6-MSA synthesis, the condensation of acetate and malonate leads to the formation of acetoacetate bound to the acyl carrier protein component of the particular multienzyme complex. Due to the specificity of the reducing enzyme component of fatty acid synthetase, the acetoacetate is rapidly reduced to ß-hydroxy-butyrate which then is further transformed into butyrate and, thus, channeled into the synthesis of fatty acids. In 6-MSA synthetase, however, acetoacetate is not reduced. On the contrary, it enters another condensation with malonate to form triacetic acid. Only then reduction occurs, leaving the keto group in position 5 untouched. It seems to be essential that this group, after dehydration and elongation of the carbon chain by condensation with another malonate residue, eventually enters an aldol condensation and thus leads to the formation of the benzene ring.

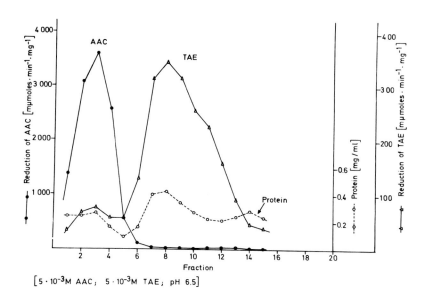

$[5 \cdot 10^{-3} M \ AAC; \ 5 \cdot 10^{-3} M \ TAE; \ pH \ 6.5]$

FIGURE 9. Reduction of S-acetoacetyl-N-acetyl cysteamine (AAC) and triacetic acid ethyl ester (TAE) by various protein fractions obtained by sucrose gradient centrifugation

It is interesting to note that the ability to
reduce triacetic acid was found to be present also
in fatty acid synthetase to a small extent. If we
now assume that by mutation of the reductase protein
component this low activity towards triacetic acid
became strongly potentiated and at the same time
activity towards acetoacetate was lost, we would
come to the conclusion that 6-MSA synthetase might
have been evolved from a precursor fatty acid synthetase in the course of evolution.

Friedrich (12) was able to support this hypothesis by immunological studies. He prepared specific
antibodies against the purified 6-MSA synthetase and
tested them with the Ouchterlony double diffusion
technique against 6-MSA synthetase, purified fatty
acid synthetase from P. patulum and purified fatty
acid synthetase from yeast. As Figure 10 illus
trates, we observed a cross reaction with fatty acid
synthetase from Penicillium but not with the one
from brewer's yeast. This observation is in good
accord with our hypothesis that fatty acid synthetase and 6-MSA synthetase have a common ancestor.

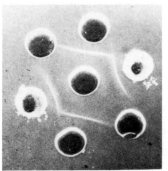

6-MSA-Synthetase

FAS (Yeast)

FAS (P.patulum)

FAS (P.patulum)

FAS (Yeast)

6-MSA-Synthetase

FIGURE 10.   Immunological comparison of 6-MSA
              synthetase, fatty acid synthetase
              (FAS) of P. patulum and FAS of yeast
              by the Ouchterlony technique.
Anti   6-MSA synthetase immunoglobulin was pi-
petted into the centre well, the various enzymes
in the outer wells as indicated in the figure.

With respect to the quaternary structure, both synthetases differ from each other. Fatty acid synthetase from P. patulum, like the one from yeast, has a molecular weight of 2.3x10⁶ Daltons and probable is built up from two polypeptides A and B, each present six times. The molecular weight of the purified 6-MSA synthetase was found to be only 760 000 Daltons (12) correcting the value of 1.1 million given by Dimroth (16) and to be composed of four subunits, having a molecular weight of 176 000 Daltons (Table V). According to the results of SDS-gel electrophoresis, these subunits appear to be identical. This would be in contrast to the situation with fatty acid synthetase. If further experiments should support this observation, we have to conclude that all the component enzyme activities of 6-MSA synthetase are present in only one multifunctional polypeptide chain which occurs four times in the purified enzyme. In agreement with this assumption, in binding experiments to the serine of acetyl/malonyl transferase, Friedrich already found 3.1 - 3.8 acetyl or malonyl residues bound per mole of enzyme (12).

TABLE V. Composition of 6-MSA synthetase

6-METHYLSALICYLATE-SYNTHETASE

	MOL.WEIGHT
NATIVE ENZYME	760 000
SUBUNITS	176 000

The dissociation of the tetrameric enzyme can be achieved by incubation with 2 M LiCl at 0° C for 4 hrs (12). Under this conditions total activity disappears completely, the partial activities for the formation of triacetic acid, the reduction step and the acyl transferase reaction, respectively, disappear only partially, or not at all. Reconstitution of the total enzymic activity can be achieved by removal of the high LiCl-concentration and incubation at 25° C in presence of dithiothreitol. Under optimal conditions 70 % of the original enzyme activity can be recovered.

In conclusion, our main results may be briefly summarized:

1. Fatty acid synthetase and 6-MSA synthetase are multienzyme complexes built from multifunctional polypeptide chains present in the complexes several times.
2. According to the results of immunological studies, both enzymes appear to have had a common ancestor and the mutation in the course of evolution has principally affected the specificity of the reducing enzyme component.
3. A structure model of fatty acid synthetase was suggested which is in good accord with the electronmicroscopic picture of the multienzyme complex.

REFERENCES

1. Oesterhelt, D., Bauer, H, and Lynen, F., Proc. Natl. Acad. Sci. U.S. 63: 1377-1382 (1969)
2. Knobling, A., Schiffmann, D., Sickinger, H.-D., and Schweizer, E., Eur. J. Biochem. 56: 359-367 (1975)
3. Engeser, H., Ph.D. Thesis, University of Munich 1978
4. Sumper, M., Oesterhelt, D., Riepertinger, C., and Lynen, F., Eur. J. Biochem. 10: 377-387 (1969)
5. Schweizer, E., Kniep, B., Castorph, H., and Holzner, U., Eur. J. Biochem. 39: 353-362 (1973)
6. Kresze, G.B., Oesterhelt, D., Lynen, F., Castorph, H., and Schweizer, E., Biochem. Biophys. Res. Comm. 69: 893-899 (1976)
7. Sumper, M., Riepertinger, C., and Lynen, F., FEBS Letters 5: 45-49 (1969)
8. Wieland, F., Ph.D. Thesis, University of Munich 1978
9. Winnewisser, W., Ph.D. Thesis, University of Munich 1978
10. Pilz, I., Herbst, M., Kratky, O., Oesterhelt, D., and Lynen, F., Eur. J. Biochem. 13: 55-64 (1970)
11. Hoppe, W., Schramm, H.J., Sturm, M., Hunsmann, N., and Gassmann, J., Z. Naturforsch. 31a: 1380-1390 (1976)
12. Friedrich, J., Ph.D. Thesis, University of Munich 1977

13. Greull, G., Ph.D. Thesis, University of Munich 1973
14. Schindlbeck, W., Ph.D. Thesis, University of Munich 1974
15. Seyffert, R., Schindlbeck, W., and Lynen, F., Abstr. 10th Meetg. Fed. Eur. Biochem. Soc. 675. Société de Chimie Biologique, Paris 1975
16. Dimroth, P., Walter, H., and Lynen, F., Eur. J. Biochem. 13: 98-110 (1970)

PYRUVATE DEHYDROGENASE COMPLEX: STRUCTURE,
FUNCTION AND REGULATION

Lester Reed[1]
Flora Pettit
Stephen Yeaman

Clayton Foundation Biochemical Institute
and Department of Chemistry
The University of Texas at Austin
Austin, Texas

I. INTRODUCTION

Pyruvate dehydrogenase systems have been isolated from
microbial and eukaryotic cells as functional units with molecular weights in the millions. The architecture, assembly,
function and regulation of these multienzyme complexes are
interesting in themselves. Moreover, it is reasonable to
suppose that cells have obtained selective advantages from the
specific ordering of their enzymes. The organization of functionally related enzymes into a complex provides possibilities
for increased efficiency, coordinate allosteric control of
more than one activity, and metabolic channeling. Complex
formation provides a means of concentrating catalysts rather
than having them randomly distributed in a cell and offers a
way of segregating enzymes that would otherwise compete for
the same metabolite. Slow dissociation of an intermediate
produced by one enzyme in a sequence could provide a high
steady state concentration for the next enzyme.

---
[1]Supported in part by NIH grant GM06590.

Copyright © 1978 by Academic Press, Inc.
All right of reproduction in any form reserved.
ISBN 0-12-660550-5

II. SUBUNIT COMPOSITION, STRUCTURE AND FUNCTION

The pyruvate dehydrogenase complexes consist of three enzymes that, acting in sequence, catalyze the reactions shown in Figure 1. The complexes are organized about a core, consisting of dihydrolipoyl transacetylase, to which the other two enzymes, pyruvate dehydrogenase and dihydrolipoyl dehydrogenase, are joined by noncovalent bonds (1).

The pyruvate dehydrogenase complex from Escherichia coli has a molecular weight of about 4,600,000. The transacetylase consists of 24 identical polypeptide chains (M_r, about 70,000) in an arrangement having octahedral (432) symmetry (Figure 2). Twelve pyruvate dehydrogenase dimers, consisting of identical chains (M_r, 96,000), appear to be located at the 12 twofold positions (i.e., on the edges) of the transacetylase cube, and 6 dihydrolipoyl dehydrogenase dimers, consisting of identical chains (M_r, 56,000), are located at the 6 fourfold positions (i.e., in the faces) (2).

The cofactor lipoic acid is attached covalently by an amide bond to a lysine residue in the transacetylase. Recent studies of the acetylation of the E. coli complex by [2-^{14}C]-pyruvate and thiamin pyrophosphate, acetylation by [1-^{14}C]-acetyl-CoA in the presence of DPNH, and the pyruvate-dependent reaction of N-ethyl[2,3-^{14}C]maleimide with the complex indicate that the transacetylase bears two functionally active lipoyl moieties on each of its 24 polypeptide chains (3-5). Charging of the 48 acetyl acceptor sites by pyruvate and thiamin pyrophosphate can occur in the presence of only a few functionally

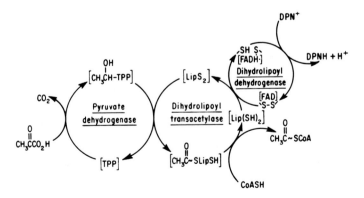

FIGURE 1.   Reaction sequence in pyruvate oxidation. TPP, thiamin pyrophosphate; $LipS_2$ and $Lip(SH)_2$, lipoyl moiety and its reduced form.

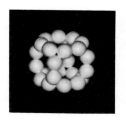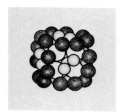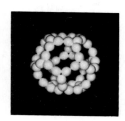

FIGURE 2. Interpretative models of the E. coli dihydrolipoyl transacetylase, the E. coli pyruvate dehydrogenase
complex, and the mammalian dihydrolipoyl transacetylase (left
to right, respectively). The 24 subunits of the E. coli transacetylase are located on the vertices of a truncated cube.
The 12 pyruvate dehydrogenase dimers are located on the edges
of the transacetylase cube, and the 6 dihydrolipoyl dehydrogenase dimers are located in the faces. The 60 subunits of the
mammalian transacetylase are located on the vertices of a pentagonal dodecahedron.

active pyruvate dehydrogenase subunits. Moreover, extensive
crosslinking of the transacetylase chains occurs when the complex is treated with pyruvate and thiamin pyrophosphate or with
DPNH in the presence of the bifunctional maleimides N,N'-o- or
p-phenylenedimaleimide, respectively (5). These findings suggest that the 48 lipoyl moieties on the transacetylase comprise an interacting network that functions as an acetyl group
and electron pair relay system through thiol-disulfide and
acetyl-transfer reactions as illustrated in Figure 3 (5,6).
The presence of this communication network suggests that a
pyruvate dehydrogenase molecule and a dihydrolipoyl dehydrogenase molecule need not be in juxtaposition to a particular

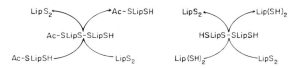

FIGURE 3. Scheme illustrating thiol-disulfide inter-
change and acetyl-transfer reactions among lipoyl moieties.

lipoyl moiety for the overall reaction to occur. This network
of interacting lipoyl moieties may have conferred some selective advantage on the organization of the transacetylase
chains into a large cube-like structure.

   In eukaryotic cells the pyruvate dehydrogenase complex is
located in mitochondria, apparently in the matrix space. The
pyruvate dehydrogenase complexes from bovine kidney and heart
have molecular weights of about 7,000,000 and 8,500,000, respectively. The components of the two complexes are very similar, if not identical. The pyruvate dehydrogenase component
has a molecular weight of about 154,000 and possesses the
subunit composition $\alpha_2\beta_2$ (7). The molecular weights of the
two subunits are about 41,000 and 36,000, respectively. The
core enzyme, dihydrolipoyl transacetylase, consists of 60
apparently identical polypeptide chains of molecular weight
about 52,000. The dihydrolipoyl dehydrogenase has a molecular
weight of about 110,000 and contains two identical polypeptide
chains and two molecules of FAD. The subunit composition of
the bovine kidney and heart pyruvate dehydrogenase complexes
is 60 transacetylase chains, 20 (kidney complex) or 30 (heart
complex) pyruvate dehydrogenase tetramers, and 5 or 6 flavoprotein dimers. A distinctive feature of the pyruvate dehydrogenase complex from mammalian cells, and apparently from other
eukaryotic cells as well, is the presence of two regulatory
components, a kinase and a phosphatase, in addition to the
three catalytic components (8). The kinase is tightly bound
to the transacetylase, whereas the phosphatase is loosely
attached. In fact, the association of the phosphatase and the
transacetylase is dependent on the presence of Ca^{2+} ions (9).
The apparent numbers of kinase and phosphatase molecules per
molecule of complex are small, about five of each. The appearance of the mammalian dihydrolipoyl transacetylase in the
electron microscope is that of a pentagonal dodecahedron, and
its design is apparently based on icosahedral (532) symmetry
(10) (Figure 2). The flavoprotein molecules appear to be located in the faces of the pentagonal dodecahedron, and the pyruvate dehydrogenase molecules are located on the edges. The
locations of the kinase and the phosphatase on the transacetylase are not yet known.

III. REGULATION OF THE MAMMALIAN PYRUVATE DEHYDROGENASE
     COMPLEX

   The pyruvate dehydrogenase multienzyme system catalyzes
a complex process linking glycolysis and the tricarboxylic
acid cycle, two of the most central metabolic pathways. The

glycolytic pathway oxidizes carbohydrates to pyruvate. Conversion of pyruvate to acetyl-CoA and oxidation of the latter substance via the tricarboxylic acid cycle is a major source of energy. In adipose tissue, the conversion of pyruvate to acetyl-CoA is regarded as the committed step in lipogenesis, since a large fraction of the acetyl-CoA generated by the pyruvate dehydrogenase system is converted into fatty acids. Therefore, regulation of the flux of carbon through the pyruvate dehydrogenase system plays an essential role in the control of energy metabolism and of lipogenesis.

Two mechanisms for modulation of the activity of the mammalian pyruvate dehydrogenase complex have been well documented: (i) product inhibition and (ii) a phosphorylation-dephosphorylation cycle. The activity of the complex is inhibited by acetyl-CoA and by DPNH, and these inhibitions are competitive with respect to CoA and DPN, respectively (11,12). The sites of acetyl-CoA and DPNH inhibition are the transacetylase and flavoprotein components of the complex, respectively. These observations have led to suggestions that the activity of the pyruvate dehydrogenase complex may be regulated in vivo, at least in part, by the intramitochondrial acetyl-CoA/CoA and DPNH/DPN molar ratios.

Another regulatory mechanism, involving phosphorylation and dephosphorylation of the mammalian pyruvate dehydrogenase complex, was first demonstrated in this laboratory (13,14). Phosphorylation and concomitant inactivation of the complex is catalyzed by a MgATP^{2-}-dependent kinase, and dephosphorylation and concomitant reactivation is catalyzed by a Mg^{2+}-dependent phosphatase. The site of this covalent regulation is the pyruvate dehydrogenase component of the complex. Phosphorylation occurs on three serine residues in the α subunit of bovine kidney and heart pyruvate dehydrogenase (7,15). Tryptic digestion of the ^{32}P-labeled pyruvate dehydrogenase yielded three phosphopeptides, a mono(Site 1)- and a di(Sites 1 and 2)-phosphorylated tetradecapeptide, and a monophosphorylated nonapeptide(Site 3) (S. J. Yeaman, E. T. Hutcheson, T. E. Roche, F. H. Pettit, J. R. Brown, and L. J. Reed, in preparation). These sequences do not bear any obvious similarities to primary sequences at sites on other proteins which are phosphorylated by protein kinases. However, Small et al. pointed out recently that about 80% of the phosphorylated residues in 14 different proteins occur within regions pre-

Site 1   Site 2
Tyr-His-Gly-His-Ser(P)-Met-Ser-Asn-Pro-Gly-Val-Ser(P)-Tyr-Arg

Site 3
Tyr-Gly-Met-Gly-Thr-Ser(P)-Val-Glu-Arg

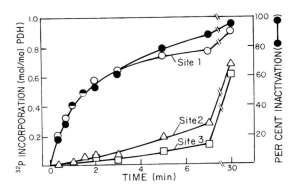

FIGURE 4. Relationship between inactivation and phosphorylation of bovine kidney pyruvate dehydrogenase complex.

dicted as β-turns, and they suggested the possible recognition of a specific secondary structure by protein kinases (16).
     Phosphorylation proceeds markedly faster at Site 1 than
at Sites 2 and 3, and phosphorylation at Site 1 correlates
closely with inactivation of pyruvate dehydrogenase (Figure
4). The functional role, if any, of phosphorylation Sites 2
and 3 is not known. Phosphorylation at Site 2 apparently requires prior phosphorylation at Site 1. However, it is not
clear whether phosphorylation at Site 3 requires prior phosphorylation at Sites 1 and 2. Also, the location of Site 3 in
the primary sequence of pyruvate dehydrogenase in relation to
Sites 1 and 2 is not known. With some preparations of uncomplexed pyruvate dehydrogenase and of the pyruvate dehydrogenase complex, phosphorylation of half of the α subunits at
Site 1 was sufficient to block the enzymatic activity completely, whereas the other half did not undergo phosphorylation. However, with other preparations complete inactivation
was associated with incorporation at Site 1 of more than 1.0
but less than 2.0 moles of phosphoryl groups per mole of pyruvate dehydrogenase. Although the molecular basis of this difference is not known, it appears that the subunits of pyruvate dehydrogenase tetramers exhibit cooperativity, possibly
half-site reactivity, with respect to phosphorylation at Site
1 and inactivation.
     The pyruvate dehydrogenase system is well designed for
fine regulation of its activity. Interconversion of the active

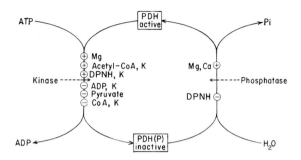

FIGURE 5. Schematic representation of the covalent modification of pyruvate dehydrogenase and its control by various
metabolites.

and inactive, phosphorylated forms of pyruvate dehydrogenase
is a dynamic process. The system is endowed with an unusual
capacity to be regulated by multiple metabolites, and it is
remarkably flexible with respect to increasing concentrations
of individual effectors. Pyruvate dehydrogenase and the two
converter enzymes, the kinase and the phosphatase, comprise a
prototype for the monocyclic interconvertible enzyme cascade
model of Stadtman and Chock (17). Figure 5 summarizes the
control of kinase and phosphatase activities by various metabolites and metal ions, observed with the purified pyruvate
dehydrogenase system. These findings have been confirmed and
extended with isolated mitochondria, hepatocytes and perfused
organs (18-22). Mg^{2+} is required by both the kinase and the
phosphatase. However, the apparent $\underline{K}_m$ of the phosphatase for
Mg^{2+} (about 2 mM) is about 100 times the apparent $\underline{K}_m$ of the
kinase for Mg^{2+}. Ca^{2+} markedly stimulates phosphatase activity. In the presence of Ca^{2+} the phosphatase binds to the
transacetylase, thereby facilitating the Mg^{2+}-dependent dephosphorylation of the phosphorylated pyruvate dehydrogenase.
Kinase activity is stimulated by acetyl-CoA and by DPNH, provided K^+ or NH_4^+ ions are present, and kinase activity is inhibited by ADP, pyruvate and CoA. ADP is competitive with
respect to ATP, and this inhibition requires the presence of
monovalent cation. Phosphatase activity is inhibited by DPNH,
and this inhibition is reversed by DPN.

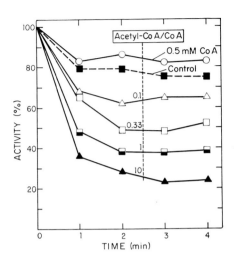

FIGURE 6.   Effect of changes in acetyl–CoA/CoA ratio on
the steady–state activity of the bovine kidney pyruvate dehydrogenase complex (25).

In the presence of functional kinase and phosphatase, the
pyruvate dehydrogenase complex reaches a steady–state level
of activity within a few minutes. The steady–state level of
activity can be varied progressively over a wide range by
varying the concentrations or molar ratios of the different
effectors (Figure 6). Shifts in the steady–state activity of
the complex reflect changes in the distribution of the pyruvate dehydrogenase component between its active form and its
inactive, phosphorylated form. Thus, the steady–state activity of the complex is affected markedly by varying the concentration of Mg^{2+} or Ca^{2+} and thereby changing the activity
of the phosphatase (23). On the other hand, at optimum Mg^{2+}
and Ca^{2+} concentrations, the steady–state activity is affected
markedly by varying the concentration of K^+ at a fixed ADP/ATP
molar ratio or by varying the ADP/ATP ratio at a fixed concentration of K^+, and thereby changing the activity of the
kinase (24). The steady–state activity of the complex is also
sensitive to the acetyl–CoA/CoA and to the DPNH/DPN molar
ratios (25). An increase in either ratio decreases the steady–
state activity by increasing the proportion of the phosphorylated, inactive form of pyruvate dehydrogenase.

It is apparent that each of the three enzymes that comprise this interconvertible enzyme system, i.e., pyruvate dehydrogenase, the kinase and the phosphatase, can be a separate target for one or more of the effectors. That the conformation of pyruvate dehydrogenase itself is an important factor in the regulation of its activity is indicated by the finding that binding of the coenzyme thiamin pyrophosphate, and particularly the transition state analog thiamin thiazolone pyrophosphate, to the catalytic site of this enzyme decreases markedly the rate of its phosphorylation by the kinase, apparently by altering the conformation about phosphorylation Site 1 so that the serine hydroxyl group is less accessible to the kinase (26).

The phosphopeptides produced by tryptic digestion of ^{32}P-labeled pyruvate dehydrogenase are effective substrates for the phosphatase, and the dephosphotetradecapeptide can serve as a substrate for the kinase (27). These findings indicate that the kinase and the phosphatase do not require an intact tertiary structure in pyruvate dehydrogenase, but apparently recognize components of the local primary sequence or the secondary structure around the phosphorylation sites. The availability of these peptide substrates should facilitate elucidation of the site and mechanism of action of the modifiers of the kinase and phosphatase activities. Preliminary experiments indicate that acetyl-CoA, DPNH, ADP and pyruvate interact with the kinase.

REFERENCES

1. Reed, L. J., and Oliver, R. M., Brookhaven Symp. Biol. 21:397 (1968).
2. Reed, L. J., Pettit, F. H., Eley, M. H., Hamilton, L., Collins, J. H., and Oliver, R. M., Proc. Nat. Acad. Sci. USA 72:3068 (1975).
3. Danson, M. J., and Perham, R. N., Biochem. J. 159:677 (1976).
4. Speckhard, D. C., Ikeda, B. H., Wong, S. S., and Frey, P. A., Biochem. Biophys. Res. Commun. 77:708 (1977).
5. Collins, J. H., and Reed, L. J., Proc. Nat. Acad. Sci. USA 74:4223 (1977).
6. Bates, D. L., Danson, M. J., Hale, G., Hooper, E. A., and Perham, R. N., Nature 268:313 (1977).
7. Barrera, C. R., Namihira, G., Hamilton, L., Munk, P., Eley, M. H., Linn, T. C., and Reed, L. J., Arch. Biochem. Biophys. 148:343 (1972).

8. Linn, T. C., Pelley, J. W., Pettit, F. H., Hucho, F., Randall, D. D., and Reed, L. J., Arch. Biochem. Biophys. 148:327 (1972).
9. Pettit, F. H., Roche, T. E., and Reed, L. J., Biochem. Biophys. Res. Commun. 49:563 (1972).
10. Reed, L. J., Acc. Chem. Res. 7:40 (1974).
11. Garland, P. B., and Randle, P. J., Biochem. J. 91:6c (1964).
12. Tsai, C. S., Burgett, M. W., and Reed, L. J., J. Biol. Chem. 248:8348 (1973).
13. Linn, T. C., Pettit, F. H., and Reed, L. J., Proc. Nat. Acad. Sci. USA 62:234 (1969).
14. Linn, T. C., Pettit, F. H., Hucho, F., and Reed, L. J.. Proc. Nat. Acad. Sci. USA 64:227 (1969).
15. Hutcheson, E. T., Doctoral Dissertation, The University of Texas at Austin, 1971.
16. Small, D., Chou, P. Y., and Fasman, G. D., Biochem. Biophys. Res. Commun. 79:341 (1977).
17. Stadtman, E. R., and Chock, P. B., Proc. Nat. Acad. Sci. USA 74:2761 (1977).
18. Denton, R. M., Randle, P. J., Bridges, B. J., Cooper, R. H., Kerbey, A. L., Pask, H. T., Severson, D. L., Stansbie, D., and Whitehouse, S., Mol. Cell. Biochem. 9:27 (1975).
19. Taylor, S. I., Mukherjee, C., and Jungas, R. L., J. Biol. Chem. 250:2028 (1975).
20. Wieland, O. H., and Portenhauser, R., Eur. J. Biochem. 45:577 (1974).
21. Batenburg, J. J., and Olson, M. S., J. Biol. Chem. 251:1364 (1976).
22. Hansford, R. G., J. Biol. Chem. 251:5483 (1976).
23. Reed, L. J., Pettit, F. H., Roche, T. E., and Butterworth, P. J., in "Protein Phosphorylation in Control Mechanisms" (F. Huijing and E. Y. C. Lee, eds.), p. 83. Academic Press, New York, 1973.
24. Roche, T. E., and Reed, L. J., Biochem. Biophys. Res. Commun. 59:1341 (1974).
25. Pettit, F. H., Pelley, J. W., and Reed, L. J., Biochem. Biophys. Res. Commun. 65:575 (1975).
26. Butler, J. R., Pettit, F. H., Davis, P. F., and Reed, L. J., Biochem. Biophys. Res. Commun. 74:1667 (1977).
27. Davis, P. F., Pettit, F. H., and Reed, L. J., Biochem. Biophys. Res. Commun. 75:541 (1977).

DISCUSSION

F. LIPMANN: The acetyl group comes from the dehydrogenase and is transferred to the transacetylase. Didn't you say there are something like 40 acetyl groups on the transacetylase. What is the stoichiometry of the separate subunits?

L. REED: The E. coli pyruvate dehydrogenase complex consists of 24 transacetylase polypeptide chains, 24 pyruvate dehydrogenase chains (i.e., 12 dimers), and 12 flavoprotein chains (i.e., 6 dimers). Each transacetylase chain apparently bears two functionally active lipoyl moieties. This finding provides a possible molecular basis for the observation of Moe et al. [Moe, O. A., Jr., Lerner, D. A., and Hammes, G.G., Biochemistry 13: 2552 (1974)], from fluorescence energy transfer experiments, that the apparent distance between FAD and thiamin pyrophosphate binding sites on the pyruvate dehydrogenase complex is more than 30 Å and probably close to 45 Å. This distance is considerably larger than the 28 Å predicted by our model of a single rotating lipoyl moiety interacting with successive active sites on the complex. However, the results of Moe et al. are compatible with the distances expected for the model (Figure 3) involving transfer of acetyl groups and electron pairs among the lipoyl moieties.

F. LIPMANN: Does the coenzyme A pick up the acetyl eventually?

L. REED: Yes, coenzyme A picks up the acetyl group from the S-acetyldihydrolipoyl moiety.

J. WILLIAMSON: Can you say something about the relative importance or how you can distinguish between the direct product inhibition by NADH and acetyl-CoA versus their effects on interconversion by phosphorylation of pyruvate dehydrogenase.

L. REED: We have not conducted experiments of that nature. However, Merle Olson and other investigators have observed that in the oxidation of pyruvate by intact mitochondria and perfused organs in the presence of fatty acids, product inhibition by acetyl-CoA and DPNH apparently plays an important role in the regulation of the activity of the pyruvate dehydrogenase complex.

J. WILLIAMSON: The point of my question to you is whether you know where NADH or acetyl-CoA might bind? A product inhibitor would be on the active site of the enzyme. I wonder if you have done any physical studies in relation to that.

L. REED: With respect to product inhibition of the mammalian pyruvate dehydrogenase complex, the sites of acetyl-CoA and DPNH inhibition are the transacetylase and flavoprotein components of the complex, respectively. However, as I indicated, acetyl-CoA and DPNH also stimulate the activity of the kinase, and DPNH inhibits the activity of the phosphatase. Perhaps Dr. Olson will comment on the relative importance of these two regulatory mechanisms.

M. OLSON: I would like to ask two questions and then I will comment with regard to feedback inhibition. The two questions are; what is the evidence that pyruvate dehydrogenase is a matrix enzyme? Is it freely soluble in the matrix or is it bound to the inner membrane?

L. REED: In our isolation procedure, mitochondria are washed several times with 0.02 M potassium phosphate buffer, pH 6.5, and then frozen and thawed. NaCl (0.05 M) is added, and the membrane fraction is removed by centrifugation. The pyruvate dehydrogenase complex is present in the supernatant fluid. This observation indicates that the complex is not tightly bound to the membranes.

M. OLSON: The second question is: You said that the kinase-phosphatase control is a fine control on the pyruvate dehydrogenase. That statement implies that there is a coarse control. Could you elaborate on what you think is fine control and coarse control of the enzyme complex.

L. REED: I said what?

M. OLSON: During your talk your suggested that the kinase-phosphatase control, the interconversion of the enzymes, is a fine control.

L. REED: I said that the pyruvate dehydrogenase system is well designed for fine regulation of its activity.

M. OLSON: Right. Is there a coarse control on the enzyme in mammalian systems?

L. REED: Our studies with the purified pyruvate dehydrogenase system do not provide an answer to this question. However, I think experiments with intact mitochondria and with perfused organs have addressed this question.

M. OLSON: I would like to comment briefly on John Williamson's question. We have been doing a lot of experiments with perfused hearts and perfused livers in which we have been measuring the metabolic flux through pyruvate dehydrogenase in these intact organs and at that same time we have been determining whether changes in the interconversion of the enzyme complex between its active and inactive forms occurs during reasonable metabolic state changes. When you add fatty acids, which have been long known to inhibit and inactivate pyruvate dehydrogenase in most organs, not only do you see an interconversion of the enzyme from the active to the inactive form but you also observe an extensive inhibition of active pyruvate dehydrogenase. The evidence is based on the fact that we see up to a 90% inhibition of metabolic flux through pyruvate dehydrogenase in the perfused heart when we add something like acetate or even oleate and you can't explain this large inhibition merely by interconversion. You can only see a 40 to 50% change in the active form of pyruvate dehydrogenase. If you add dichloracetate to the perfused heart, dichloracetate is a potent inhibitor of the pyruvate dehydrogenase kinase, you can lock the enzyme in completely the active form and you have no chance for interconversion. In that case when you add acetate or medium chain fatty acids you can still see up to 40% inhibition of the flux through pyruvate dehydrogenase. This indicates that we shouldn't forget about the feedback effects on this active enzyme. Hence, we believe that metabolic flux changes in this reaction occur not only by interconversion of pyruvate dehydrogenase between its active and inactive forms but also by direct effects of various molecular species on the active form.

J. BLUM: In the experiments where you adjusted the level of active and inactive kinase by varying the relative activity of the kinase and of the phosphatase, you are essentially operating an ATPase activity by the joint action of the kinase and phosphatase. This is a sort of futile cycle. I was wondering if you have any measurements on the amount of "ATPase" activity in that system.

L. REED: The molecular activities of the kinase and the phosphatase appear to be relatively low, i.e., about 5 moles/min/mole of enzyme [Hucho, F., Randall, D. D., Roche, T. E., Burgett, M. W., Pelley, J. W., and Reed, L. J. Arch. Biochem. Biophys. 151: 328 (1972]. Therefore, it seems that the resultant "ATPase activity" of this system is insignificant. I should also point out that Newsholme [Newsholme, E. A., and Gevers, W., Vitamins Hormones 25:1

(1967)] and other investigators have emphasized that at least
some so-called futile cycles may confer significant regulatory
advantages on cells (see also Ref. 17).

J. BLUM: I might comment that some theoretical analysis that
we have done of futile cycles at a crossover point would indicate that the conclusions which have been reached by
Newsholme and Start (see reference in R. Stein and J. J. Blum,
J. Theor. Biol., 1978, in press) are considerably oversimplified. It is not at all clear that one does gain a regulatory
advantage by a futile cycle in the sense that has been so
far indicated.

T. ROCHE: I want to comment on a mechanism for the regulation
of pyruvate dehydrogenase kinase activity by several modulators that are also substrates or products of the reaction catalyzed by the pyruvate dehydrogenase complex. As indicated
in Lester Reed's talk, PDH kinase activity is stimulated by
acetyl-CoA and NADH. We have presented evidence, supporting
the mechanism shown in Figure 1, in which the stimulation of
this enzyme may be mediated by the acetylated and reduced
forms of lipoic acid (Roche, T. E. and Cate, R. L. (1976)
Biochem. Biophys. Res. Commun. 72, 1375-1383). Thus the type
of shuttling of acetyl groups and electrons between lipoyl
moieties that Lester Reed talked about may be of importance
in this mechanism. An early observation that initiated our
interest was that stimulation by acetyl-CoA did not occur if
acetyl-CoA alone was added. We showed that a reducing substance such as dithiothreitol was required and that low concentrations of NADH could replace this requirement. I want to
point out a couple of subsequent observations. One is that
very low concentrations of free reduced lipoamide stimulates
PDH kinase activity. Regarding the second observation I must
first note that, in addition to pyruvate inhibiting PDH kinase
activity under some conditions, low concentrations of pyruvate, under direct conditions, stimulates PDH_a kinase activity. We have shown that, if you treat the pyruvate dehydrogenase complex with pyruvate and then separate the pyruvate
by gel filtration chromatography, the stimulation of PDH_a
kinase activity persists and that addition of NADH or acetyl-
CoA then gives no stimulation. So the stimulatory effect seems
to be saturated. I understand from Lester Reed that he has
evidence from his peptide work that some of these stimulations
can be observed in the absence of an intact complex. This
would not be consistent with our proposed mechanism. I would
like to ask Dr. Reed a couple of questions: First, have you
shown that pyruvate stimulation occurs in the peptide system?
Also have you tested whether free reduced lipoamide stimulates
with the peptide assay?

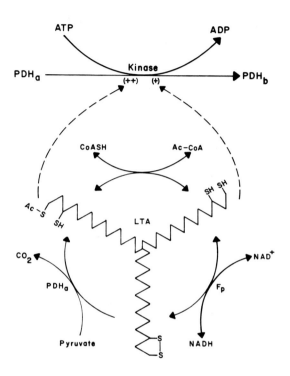

Figure 1. Mechanism for lipoic acid mediated stimulation of PDH_a kinase activity. Fp, dihydrolipoyl dehydrogenase (a flavoprotein); LTA, dihydrolipoyl transacetylase. The proposed mechanism is that reduction by
NADH or acetylation by acetyl–CoA or pyruvate of the
lipoyl moiety of the transacetylase component of the complex is required for stimulation of PDH_a kinase by these
effectors (Cate, R. L. and Roche, T. E. (1978) J. Biol.
Chem. <u>253</u>, 496–503).

L. REED: Dr. Roche has referred to our finding that a phosphorylated tetradecapeptide derived from the phosphorylated,
inactive pyruvate dehydrogenase can serve as a substrate
for pyruvate dehydrogenase phosphatase, and the dephosphotetradecapeptide is an effective substrate for the kinase
(Ref. 27). In this simplified system, pyruvate, at a con-

centration of 0.5 mM, inhibited kinase activity, and dihydro-lipoamide did not stimulate kinase activity. Since this investigation is in a preliminary stage, I do not think it would be profitable to discuss our results further at this time.

B. CHANCE: Well, perhaps my question is irrelevant and maybe it isn't even a question. We are supposed to identify whether these macromolecular complexes are associated with microenvironments of the Srere and not the Veech type. Maybe I could throw out the suggestion that in a micro-environment, substrates must be out of diffusion equili-brium with the surrounding macroenvironment. This suggests that you have established concentration gradients. Is there any evidence that this magnificent 900 KILO dalton complex has concentration gradients around it? Is there a microenvironment of the external components? Not the obvious intermediates as you indicate, which will be in their own microenvironment, but as a whole does this accumu-late intermediates out of equilibrium with the surrounding substrates? Perhaps this question is just as appropriate for Paul Srere. I think we should come to grips with the issue of macromolecules at some point in this Symposium.

L. REED: As I recall, Gordin Kaplan, in studies with an en-zyme system from yeast, obtained data indicating that there was no exchange between an intermediate noncovalently bound to the enzyme system and the macroenvironment. Does anyone remember details of this investigation?

P. SRERE: The question is: If we have a multienzyme system and the substrates are not bound then that is really not a microenvironment because you are going from one active site to another.

B. CHANCE: Yes, I would call those intermediates.

P. SRERE: There are two systems. I think Mary Ellen's system is one and I think the one by P. F. Lue and J. G. Kaplan, Biochem. Biophysica Acta. 220, 365 (1970), is another one.

R. DAVIS: I think that the work of Lue and Kaplan was the one concerning the binding of carbamylphosphate to carbamyl-phosphate synthetase–ATCase complex in yeast. I think simi-lar data has been obtained for the tryptophan synthetase reaction by Matchett (J. Biol. Chem. 249, 4041, 1974) and DeMoss (Biochem. Biophys. Acta 62, 279, 1962). These are two good examples. Probably the next part of the Symposium will go into that in the pentafunctional <u>arom</u> complex. I think the question is whether intermediates have to be covalently bound or not. I don't think they do.

B. CHANCE: Of course, that would certainly satisfy my concept of out of diffusion equilibrium, but that is over binding. I do think we have to think of diffusion gradients within the matrix space of the mitochondria.

R. DAVIS: Well the fact that the degree of channeling is dependent on the concentration of a competitor indicates that there is a gradient.

J. LOWENSTEIN: I would like to ask Dr. Reed a quick question. You said that phosphorylation at site 1 correlates well with inactivation and that the function of phosphorylation, at what you call sites 2 and 3, is not well understood. Have you considered the analogy with phosphorylase b kinase which has two phosphorylation sites. It has been shown rather elegantly by P. Cohen <u>et</u> <u>al</u>. (Eur. J. Biochem. (1973) <u>34</u>, 1-14: (1975) <u>51</u>, 79-92, 93104), that after the first site is phosphorylated, phosphorylase b kinase phosphatase attacks this form only very slowly. Two sites have to be phosphorylated before the enzyme can be converted back readily to the dephospho form. Have you done such studies with the pyruvate dehydrogenase complex?

L. REED: We have investigated the phosphorylation and dephosphorylation at Sites 1, 2 and 3, but as yet we have not found any function for phosphorylation Sites 2, and 3.

ENZYME ORGANIZATION IN VIVO:
THERMODYNAMIC-KINETIC PERSPECTIVES

G. Rickey Welch[1]
John A. DeMoss

Department of Biochemistry
and Molecular Biology
University of Texas Medical School
Houston, Texas

I. INTRODUCTION

Stripped of all its trappings and finery, the question at the heart of this Symposium is that of how does proto-plasm work? Protoplasm, the living substance, appears superficially as a rather amorphous state of matter. The physiologist C. Bernard termed protoplasm "non-determinate life", life in the "naked state" (1). Accordingly, "here are to be found all the essential properties of which the mani-festations of the higher beings are only diversified and definite expressions, or higher modalities". Protoplasm is a microcosm of life we see in the macroscopic world around us.

It is a trite statement today to assert that a cell is not simply a "bag" containing an aqueous solution uniformly dispersed with enzymes and freely-diffusing metabolites. Indeed, it is rather tautological to say that living systems possess a high degree of spatial order. But, we are only beginning to grasp the implications of this tautology at the level of the single cell. If we accept Bernard's view of the nature of protoplasm, we should be able to look at the biological world around us -- the world we can see, feel and readily appreciate, to take relationships which we observe between interacting components in this macroscopic world and

---

[1]Address after June 1, 1978: Department of Biological Sciences, University of New Orleans, New Orleans, Louisiana.

323

Copyright © 1978 by Academic Press, Inc.
All right of reproduction in any form reserved.
ISBN 0-12-660550-5

project those relationships into the function of protoplasm.
Our license to act in this manner may be found in a principle enunciated by N. Rashevsky: the principle of relational
invariance, which expresses the fact that in spite of all
the quantitative differences, all organisms are invariant
with respect to some qualitative relations within them (2).
The qualitative relations between such phenomena as loco-
motion, attainment of nutrient, ingestion of nutrient,
defense of nutrient supply, etc., remain the same throughout
the spectrum of life. Hence, a living organism becomes
completely analogous to a society (3).

Such a conceptualization is of significant heuristic
value. It leads us to believe that a far greater degree of
correlation of interacting components in time and in space
must exist in vivo, than what we might suppose from in vitro
studies of isolated components. These considerations are
particularly relevant to sequences of enzymes involved in
intermediary metabolism. A diversity of experimental findings strongly suggests that the metabolic machinery of the
cell exists in a state of spatial organization not only at
the organellar level but, more interestingly, also at the
subcytoplasmic level. For example, whole-cell centrifugation
studies with Euglena gracilis (4) and Neurospora crassa (5)
indicated that most so-called "soluble" proteins do not
exist as such in vivo, and that the association of the
entire cytoplasmic macromolecular apparatus, encompassing
all biochemical processes, with large particulates may be a
basic structure of cellular organization (cf. refs. 6,7).
Moreover, with the development of gentler methods of extraction, enzymes catalyzing multiple sequential reactions have
been isolated as "soluble" multienzyme aggregates or as
"particulate" membrane-bound systems (see ref.3 and others
cited therein). Such clusters of enzymes usually exhibit
quite unique kinetic and/or regulatory features, in comparison with the non-associated state.

In the present article we wish to treat, in general
terms, certain advantageous features associated with enzyme
organization, and to discuss a rather model system for
studying functional aspects of such organization. In conclusion, the relevance of these views to the topic of this
Symposium is presented.

II.   THE FABRIC OF CELLULAR METABOLISM

It may be said that the "first principle" of intracellular organization is that certain enzymes are associated
together and separated from others. Nonetheless, with the

exception of certain multienzyme systems specifically associated with organelles (e.g., mitochondrion, nucleus, Golgi
apparatus, etc.), a host of intermediary metabolic processes
have been relegated conveniently to a homogeneous existence
in the cytoplasmic space. Such a prejudice is coming into
conflict with the increasing volume of information, like
that referenced above, intimating that cytoplasm has an
infrastructure all of its own. What do we make of the clues
offered by the isolable fragments ("mesoforms") of the
catalytic machinery of cellular metabolism? The answer to
this question must lie in our appreciation that life is more
"creative" (in the teleonomic sense) than what we might
surmise from the "isotropic chaos" in vitro.

The active, interior milieu of the cell is separated
from the exterior world by a membrane -- a barrier which
selectively screens what enters into and leaves from the
cell. But, this global structure is not sufficient, of
itself, to create the special inner conditions necessary for
the vitality of the cell. For the most part, the basic
physicochemical processes at work in the cell fall into the
following categories: chemical (enzymatic) reaction; diffusion, arising from spatial gradients of chemical (or
electrochemical) potential; and bulk motion (e.g., "pro-
toplasmic streaming"), arising, for example, from internal
states of stress. Intuitively, it would seem that these
various processes must be coupled in specific ways, in order
to generate the highly coordinated and coherent behavior
characteristic of the living cell. The existence of such
coupling can be ruled out, on physical grounds, in isotropic
systems (3). For example, simultaneous diffusion and enzyme
reaction cannot be coupled phenomenologically in a homogeneous, isotropic milieu. Thus, it may be by virtue of a
complex infrastructure (i.e., anisotropy) that these processes can, indeed, be coupled in a specific, unifying
manner in the cell.

A spatial organization of multienzyme systems implies
that we must synthesize a new conceptualization of the
fabric of cellular metabolism -- a view based perhaps on the
precedence of "surface effects" over ordinary statistical,
mass-action relationships (8), a view differing (in some
cases, radically) from our familiar in vitro description of
enzyme action. With this new synthesis must come the realization that pure biochemistry is inadequate for the task at
hand; for, as noted by the eminent topologist R. Thom, "the
whole geometrical and spatial aspect of biochemical reactions eludes the power of biochemical explanation" (9). In
biology, as a molecular science, there has been a tendency
to underestimate the dynamic and continuous nature of

"living phenomena". As purely physical and mathematical as
it may seem, the fabric of cellular metabolism (as for all
"living phenomena") must be conceived in the form of a
field -- an unique property of space-time, a geometric
object, an aspect of the "life field" (champ vital) (9). We
might view the interior workings of the cell according to a
"machine-with-slots" representation (3), as used for example
in gravitational field theory (10). An "input" slot takes a
set of concentrations and respective spatial fluxes of a
group of metabolites -- which "input" may be imposed on the
system from the environment or the remainder of the cell
interior. The "output" is a set of concentrations and respective spatial fluxes of a group of metabolites maintained
at localized sites by the given metabolic processes specific
for those sites. Thus, the "machinery" of the cell takes
concentrations and fluxes of various substances (e.g.,
biosynthetic precursors), "localizes" them, and transforms
them into pools and fluxes specific to given metabolic
processes. The basic question is how to characterize mathe-
matically the flow of matter within the organized multienzyme systems which form the meshwork of this "machinery".
Normally, one attempts to describe macroscopically the
spatiotemporal behavior of the concentration of an intermediate substrate by setting up a mass-balance relation
(differential equation), which takes into consideration the
diffusion (or electrodiffusion) of that substrate in the
medium plus any relevant chemical reaction terms (3). However, such a formalism has some serious technical limitations, e.g., a frequent restriction to time-independent
(steady) states and linear relations, and the difficulty in
providing a macroscopic description when the system exhibits
inhomogeneity and anisotropy (3,11). It appears that the
theory of network thermodynamics (11,12) is the most suited
to date for depicting the interrelationships between dynamic
processes and organizational complexity in the living cell.
This theory is not subject to the above limitations. Moreover, its approach is based on system topology; or, as noted
by Oster et.al. (11), "in the network approach we 'pull
apart' the continuum, revealing the implicit topological
relations". Bunow and Aris (13) have presented a matrix
method, formally similar to the network theory, which may be
of particular value in picturing the "machine-with-slots"
operation of structured enzyme systems (3). It is anticipated that further work in this area will be forthcoming.

III. ENERGETIC ECONOMY IN THE DESIGN OF THE METABOLIC MACHINERY

Let us consider some general aspects of the "energy budget" of a living organism. Following the formulation of León (14), we suppose that at age (or, perhaps, time) t the phenotype of the organism can be described (at the level of organization of interest) by a set of n functions $Y_i(t)$ ($i = 1,2,...,n$), composing the (column) phenotype vector $Y_F = [Y_1(t),..., Y_n(t)]^T$ (where "T" indicates transposition). For example, the Y's might be weights of appropriate subsystems (e.g., metabolic processes) of the organism. Now, let $\dot{E}_C$ be the rate of energy (say, free energy) intake by the organism and $\dot{E}_A$ the rate at which it is expended for an activity A. The basic activities are survival S, maintenance M, growth G and reproduction R. Each "growing" subsystem i has its share $\dot{E}_i$ of $\dot{E}_G$, so that

$$\dot{E}_G = \sum_{i=1}^{n} \dot{E}_i .$$

This leads to the definition of a time (age)-dependent "vector of energetic investments":

$$E = [\dot{E}_0(t), \dot{E}_1(t),..., \dot{E}_n(t)]^T,$$

where $\dot{E}_0$ denotes $\dot{E}_S$ (14). Clearly, at any age (or time) the organism is constrained by an instantaneous energy budget:

$$\dot{E}_C(Y_F) = \dot{E}_M(Y_F) + \dot{E}_R + 1^T E,$$

where 1 is the identity column vector, and $1^T E$ is just the sum of the individual "investment rates".

For a certain organism, situated in a stable environment, we can assume that $\dot{E}_C$ is a maximum compatible with the phenotype of that organism. Suppose another similar type of organism coinhabits the same niche and exhibits quantitatively the same value of $\dot{E}_C$ as for the other type. Obviously, the organism which is capable of apportioning more energy to $1^T E$ and/or $\dot{E}_R$ at the appropriate time, at the expense of the metabolic cost ($\dot{E}_M$) of running the organism, might be favored in the struggle for existence (14). This

argument is tenable on the simple ground of efficiency.[2]
[As an additional refinement, we might assume, as did
Huxley (15), that survival selection is more important in
the process of biological evolution than reproductive
selection. Hence, the energetic investments directed toward
the various phenotypic functions concerned with growth,
maintenance, and survival are more sensitive to the forces
of natural selection than the investments related strictly
to reproduction (16).]

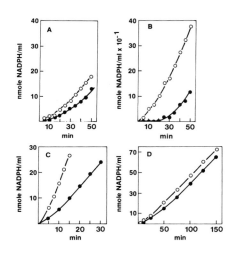

FIGURE 1. Graphical illustration of the formation of
product (NADPH) plotted against time for matrix-bound hexokinase (HK) + glucose-6-phosphate dehydrogenase (G-6-PDH)
preparations (O) and the corresponding soluble systems
(●). A.(I) Sepharose-bound HK + G-6-PDH; B. HK + G-6-PDH
bound to crosslinked co-polymer of acrylamide-acrylic acid;
C. HK + G-6-PDH entrapped in polyacrylamide; D. (II)
Sepharose-bound HK + G-6-PDH. [Reproduced from Mosbach, K.,
and Mattiasson, B. (1970) Acta Chem. Scand. 24, 2093, with
the kind permission of the authors.]

---

[2]As another avenue for evolutionary improvement, the
flux E_C may be increased via evolutionary alterations in the
phenotype Y_F. The latter factor is treated elsewhere (3).

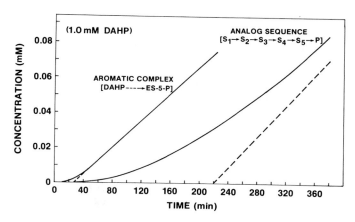

FIGURE 2. Comparison of the overall activity of the "aromatic cluster" and that predicted by computer for the hypothetical, analogous multienzyme sequence, with 1.0mM initial condition. Abbreviations: DAHP, 3-deoxy-D-arabino-heptulosonate 7-phosphate; ES-3-P, 5-enolpyruvylshikimate 3-phosphate. (See ref.3 for details.)

The value of enzyme organization in the economy of cellular metabolism can be seen from various angles. The most overbearing condition with which life processes must contend continually is that posed by the random field in their environment. Teleonomically speaking, life as an emergent and evolving phenomenon has had to combat against the random field at some levels and couple to it at other levels of complexity (17). At the level of multienzyme clusters, we find that physical association of metabolically consecutive enzymes is a most efficient means for precluding the degradation of the chemical potential of intermediate substrates by a "random field" which might prevail otherwise (3). Naturally, this organization can affect in a number of ways the energetic economy of cellular metabolism.

A notable example is the reduction of transient time (τ) in steady-state transitions. This lag phase represents the time required for intermediate substrates to accumulate to levels necessary to sustain a given steady-state flux in a sequence of reactions. In general, τ will depend on enzyme concentration, medium viscosity (or substrate diffusion coefficients), and Boltzmann energy term (relating the activation energies for the various steps in enzyme catalysis) (16). Reduction of transient time has been observed both for immobilized (18) (Fig.1) and for naturally-occurring (3,19)

(Fig.2) multienzyme systems. As expected, the free-energy "cost of transition" is proportional to τ; and the calculated value of τ is found to be unrealistically high for in vivo situations -- if one assumes no spatial organization (16).

Reduction of transient time in structured multienzyme systems (particularly, membrane-bound arrays) is usually attributed to such factors as maintenance of high local concentrations of enzymes (and substrates) and restriction on the out-diffusion of intermediate substrates. However, activation energy may be another factor, which is more subtle and yet of importance in the overall economy of metabolic sequences. Indeed, this element stands on its own, aside from its influence on transient time, as contributing to the evolution of enzyme organization. Boltzmann's relation tells us that the fraction of molecules in a given population having activation energy E_A will be $\exp(-E_A/k_BT)$. The higher the value of E_A, the greater the concentration of the intermediate substrate necessary to maintain the metabolic process at a requisite rate (20).

One of the most outstanding characteristics of a living cell, as distinct from a corresponding in vitro mixture of the same chemical reactants and products, is the rapidity of reaction evident in the former. Of course, this is due to the presence of specific enzyme catalysts, whose role is to supply paths of chemical transformation with lowered activation-energy barriers. But, evolution has not stopped with this singular thermodynamic-kinetic feature in the optimization of metabolic processes. For example, Atkinson (21) points to the role of activated intermediates (formed via cofactors such as coenzyme A, thiamine pyrophosphate, lipoic acid, etc.) ubiquitous in metabolic pathways. (Activation of intermediates, in effect, raises free-energy "pits".) We contend that this "smoothing" effect on the free-energy profile for reaction sequences extends to higher levels of complexity.

At the level of the component enzymes, catalytic facilitation in organized systems may relate to a number of specific contributions to the free energy of activation, $\Delta G^{\ddagger}$. We enumerate below some factors, which are discussed in detail elsewhere (3):

1) Various "steric" and enthalpic factors arising from activation effects in aggregated systems.

2) "Structural effects" of Laidler and Bunting (22). Many enzymes undergo a reversible conformational change during the course of the reaction process.

(Perhaps a slightly unfolded state makes the active site more available to the substrate.) In enzyme aggregates the individual proteins might be stabilized in optimally "open" configurations, obviating some postcatalytic refolding.

3) The "entatic state" (23). Certain types of enzymes can be energetically poised for catalytic action in the absence of substrate. Thus, the geometry of the active center can generate "internal activation", due to conformational stress. A substrate molecule entering such a domain would find itself under attack by unusually activated groups. Again, in the aggregated state, there is greater potential for component enzymes to be stabilized in "entatic" conformations.

4) Protein configurational fluctuation (e.g.,ref.24). Many individual proteins, particularly components of interacting systems, can exist in solution as an equilibrium mixture of a number of configurations of approximately equal energy. In many such cases (involving enzyme reaction), it is observed that only one configuration is optimal for catalytic function. Consequently, we must associate with the activated state of the enzyme-substrate complex not only a requisite energetic fluctuation, but also a specific configurational fluctuation in the protein. The latter feature yields a negative contribution to the activation entropy for the enzyme-catalyzed reaction. Notably, it has been found for some such "fluctuating" systems that the formation of a multi-enzyme aggregate can "freeze" each component protein into a single (optimal) configuration for catalysis.

5) Chemical activation (25). Essentially every type of elementary chemical reaction yields products, initially, with a nonequilibrium energy distribution (e.g., excited internal vibrational states). For homogeneous systems in solution, the fate of such excited states is rapid relaxation (e.g., via collisional deactivation). However, in physically associated enzyme systems, a portion of this energy released by the chemical subsystem may be retained within the protein structure for specific utilization in subsequent catalytic events.

6) Electrostatic contributions (22). Consider the
enzyme and substrate as ions. For reactions in ionic
solution, the free energy of activation for the
formation of an activated complex from two ions will
contain a part $\Delta G_{es}^{\ddagger}$, due to the free-energy change
associated with the electrostatic forces between the
two reactants as they are brought together. This has
the form

$$\Delta G_{es}^{\ddagger} = \frac{Z_1 \, Z_2 \, e^2}{\varepsilon r^{\ddagger}} \quad ,$$

where Z_1 and Z_2 are the number of charges on the
respective ions, e the electronic charge, ε the
dielectric constant of the medium, and $r^{\ddagger}$ some
critical distance between the two ions. For the
formation of an enzyme-substrate complex in solution, the net charge of the protein will affect the
overall interaction potential. Hence, in general,
$\Delta G_{es}^{\ddagger}$ will not be negative (rate-ehancing). Within
the confinement of a multienzyme cluster, a nascent
intermediate-substrate molecule might not "see" the
overall charge of the protein (or matrix structure),
but only that in the vicinity of the active center.
Also, the value of ε might be significantly lower
(than for water) in structured regimes. Then, a
negative value of $\Delta G_{es}^{\ddagger}$ might be a "built-in" feature
of the organized state.

The potential influence on $\Delta G^{\ddagger}$ of these combined factors, resulting from aggregation, is illustrated in Fig.3.
Some features (e.g., 1,4 and 6 above) might lower $\Delta G^{\ddagger}$,
while other (e.g., 2,3 and 5) might elevate the free-energy
"valley", or "pit" (See $\Delta G_i^{\ddagger}$ and $\Delta G_{i+1}^{\ddagger}$ in Fig.3).
Employing the "complementarity" concept proposed by
Lumry and Biltonen (26), it may be envisaged that free-
energy complementarity along the reaction coordinate of the
total system (i.e., chemical subsystem plus protein configuration) is the real entity that is being optimized in
enzyme evolution (Fig.4). We adopt, as did the previous
authors (26), the view that a metabolic pathway, consisting
of a sequence of enzymes, must be evolutionarily adapted as
a unit. Physical association of related enzymes offers a
unification, a way of extending "complementarity" over a
large system of functionally coupled macromolecules. For
such systems the term "super-complementarity" is most
appropriate (3,26). Some time ago, the principle was stated
that "biological systems tend to perform at an optimum
efficiency for maximum power output" (27). Enzyme organi-

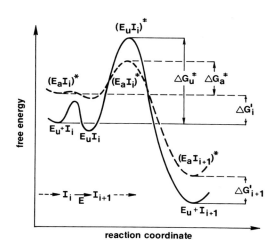

FIGURE 3. Potential effects of enzyme clustering on
the free-energy profile of the reactions of intermediary
metabolism. As discussed in the text, catalytic facilitation
by structured multienzyme systems may entail a "smoothing"
effect on the overall profile, resulting from a lowering of
energy barriers and/or a raising of energy valleys. In the
example above, the enzyme E (structured, a, or unstructured,
u) catalyzes the reaction $I_i \to I_{i+1}$ among metabolic intermediates. (See text for further details.) [Reproduced from
ref. 3, with the kind permission of Pergamon Press, Inc.]

zation in the living cell seems a fitting example of this
tendency. In this context, it appears that "the general
evolutionary trend toward complexity is thus a direct manifestation of the success of modifications which maintain
speed but increase efficiency, or increase speed without
loss of efficiency" (26).

IV. THE AROMATIC-TRYPTOPHAN BIOSYNTHETIC PATHWAY: A CASE IN POINT

A metabolic segment exhibiting rather extensive spatial
organization of component enzymes is represented by the
aromatic-tryptophan pathway in microorganisms (and in higher
plants) (3). This pathway is composed of a multienzyme

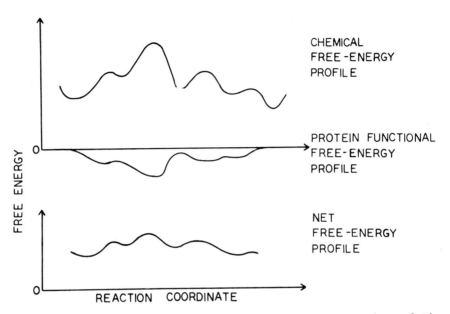

FIGURE 4. Simplified example of the flattening of the net free-energy profile through "complementarity" developed between the chemical parts of the protein-supported process and the conformational contribution from the functional conformation process of the protein. (See text for more details.) [Reproduced from ref.26, with the kind permission of Marcel Dekker, Inc., and of the authors.]

system catalyzing a total of 13 reactions (Fig.5A). Steps 1-7 (the "polyaromatic" pathway) convert the glycolytic by-products, phosphoenolpyruvate and erythrose 4-phosphate, to the branch-point intermediate chorismate (CA); and this sequence is common to the synthesis of all aromatic amino acids and certain vitamins as well (Fig.5B). The potential structural-functional unity of the aromatic biosynthetic system was first emphasized by Doy (28). He speculated on physiological grounds that the physical arrangement of aromatic biosynthetic enzymes into "natural units of organization" might extend to the case of interaction of activities controlling both synthesis and utilization of the branch-point intermediate, chorismate. That such a conjectural notion may be correct is seen from the following observations.

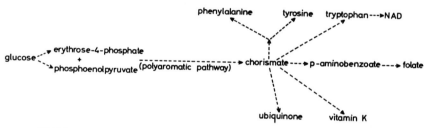

FIGURE 5. Biosynthesis of aromatic substances in microorganisms. A. The polyaromatic-tryptophan biosynthetic pathway. B. Illustration of the primary biosynthetic routes for the aromatic amino acids and various other aromatic compounds. The "polyaromatic pathway" is common to the synthesis of all such substances. (See ref.3 for abbreviations.) [Reproduced from ref.3, with the kind permission of Pergamon Press, Inc.]

Figure 6 gives a phylogenetic comparison of the presently-known (in vitro) state of organization of the polyaromatic-tryptophan pathway. In Neurospora crassa, for example, ten of the 13 enzymic activities are readily isolable in vitro as three distinct multienzyme clusters (arom "conjugate", anthranilate synthase "complex", and tryptophan synthase "conjugate"); and the three remaining activities are found separately in vitro (29). Importantly, each of the

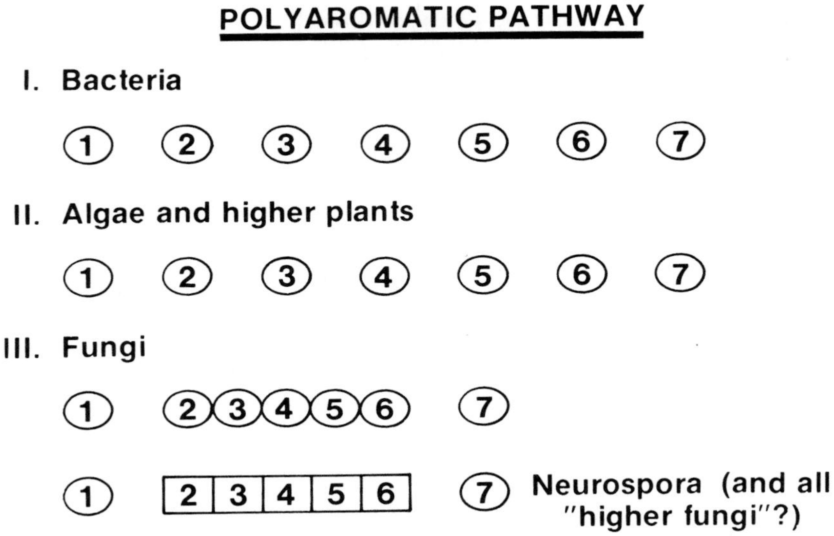

POLYAROMATIC PATHWAY

I. Bacteria

① ② ③ ④ ⑤ ⑥ ⑦

II. Algae and higher plants

① ② ③ ④ ⑤ ⑥ ⑦

III. Fungi

① ②③④⑤⑥ ⑦

① [2 3 4 5 6] ⑦ **Neurospora (and all "higher fungi"?)**

FIGURE 6. A phylogenetic comparison of the (in vitro) state of enzyme organization in the polyaromatic-tryptophan biosynthetic pathway. "Ovals" represent physically distinct enzyme activities. Conjoined "squares" represent multienzyme conjugates, i.e., fused polypeptides (49). Conjoined "ovals" and conjoined "oval-square" assemblies represent multienzyme complexes. [Numbers refer to respective pathway steps in Fig. 5. The "G" subunit confers glutamine amidotransferase activity on step 8.]

three enzyme clusters exhibits unique kinetic and/or regulatory properties, e.g., metabolite "channeling" and coordinate activation (3). Furthermore, preliminary results (30) from sucrose density-gradient centrifugation studies with a strain lysed under very gentle conditions indicate a more extensive association of the respective enzymic components. (In this case, extracts were prepared and analyzed under stringently anaerobic conditions from osmotic lysates of a wall-less variant of N. crassa [slime].) In addition, the catalytic activity of purified tryptophan-synthase cluster from N. crassa was found to be stimulated by proteins such as serum albumin (31). The latter authors interpreted this phenomenon in terms of "intermolecular cooperativity" which might exist in situ between this enzyme

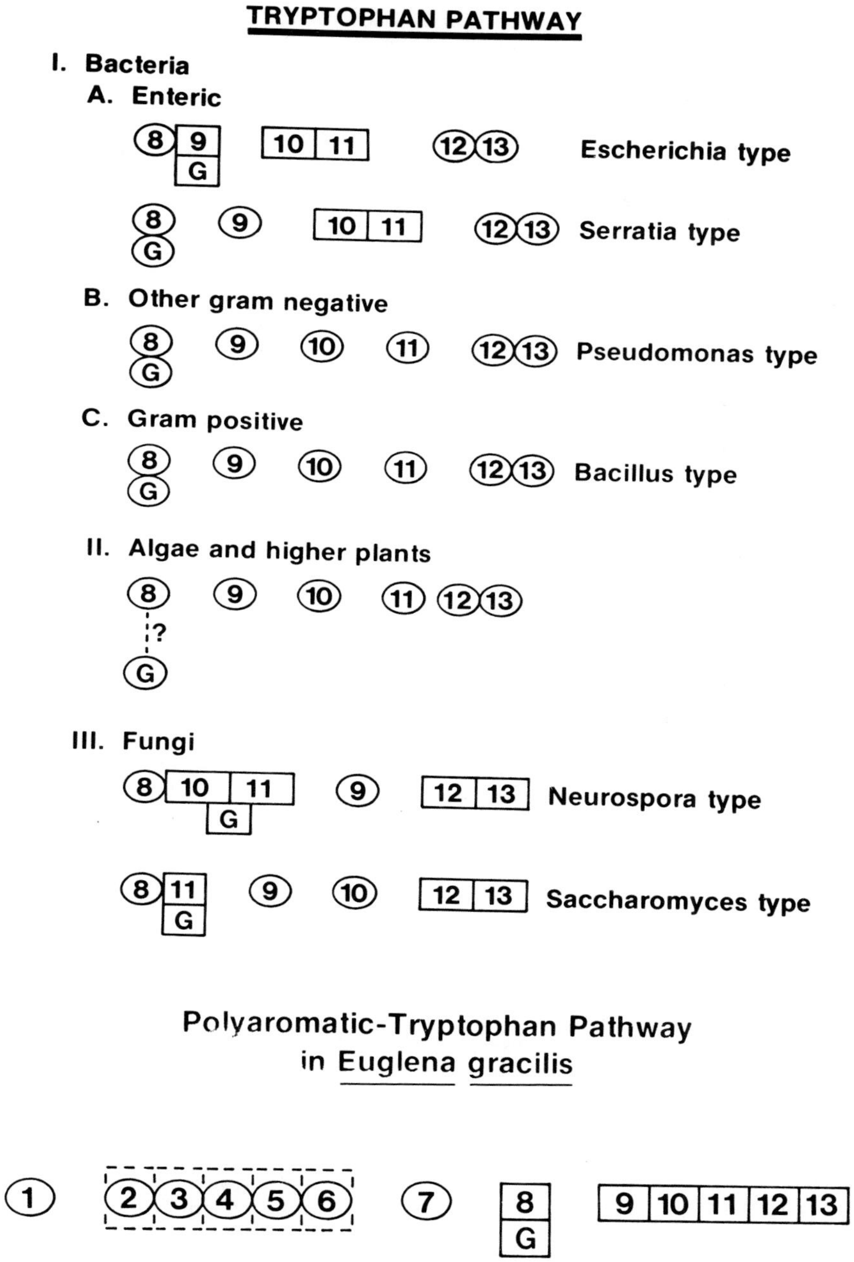
TRYPTOPHAN PATHWAY
I. Bacteria
A. Enteric
8 9 G 10 11 12 13 Escherichia type
8 G 9 10 11 12 13 Serratia type
B. Other gram negative
8 G 9 10 11 12 13 Pseudomonas type
C. Gram positive
8 G 9 10 11 12 13 Bacillus type
II. Algae and higher plants
8 ? G 9 10 11 12 13
III. Fungi
8 10 11 G 9 12 13 Neurospora type
8 11 G 9 10 12 13 Saccharomyces type
Polyaromatic-Tryptophan Pathway
in Euglena gracilis
1 2 3 4 5 6 7 8 G 9 10 11 12 13

FIGURE 6. (continued)

cluster and other enzymic components of the tryptophan
pathway. Also, Welch et al. (32) found that catalytically-
active chorismate synthase is highly unstable in the absence
of albumin (or other proteins). Moreover, recent chromatographic studies (33) are indicative of a possible interaction between this enzyme and other pathway components. In
this regard, Doy (34) cited evidence showing that properties
of N. crassa 3-deoxy-D-arabino-heptulosonate-7-phosphate
(DAHP) synthase (step 1) are altered by mutations originally
thought to affect only the activities of the arom cluster
and chorismate synthase.

Recent findings from the flagellated photosynthetic
organism, Euglena gracilis, have given even more credibility
to the existence of the hypothetical "units". While eugle-
noids share many morphological features in common with algal
and protozoan species, they apparently also share certain
biochemical characteristics otherwise restricted to higher
organisms. For example, E. gracilis possesses an arom
cluster quite similar in structure to that in fungi (35).
Also, the tryptophan synthase cluster in E. gracilis closely
resembles that in fungi with respect to structural and
kinetic features. Of significance in the case of Euglena,
however, was the discovery (36) that the tryptophan synthase
system is also clustered with three other metabolically
proximal enzymes in the tryptophan pathway. Thus, in this
organism it appears that at least ten of the 13 enzymes in
the entire pathway of tryptophan biosynthesis exist in only
two separate isolable clusters. At least two of the remaining three activities --DAHP synthase, chorismate synthase,
and anthranilate synthase -- have been seen to interact with
various pathway components in a number of other physio-
logically-related species (28,34,37,38). Consequently, Lara
and Mills (39) were led to offer the prospect that in vivo
there exists a "pathway particle" consisting of all 13,
perhaps loosely (or transiently) bound, enzymic activities
(cf. ref.40).

The aromatic-tryptophan pathway yields perhaps the
greatest degree of organizational complexity for any multienzyme system of a non-membranous (or non-organellar)
nature. (It remains to be seen whether or not this system is
anchored in vivo to intracellular particulates [41].) Moreover, the coincidence of the organized state with the novel
kinetic and/or regulatory properties displayed by the constituent aggregated entities in this pathway should avail as
an initiative for the elucidation of more such structural-
functional relationships potentially existent in other
systems. Pathways of amino acid biosynthesis have proved
particularly rich sources in this respect. We fully antici-

pate that the general concepts discussed above will provide a broader basis for analyzing and/or determining the overall physiological and evolutionary significance of such "pathway particles".

V. CONCLUDING REMARKS

We shall close in a somewhat philosophical (epistemological) tone. We began on a note from C. Bernard; let us end on one from the same. According to Bernard (1), the "man of science" shies from discussions of "final causes" (intentional purpose) and concentrates on the "efficient cause" within the object at hand. With this particular finality (or "intraorganic teleology", as Bernard terms it) comes the realization that the living organism is a microcosm, "a little world where things are made one for another, and the relationship can be comprehended because one can embrace the natural whole of these things". This view has guided us in the present work.

Nature has a logic of its own, a logic which does not necessarily coincide with man's logic. Man uses his own logic to construct the way things "ought to" behave, and then he submits it for approval to Nature. Man's personal conceptualization is very important. It governs not only the behavior he expects to find in Nature, but also the methods and approaches he uses to explore that behavior. We find a good example here. The present Symposium deals with a profound question, viz., the role of organization and compartmentation in cellular metabolism. As is evident from the variety of papers and the discussion comments, the same piece of experimental data can be interpreted in different ways depending on one's point of view. The question of the role of compartmentation will certainly not be resolved with unanimity in the short period of this Symposium. But, the Symposium will have served a worthwhile purpose if it heightens interest and focuses attention on this important issue.

There are those who are resigned to the impossibility of knowing how protoplasm works -- until the very day when we can take apart the cell, piece by piece, and put it together again into a functional whole. Is the life process so illusory as to deserve such resignation? We think not. In particular, we are of the opinion that the metabolic fragments (multienzyme clusters), which are being extracted from the cell with ever-increasing frequency, are "mesoforms" -- parts of an integrated, interlocking mosaic in vivo (42). In

order to construct a picture of cellular infrastructure --
in order to unify enzymology and cell biology, from the
clues offered by these isolated fragments, we must start
from some "first principles" like the following:

1) "1 + 1 $\neq$ 2" law -- P. Weiss. This is the precise
   statement of anti-reductionism. Life is a web, not
   a jigsaw puzzle (43).

2) la logique du vivant -- F. Jacob. Life does, indeed,
   have a logic. It is a logic of a crystal in three
   dimensions, of integrative levels of complexity
   (44).

3) life as "dissipative structure" -- I. Prigogine.
   This notion, in a very real sense, establishes the
   causal link between the concept of the living
   organism as a thermodynamically open system and that
   of the living organism as an unique space-time
   structure. The theory of "dissipative structures"
   shows that under certain nonequilibrium conditions,
   the equations describing the chemical kinetics together with diffusion may lead to a new long-range
   order -- which transcends the relatively short-range
   interactions dominating our physicochemical thinking. In short, "the coherence introduced by 'dissipative structures' is always characterized by a
   supermolecular scale that leads to a modification of
   the 'space-time structure' in which the molecules
   are embedded" (45).

4) a "there-must-be" approach -- C. Asensio. "We now
   have available a cohesive frame of biological
   thought that allows us to jump, to make short cuts
   in order to pick new concepts and facts for which
   real evidence is patently absent" (46).

     T. Kuhn (47), in his theory of scientific revolutions,
suggests that in doing science we choose a paradigm, with an
appropriate set of metaphors, which guides our whole outlook
to our respective scientific work. We have chosen our paradigm. It is based on a belief that the living cell possesses
an almost intangible beauty far beyond that indicated by our
in vitro preconceptions. Our metaphors are crystals, fabrics, and fields (48).

REFERENCES

1. Bernard, C., "Lectures on the Phenomena of Life Common to Animals and Plants" (translation of the 1878 French edition by H.E. Hoff, R. Guillemin and L. Guillemin), Charles C. Thomas Publisher, Springfield, Illinois, 1974.
2. Rashevsky, N., in "Foundations of Mathematical Biology", Vol. 3 (R. Rosen, ed.), p. 177. Academic Press, New York, 1973.
3. Welch, G.R., Prog. Biophys. Mol. Biol. 32:103 (1977).
4. Kempner, E.S., and Miller, J.H., Exptl. Cell Res. 51:150 (1968).
5. Zalokar, M., Exptl. Cell Res. 19:114 (1960).
6. Sjöstrand, F.S., in "Cytology and Cell Physiology" (G. H. Bourne, ed.), p. 311. Academic Press, New York, 1964.
7. Coleman, R., Biochim. Biophys. Acta 300:1 (1973).
8. Peters, R.A., Trans. Faraday Soc. 26:797 (1930).
9. Thom, R., "Structural Stability and Morphogenesis", W.A. Benjamin, Reading, Massachusetts, 1975.
10. Misner, C.W., Thorne, K.S., and Wheeler, J.A., "Gravitation", W.H. Freeman, San Francisco, 1973.
11. Oster, G., Perelson, A., and Katchalsky, A., Nature (London) 234:393 (1971).
12. Oster, G., Perelson, A., and Katchalsky, A., Quart. Rev. Biophys. 6:1 (1973).
13. Bunow, B., and Aris, R., Math. Biosci. 26:157 (1975).
14. León, J.A., J. Theor. Biol. 60:301 (1976).
15. Huxley, J., "Evolution: The Modern Synthesis", Allen and Unwin, London, 1963.
16. Welch, G.R., J. Theor. Biol. 68:267 (1977).
17. Welch, G.R., in "Enzyme Engineering", Vol. 4 (G.R. Broun, G. Manecke, and L.B. Wingard, Jr., eds.), Plenum Press, New York, 1978 (in press).
18. Mosbach, K., FEBS Letters (Suppl.) 62:E80 (1976).
19. Reddy, G.P.V., Singh, A., Stafford, M.E., and Matthews, C.K., Proc. Natl. Acad. Sci. USA 74:3152 (1977).
20. Pollard, E., J. Theor. Biol. 4:98 (1963).
21. Atkinson, D.E., "Cellular Energy Metabolism and Its Regulation", Academic Press, New York, 1977.
22. Laidler, K.J., and Bunting, P.S., "The Chemical Kinetics of Enzyme Action" (2nd ed.), Oxford University Press, London, 1973.
23. Vallee, B.L., and Williams, R.J.P., Proc. Natl. Acad. Sci. USA 59:498 (1968).
24. Karush, F., J. Amer. Chem. Soc. 72:2705 (1950).

25. Rabinovitch, B.S., and Flowers, M.C., Quart. Rev. Chem. Soc. (London) 18:122 (1964).
26. Lumry, R., and Biltonen, R., in "Structure and Stability of Biological Macromolecules" (S.N. Timasheff and G.D. Fasman, eds.), p. 65. Marcel Dekker, New York, 1969.
27. Odum, H.T., and Pinkerton, R.C., Amer. Sci. 43:331 (1955).
28. Doy, C.H., Rev. Pure Appl. Chem. 18:41 (1968).
29. Gaertner, F.H., and DeMoss, J.A., Methods Enzymol. 17:386 (1970).
30. Gaertner, F.H., and Leef, J.L., Biochem. Biophys. Res. Comm. 41:1192 (1970).
31. Tsai, H., and Suskind, S.R., Biochim. Biophys. Acta 284:324 (1972).
32. Welch, G.R., Cole, K.W., and Gaertner, F.H., Arch. Biochem. Biophys. 165:505 (1974).
33. Cole, K.W., and Gaertner, F.H., Biochem. Biophys. Res. Comm. 67:170 (1975).
34. Doy, C.H., Biochim. Biophys. Acta 198:364 (1970).
35. Berlyn, M.B., Ahmed, S.I., and Giles, N.H., J. Bacteriol. 104:768 (1970).
36. Hankins, C.N., and Mills, S.E., J. Biol. Chem. 252:235 (1977).
37. Crawford, I.P., Bacteriol. Rev. 39:87 (1975).
38. Hütter, R., and DeMoss, J.A., J. Bacteriol. 94:1896 (1967).
39. Lara, J.C., and Mills, S.E., J. Bacteriol. 110:1100 (1972).
40. Bearden, L., and Moses, V., Biochim. Biophys. Acta 279:513 (1972).
41. Balinsky, D., and Davies, D.D., J. Exp. Bot. 13:414 (1962).
42. Novikoff, A.B., in "Interrelations: The Biological and Physical Sciences" (R.T. Blackburn, ed.), p. 161. Scott, Foresman and Company, Chicago, 1966.
43. Weiss, P., in "The Neurosciences: A Study Program" (G.C. Quarton, T. Melnechuk, and F.O. Schmitt, eds.), p. 801. Rockefeller University Press, New York, 1967.
44. Jacob, F., "La Logique du Vivant", Gallimard, Paris, 1970.
45. Nicolis, G., and Prigogine, I., "Self-Organization in Nonequilibrium Systems", Wiley-Interscience, New York, 1977.
46. Asensio, C., in "Reflections on Biochemistry" (A. Kornberg, B.L. Horecker, L. Cornudella, and J. Oro, eds.), p. 235. Pergamon Press, Oxford, 1976.

47. Kuhn, T., "The Structure of Scientific Revolutions" (2nd ed.), International Encyclopedia of Science, University of Chicago Press, Chicago, 1970.
48. Haraway, D.J., "Crystals, Fabrics, and Fields: Metaphors of Organicism in Twentieth-Century Developmental Biology", Yale University Press, New Haven, Connecticut, 1976.
49. Gaertner, F.H., Trends Biochem. Sci., 1978 (in press).

DISCUSSION

B. CHANCE: Just a brief comment. I think one leap in logic that we should not take would be to ignore glycolysis. The transient time idea is not one that would stand up against the fact that glycolysis is made to get reducing equivalents from glucose into the mitochondria in a hurry or out to lactate or alcohol. I do not think that Hess' work (in Protein-Protein Interactions, ed. R. Jaenicke and E. Helmreich, pg. 271-297, New York, Springer, 1972) on the stoichiometric ratios should be ignored. Maybe the system is designed to ignore the microenvironment hypothesis or at least to keep the pool so small compared to the enzyme concentrations that their build up and decay is small compared to the enzymatic reactions. There is no more striking experiment that you can do experimentally than to add glucose to a suspension of yeast cells and observe that within tens and twenty's of milliseconds that cytochrome b undergoes reduction. The whole process has gone through to the mitochondrial space in a very short time. Perhaps many of these problems may derive from inadequate studies of yeast cells. (Incidentally put my Er term to zero).

R. WELCH: First, let me say that I did not mean to criticize the results from studies on glycolysis. Indeed, glycolysis represents a beautiful model system for doing both theoretical and experimental work. It is quite true that the overall transient time is of the order of milliseconds for glycolysis, because the respective enzyme concentrations are very high -- at least in yeast cells [cf. Hubscher, G., Mayer, R. J. and Hansen, H. J. M., Bioenergetics 2, 115 (1971)]. This is a well-established fact. Glycolysis is perhaps the most "central" pathway in all of metabolism. Reduction of the overall transient time may be an important teleonomic reason for such high enzyme concentrations.

However, my point of emphasis is that glycolysis is an exception. In general, enzymes of intermediary metabolism do not exist in 10^{-5} to 10^{-4} M whole cell concentrations. And, it takes only one low enzyme concentration (i.e., one long component transient time) at a given step in a metabolic pathway to give an additive effect on the overall transient time [Welch, G. R., J. Theor. Biol. 68, 267 (1977)]. Moreover, reduction of the transient time is not the sole advantageous feature of enzyme organization. In fact, there are reasons, irrespective of the transient-time argument, for believing that an organization of the glycolytic multienzyme system in vivo may be important [Welch, G. R., Prog. Biophys. Mol. Biol. 32, 103 (1977)].

CATALYTIC AND STRUCTURAL PROPERTIES OF THE PENTAFUNCTIONAL arom ENZYME CONJUGATE[1]

F. H. Gaertner

The University of Tennessee—Oak Ridge
Graduate School of Biomedical Sciences and,
Biology Division, Oak Ridge National Laboratory,
Oak Ridge, Tennessee

Although it is a foregone conclusion that much of the molecular organization of a cell is lost when it is disrupted in the process of extracting enzymes or other cellular constituents, the nature, extent, and physiological function of this organization remain open questions. In addition to the organization lost due to the mechanical separation of weak noncovalent macromolecular associations, it has recently been emphasized that even strong covalent associations are at risk. It is now clear that the action of resident proteases released during extraction and purification procedures can lead to the formation of artificial subunit structures for a number of enzyme systems (1–4). For example, it has been known for more than 10 years that five of the enzymes in the central pathway leading to the biosynthesis of the aromatic amino acids in Neurospora crassa are physically associated (5). However, until recently it was thought that this enzyme system was a clear-cut example of a multienzyme complex or enzyme aggregate, with most, if not all, of the five sequential enzymes associated solely by noncovalent forces (6, 7). Instead, it is now known that the "complex" is an artifact produced by one or more endogenous proteases (1), and that in actuality all

---

[1]Research supported in part by Grant No. PCM76-80227 from the National Science Foundation, and by the Department of Energy under contract with the Union Carbide Corporation.

Copyright © 1978 by Academic Press, Inc.
All right of reproduction in any form reserved.
ISBN 0-12-660550-5

five activities reside on a single polypeptide chain (8, 9).   Since it is
no longer appropriate to refer to this multifunctional protein as a multienzyme complex, the term multienzyme conjugate[2] has been chosen to
denote this structure (10).   Hence, the arom complex is renamed here
the arom conjugate.   Also, based on the one gene–one polypeptide
hypothesis, the arom gene region can no longer be considered a con-
tiguous set of five separate genes, but is rather a single genetic element
(Figure 1) which we have termed a cluster-gene (8).

Structural Properties of the arom Conjugate

The native arom conjugate has a molecular weight of about 300,000
daltons as determined by analytical ultracentrifugation (6) and a subunit
molecular weight of ~150,000 daltons (1, 8) as determined by gel electrophoresis under denaturing conditions with dodecyl sulfate (1, 8), thus
it is a dimer of 150,000-dalton polypeptides.   That these peptides must
be identical is established by the fact that two of the enzymes of this
system, dehydroquinate synthase and dehydroshikimate reductase
(shikimate:NADP$^+$ oxidoreductase, EC 1.1.1.25), exhibit allelic com-
plementation.   Interestingly, by genetic analysis (11), these two enzymes appear to be, respectively, the aminoterminal and carboxyterminal enzymes of the peptide (Figure 1).   The above results concerning
the structure of the arom conjugate have been essentially confirmed by
Lumsden and Coggins (9), except that they report a slightly higher
molecular weight for the subunit of the homo-dimer.   In addition,
electron micrographs of the purified conjugate are consistent with such
a structure (Allison and Gaertner, in preparation).

Catalytic Properties of the arom Conjugate

Coordinate Activation.   When the purified arom conjugate is incubated with its first substrate (3-deoxy-D-arabino heptulosonate-7 phosphate, DAHP), four of the five activities are activated (12).   As shown

---

[2]The term multifunctional enzyme also has been used to denote covalently associated enzyme systems (2).   However, such terminology is
ambiguous as it can also be used to designate a single catalyst capable
of more than one physiological function.

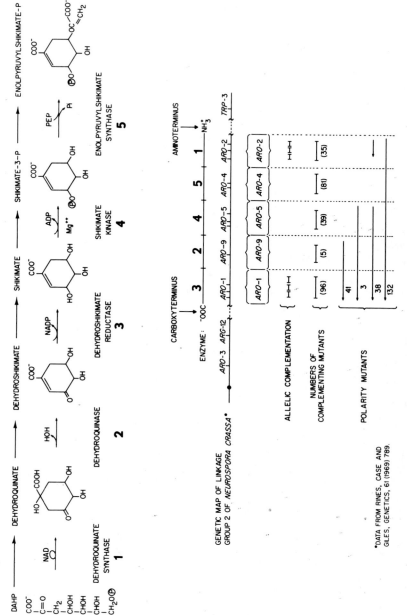

FIGURE 1: The polyaromatic pathway and the arom cluster gene.
*Data from Rines, Case, and Giles, Genetics 61: 789, 1969.

in Table I, all but shikimate kinase — the fourth enzyme in the sequence, show decreased values of $\underline{K}_m$ after such incubation, and the first enzyme, dehydroquinate synthase, also shows a twofold increase in $\underline{V}_{max}$. It has been suggested (12) that this coordinate activation may play a physiological role in controlling the flow of intermediates through the polyaromatic biosynthetic pathway such that, when the system is activated, ATP-dependent fourth enzyme becomes rate-limiting and thereby more sensitive to regulation by the energy demands of the cell.   Under this hypothesis, when the energy charge is low, existing pools of aromatic intermediates [possibly contained in vesicles (13)] could be shunted to an existing catabolic, energy-producing quinate pathway (5). Huang et al. (14) have independently suggested a similar type of regulation for the polyaromatic pathway of Bacillus subtilis.

Coordinate Protection.   We have also found that, when the first substrate (DAHP) is incubated with the arom conjugate, all five activities are protected from proteolytic attack (15).   This observation demonstrates the rather extensive conformational change that must occur when the first substrate binds to the conjugate.   It also suggests an additional physiological role for the organization of the five activities on a single polypeptide chain.   The order of sensitivity of the five activities to proteolysis is: shikimate kinase, dehydroquinate synthase, dehydroquinase, dehydroquinate reductase, and enolpyruvylshikimate

TABLE I. Effect of Activation by DAHP on Rate Parameters
of the arom Conjugate

Enzyme	$\underline{V}$		$\underline{K}_m$ (µM)	
	Not activated	Activated	Not activated	Activated
Dehydroquinate synthase	1	2	60	<12
Dehydroquinase	20	20	100	20
Dehydroshikimate reductase	4	4	40	20
Shikimate kinase	2	2	100	100
ES-3-P synthase	5	5	100	10

(From Welch and Gaertner, Arch. Biochem. Biophys. 172: 485, 1976.)

synthase (15).   Since shikimate kinase is implicated as the site of regulation for the control of the flow of carbon through either the biosynthetic or the catabolic pathways, degradation of this enzyme first is
consistent with satisfying the cellular metabolic requirements in times
of energy deficit.

Transient Time.   With a physically unassociated set of enzymes, the
product of one reaction would be required to diffuse to the site of the
subsequent enzyme.   Thus, the intermediate would accumulate in an
in vitro reaction mixture or in the cell until a concentration was
achieved sufficient to allow the subsequent enzyme to catalyze its
reaction at the same rate as the one before it.   The resultant lag, also
known as the transition time (16) or transient time (17), can be simply
expressed as the time (τ) required for the system to achieve ~63% of the
final steady-state rate.   With the simplifying assumptions that (i) the
K_m is much greater than the concentration of intermediate substrate and
that (ii) the final steady-state rate does not equal V_{max} (where K_m and
V_{max} are the rate constants of the subsequent enzyme), Easterby (17)
has shown that τ is simply equal to K_m/V_{max}.   It is also easy to show
that, with a sequence of more than two enzymes, the τ's will be additive.   Welch and Gaertner (18) have analyzed the overall τ for the
arom conjugate under various conditions in vitro with the use of the
analog computer.   In the simulation it was assumed that the system behaved as a set of five independent, physically unassociated enzymes.
Under these conditions the computer predicted that τ's of 125 to 200 min
would be obtained.   However, in actual experiments, the overall
reaction exhibited a τ of 12 to 20 min, 10 to 15 times less than that
expected.   These results are most readily interpreted as an indication
that the intermediates do not accumulate extensively in the reaction
mixture, but rather are in some manner confined within the enzyme system or on its surface.   Containment of this type would greatly reduce
the time required to achieve the necessary intermediate concentrations.
It is likely that rapid transition from one steady state to another is a
requirement for efficient cellular function.   Therefore, it is also likely
that this requirement is one of the major evolutionary selective pressures
which brought about such organized enzyme systems (19).

It is also possible that compartmentation of intermediates by the arom
conjugate has another important physiological role.   Giles et al. (5)
have suggested that the intermediates are "channeled" as a mechanism
to separate the polyaromatic biosynthetic pathway from a competing
inducible catabolic system of enzymes.   Since dehydroquinate (an
intermediate of both the biosynthetic polyaromatic pathway and the
catabolic quinate pathway) can induce the catabolic system (20), it is

especially critical that this intermediate not be allowed to diffuse freely and thereby accumulate in the cell under conditions favorable for the biosynthesis of aromatic amino acids.   On the other hand, under conditions of energy deficit, as has already been suggested, the channel may be broken and the cell can then use the catabolic pathway for energy production (see Coordinate Activation above).

   Rate Enhancement.   It is possible that the physical association of the enzymes in the arom conjugate permits an inherent improvement in the rate constants of the constituent enzymes.   For example, the rate of diffusion, also termed the transit time (16), could be rate limiting.   If this is the case and a given intermediate is completely compartmentalized, the K_m of the constituent enzymes, or the V_{max}, or both, interacting with an internal intermediate substrate, may be inherently better than the constants measured with the use of external intermediate substrates.   Also, intermediates may pass from one active site to the next by some direct mechanism rather than by a random thermal process, again bringing about an inherent facilitation of the catalytic process. The best evidence that such rate enhancement might occur in the arom conjugate was suggested by the observation that the overall reaction was catalyzed at a rate greater than could be achieved with an intermediate substrate (21).   However, it is possible that this effect was due primarily, if not totally, to activation of the system by the first substrate.   Whether true rate enhancement occurs with this system, or with any other, remains to be determined.   It does not appear that this will be an easy parameter to measure.

Summary

   The arom enzyme conjugate exhibits several unique catalytic and structural features which may provide the system with various physiological advantages.   The presence of all five activities on a single polypeptide chain may be important in both the coordinate activation and coordinate protection of the arom conjugate.   The physical association of the enzymes may (i) enable the system to respond rapidly with little or no transient to changes in metabolic flux, (ii) provide an inherent increase in the catalytic capacity of the individual enzymes and (iii) allow for the channeling of intermediate substrates, thereby sequestering them from a competing catabolic pathway.

REFERENCES

1. Gaertner, F. H., and Cole, K. W., Arch. Biochem. Biophys. 177: 566-573 (1976).
2. Kirschner, K., and Bisswanger, H., Ann. Rev. Biochem. 45: 143-166 (1976).
3. Pringle, J. R., in "Methods in Cell Biology" (D. M. Prescott, ed.), Vol. 12, pp. 149-184, Academic Press, New York, 1975.
4. Hulett, F. M., and DeMoss, J. A., J. Biol. Chem. 250: 6648-6652 (1975).
5. Giles, N. H., Case, M. E., Partridge, C. W. H., and Ahmed, S. I., Proc. Natl. Acad. Sci. USA 58: 1453-1460, 1967.
6. Gaertner, F. H., Arch. Biochem. Biophys. 151: 277-284, 1972.
7. Jacobson, J. W., Hart, B. A., Doy, C. H., and Giles, N. H., Biochim. Biophys. Acta 289: 1-12, 1972.
8. Gaertner, F. H., and Cole, K. W., Biochem. Biophys. Res. Commun. 75: 259-264, 1977.
9. Lumsden, J., and Coggins, J. R., Biochem. J. 161: 599-607, 1977.
10. Gaertner, F. H., Trends Biochem. Sci., in press, 1978.
11. Rhines, H. W., Case, M. E., and Giles, N. H., Genetics 61: 789-800, 1969.
12. Welch, G. R., and Gaertner, F. H., Arch. Biochem. Biophys. 172: 476-489, 1976.
13. Weiss, R. L., J. Bacteriol. 126: 1173-1179, 1976.
14. Huang, L., Montoya, A. L., and Nester, E. W., J. Biol. Chem. 250: 7675-7681, 1975.
15. Vitto, A., Cole, K. W., and Gaertner, F. H., in preparation.
16. Webb, J. L., "Enzyme and Metabolic Inhibitors," Vol. 1, pp. 373-383, Academic Press, New York, 1963.
17. Easterby, J. S., Biochim. Biophys. Acta 293: 552-558, 1973.
18. Welch, G. R., and Gaertner, F. H., Proc. Natl. Acad. Sci. USA 72: 4218-4222, 1975.
19. Welch, G. R., J. Theor. Biol. 68: 267-291, 1977.
20. Giles, N. H., Partridge, C. W. H., Ahmed, S. I., and Case, M. E., Proc. Natl. Acad. Sci. USA 58: 1930-1937, 1967.
21. Gaertner, F. H., Ericson, M. C., and DeMoss, J. A., J. Biol. Chem. 245, 595-600, 1970.

DISCUSSION

R. WEISS: Frank, do you know if other complexes (like the
histidine complex of Gerry Fink) have the same characteristics
in that there is a competing degradative pathway or is that
a unique feature of the arom complex?   In other words, are
the intermediates of the histidine complex capable of being
used by the organism in some other way?

F. GAERTNER: I am not aware of any competing pathway in the
histidine system.

R. WEISS: So that a competing degradative pathway may be
a unique feature to this complex and other features may be
more important.

F. GAERTNER: That's possible - right.

B. CHANCE: One of the approaches to finding out about the diffusion and concentration gradients of intermediates of course
is to use the simple dilution test which we have used actually to study glycolysis where an oscillating system can be observed within the cell.   It can be observed in the cell-free
glycolytic extract and of course the rates were slower.   The
factor, if I remember correctly, was about 80, so that there
is probably something about the cytosol that gives it apparently greater retention of concentration gradients.   Have
you done that kind of experiment with the arom complex?

F. GAERTNER: I guess the best answer to that is no. We really
have not done the type of experiment that would give us a
definite answer.

B. CHANCE: Well of course with oscillations you had something going on all the time so you can measure flux through
the system just as a function of dilution.   That I think is
a take home thought for those who want to identify localized
concentrations.

F. GAERTNER: Our situation now is that determining the
structure of the system is taking up our time.   We are concerned with getting the enzyme system under optimal conditions and it is clear that up until now we really haven't achieved that. I think we are in a much better position to do
the kinds of experiments we have been wanting to do all along
with the material that we have now. Previously what we had
was a system that had been all chopped up by proteases and
we looked at it on gels and it looked happy, healthy, normal,

but then you put it on SDS gel and it fell apart. So this conjugate is a bit different from the one we have had before and I think all the experiments that we have done before need to be redone.

F. LIPMANN: Do you get any continuing synthesis after you break the enzymes up?

F. GAERTNER· You are asking if we can break the enzymes up? The question stops right there because we can't do that. It is possible to get fragments from mutants, but so far we haven't been able to take proteases and chop it up and get active fragments. That doesn't mean that we can't do it - we just haven't been able to so far.

COMPLEXES BETWEEN GLUTAMATE DEHYDROGENASE
AND OTHER MITOCHONDRIAL ENZYMES[1]

Leonard Fahien
Edward Kmiotek

Department of Pharmacology
University of Wisconsin
Madison, Wisconsin

Kinetic and Sephadex gel filtration experiments indicate
that in the presence of palmitoyl-CoA, glutamate dehydrogenase forms a complex with mitochondrial malate dehydrogenase.
In this complex, palmitoyl-CoA is bound to glutamate dehydrogenase but is not bound to malate dehydrogenase. Consequently, palmitoyl-CoA inhibits and dissociates glutamate
dehydrogenase, while glutamate dehydrogenase completely pro-
tects malate dehydrogenase against palmitoyl-CoA inhibition.
Glutamate dehydrogenase also forms a complex with several
mitochondrial aminotransferases. However, the level of
specific ligands determines whether glutamate dehydrogenase
is bound to an aminotransferase or malate dehydrogenase.
For example, binding of glutamate dehydrogenase to ornithine
aminotransferase is enhanced by aspartate and ornithine,
while binding of glutamate dehydrogenase to malate dehydrogenase is enhanced by palmitoyl-CoA. In the presence of
palmitoyl-CoA, malate dehydrogenase, rather than an aminotransferase, would be bound to glutamate dehydrogenase.

I. INTRODUCTION

Previous experiments have demonstrated that palmitoyl-CoA
is a potent inhibitor of and dissociates glutamate dehydrogenase (1,2). Palmitoyl-CoA was also found to be an inhibitor of mitochondrial malate dehydrogenase. Inhibition was
specific for acyl-CoA derivatives with a long hydrocarbon
chain. Palmitate, coenzyme A, and acetyl-CoA did not inhibit.
Palmitoyl-pantetheine, palmitoyl-carnithine, and detergents
were poor inhibitors (1). The level of palmitoyl-CoA
required for inhibition was lower than its critical micellar

---

[1]Supported by NIH grant AM17857.

Copyright © 1978 by Academic Press, Inc.
All right of reproduction in any form reserved.
ISBN 0-12-660550-5

concentration (1-3). In view of the potential physiological
significance of this effect of palmitoyl-CoA, the study of
interaction between palmitoyl-CoA and both enzymes was undertaken.

II. MATERIALS AND METHODS

A. Enzymes and Reagents

Bovine liver mitochondrial glutamate dehydrogenase,
malate dehydrogenase, aspartate aminotransferase, and rat
liver glutamate dehydrogenase were prepared as previously
described (4-9). Pig heart mitochondrial malate dehydrogenase was obtained from Sigma or Boehringer Mannheim
Corporation. All enzymes were extensively dialyzed versus
0.025 M sodium arsenate, 0.1 mM EDTA, pH 7.8, prior to use in
these experiments.

Palmitoyl-CoA and [^{14}C] palmitoyl-CoA were obtained,
respectively, from P.L. Biochemicals and New England Nuclear.
Other substrates, enzymes, coenzymes, and reagents were
obtained from Sigma. Stock solutions of all reagents used in
assays were adjusted to the pH of the assays and prepared as
sodium salts. Solutions of coenzymes were prepared fresh
daily.

B. Enzyme Concentration

The molar concentration of glutamate dehydrogenase and
mitochondrial malate dehydrogenase is expressed in terms of
monomers using molecular weights of 5.6×10^4 (10,11) and
3.5×10^4 (12), respectively. These concentrations were calculated from spectrophotometric measurements using 8.3 (13)
and 2.5 (14,15), respectively, for the $E^{1\%}_{1cm}$ of mitochondrial,
glutamate dehydrogenase, and malate dehydrogenase. The concentration of bovine serum albumen, mitochondrial aspartate
aminotransferase, and lactate dehydrogenase was determined
with the method of Lowry et al. (16).

C. Gel Filtration

In these experiments [^{14}C] palmitoyl-CoA (specific activity 200 cpm/nmole) was incubated for 10 min. with glutamate
dehydrogenase alone or malate dehydrogenase alone or both
enzymes together in 0.025 M sodium arsenate, 0.1 mM EDTA,
pH 7.8 at 25°, and applied to Sephadex-G200 columns

(2.5 x 27 cm) which were equilibrated with the arsenate buffer. The volume of each fraction from the column was 2 ml. The columns were calibrated by adding the markers: blue dextran, yeast alcohol dehydrogenase, rabbit muscle lactate dehydrogenase, and mitochondrial aspartate aminotransferase before and after each experimental run. The elution profile of the markers was the same on all columns so the results could be directly compared. Also, adding the markers either before or after chromatography of palmitoyl-CoA plus glutamate dehydrogenase and/or malate dehydrogenase did not alter the elution profile of the markers.

D. Estimates of the Concentration of One Enzyme in the Presence of Another

In experiments where glutamate dehydrogenase and malate dehydrogenase were incubated with labeled palmitoyl-CoA and chromatographed on Sephadex G-200 columns, the concentration of palmitoyl-CoA in fractions from the column was measured by assaying radioactivity. The concentration of glutamate dehydrogenase was calculated by measuring the absorbance at 280 nm and correcting for the slight absorbance due to palmitoyl-CoA. This is apparently a valid method because in the presence of glutamate dehydrogenase and equal or lower concentrations of malate dehydrogenase, the corrected absorbance at 280 nm is essentially due only to glutamate dehydrogenase. This is because mitochondrial malate dehydrogenase is void of tryptophan (12), palmitoyl-CoA has no effect on the absorbance of either enzyme at 280 nm, and in the absence of malate dehydrogenase, estimates of glutamate dehydrogenase concentration based on the corrected absorbance at 280 nm agreed with those performed with the method of Lowry et al. (16). Also, similar results were obtained with palmitoyl-CoA, malate dehydrogenase, and $NaBH_4$-reduced pyridoxal-P glutamate dehydrogenase instead of the native enzyme. In this case, it was found that estimates of glutamate dehydrogenase concentration based on the absorbance at 320 nm (17) and the corrected absorbance at 280 nm were in agreement. Another way of determining the concentration of both enzymes was to concentrate fractions from the columns, remove aliquots, electrophorese on 5.6% polyacrylamide gels, and determine the amount of glutamate dehydrogenase and malate dehydrogenase on the gels with previously described methods (18,19). All estimates of malate dehydrogenase and glutamate dehydrogenase concentration were essentially in agreement.

E. Enzyme Assays

Measurements of the rate of DPNH oxidation were performed spectrophotometrically at 340 nm as previously described (4-6). Assays of glutamate dehydrogenase were performed with DPNH, 100 µM, NH_4Cl, 50 mM, and α-ketoglutarate, 2 mM. Assays of malate dehydrogenase activity were performed with DPNH, 100 µM, and oxalacetate, 100 µM.

It was found that if malate dehydrogenase was assayed in the presence of palmitoyl-CoA and glutamate dehydrogenase, there was an initial lag, but velocity was at a maximum after 3 min. This lag was not observed if glutamate dehydrogenase was incubated with palmitoyl-CoA plus substrates for 3 min. prior to adding malate dehydrogenase or if both enzymes were incubated for 3 min. with palmitoyl-CoA plus DPNH prior to starting the reaction with oxalacetate. The rates presented were those obtained either after this initial lag or those found after malate dehydrogenase or substrate were added to a previously incubated solution of glutamate dehydrogenase plus palmitoyl-CoA. All three rates were found to be identical. All assays were performed in 0.025 M sodium arsenate, 0.1 mM EDTA, pH 7.8, at 25°.

F. Assays of Radioactivity

These assays were performed with a Packard Tri-Carb Liquid Scintillation Spectrophotometer as previously described (20).

III. RESULTS AND DISCUSSION

A. Glutamate Dehydrogenase-Malate Dehydrogenase Complex

Glutamate dehydrogenase has a much higher affinity than mitochondrial malate dehydrogenase for palmitoyl-CoA. In our kinetic experiments, the concentration of palmitoyl-CoA required for two-fold inhibition was 0.4 and 2 µM, respectively for glutamate dehydrogenase and malate dehydrogenase. Furthermore, if [14C] palmitoyl-CoA was incubated with either enzyme alone (in ratios of 4 to 100 mols of palmitoyl-CoA per mol enzyme polypeptide chain) and chromatographed on Sephadex G-200 (in experiments similar to those described in Figs. 1 and 2 and Methods), it was found that a maximum of 9 and 25 mols of palmitoyl-CoA per mol enzyme polypeptide chain remained associated with malate dehydrogenase and glutamate dehydrogenase, respectively. It was also found that

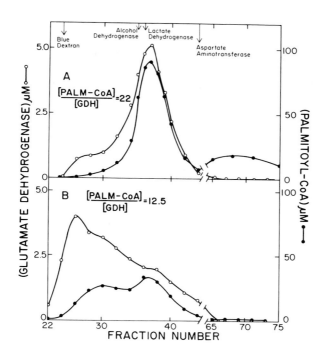

Figure 1. Sephadex G-200 chromatography of palmitoyl-CoA–glutamate dehydrogenase. In these experiments, bovine liver glutamate dehydrogenase plus [^{14}C] palmitoyl-CoA was incubated for 10 min. in 0.025 M sodium arsenate, pH 7.8, at 25°C and applied to columns of Sephadex G-200 (see Methods). The ratio of mol palmitoyl-CoA per mol glutamate dehydrogenase polypeptide chain in the incubated solution was 22 in Experiment A and 12.5 in Experiment B. The actual concentration of glutamate dehydrogenase and palmitoyl-CoA in these solutions was 59 μM and 1.3 mM in Experiment A, and 64 μM and 0.8 mM in Experiment B. The columns were calibrated by adding markers, as described in Methods.

palmitoyl-CoA completely inhibited and dissociated glutamate dehydrogenase from a hexamer into a dimer since the enzyme was eluted as a protein with an apparent molecular weight of 1.2×10^5 (Fig. 1). Alternatively, binding of palmitoyl-CoA to malate dehydrogenase increased the apparent molecular weight of this enzyme from 7×10^4 to 9×10^4, and this required 9 mols of palmitoyl-CoA per mol enzyme polypeptide chain in the incubation. If the molar ratio of palmitoyl-CoA to enzyme was less than 9, the apparent molecular weight of

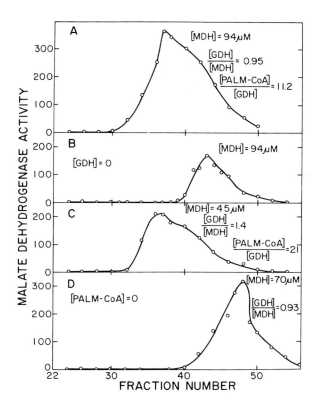

Figure 2. Sephadex G-200 chromatography of mitochondrial malate dehydrogenase. In these experiments, heart mitochondrial malate dehydrogenase was incubated for 10 min. with: A, glutamate dehydrogenase, 89 μM, plus palmitoyl-CoA, 1 mM; B, palmitoyl-CoA, 1 mM; C, glutamate dehydrogenase, 61 μM, plus palmitoyl-CoA, 1.3 mM; or D, glutamate dehydrogenase, 65 μM, and then applied to a column of Sephadex G-200 (2.5 x 27 cm). The concentration of malate dehydrogenase was: A, 94 μM; B, 94 μM; C, 45 μM; and D, 70 μM. Assays of malate dehydrogenase are expressed in units of change in optical density per min. per ml of fraction. Remaining experimental conditions are described in Methods. The columns were calibrated by adding markers, as described in Methods.

malate dehydrogenase was lower than 9×10^4 (Fig. 2, Experiments B and D). Accompanying this increase in molecular weight was a loss of malate dehydrogenase activity (Table I).
    The greater affinity of glutamate dehydrogenase than malate dehydrogenase for palmitoyl-CoA was also demonstrated

TABLE I

Effect of Palmitoyl-CoA (P-CoA) on Glutamate Dehydrogenase
(GDH) and Malate Dehydrogenase (MDH) Activity[a]

Additions			Percent Residual Enzyme Activity	
GDH	MDH	P-CoA	GDH	MDH
μM	μM	mM		
None	45	None		100
61	None	None	100	
None	45	1.3		16
61	None	1.3	0	
61	45	1.3	2	100

[a]In these experiments, enzyme was incubated (with the
additions indicated below) in 0.025 M sodium arsenate, 0.1 mM
EDTA, pH 7.8, at 25° for 10 min. At the end of the incubation, the solutions were diluted (10^3) and assayed for glutamate dehydrogenase or diluted (10^4 to 10^5) and assayed for
malate dehydrogenase activity, as described in Methods.

by incubating glutamate dehydrogenase, 16 μM, malate dehydrogenase, 107 μM, plus [^{14}C] palmitoyl-CoA, 1 mM, and chromato-
graphing on Sephadex G-200 (as described in Figs. 1 and 2 and
Methods). It was found that glutamate dehydrogenase was
almost completely dissociated and inhibited, most of the
palmitoyl-CoA was eluted with glutamate dehydrogenase, there
was 75% recovery of malate dehydrogenase activity, and the
peak of malate dehydrogenase activity was in fractions which
corresponded to a molecular weight of 7×10^4 instead of
9×10^4. Thus, in spite of the fact that the ratio of malate
dehydrogenase to glutamate dehydrogenase was 7:1, the vast
majority of the palmitoyl-CoA remained associated with glutamate dehydrogenase, and palmitoyl-CoA had little effect on
either the elution volume or activity of malate dehydrogenase.
    Since glutamate dehydrogenase has a greater affinity than
malate dehydrogenase for palmitoyl-CoA, it would be expected
that when the ratio of malate dehydrogenase to glutamate
dehydrogenase is 1:1 or lower, palmitoyl-CoA would be exclusively bound to glutamate dehydrogenase. This is the case,
for as shown in Fig. 3, under these conditions, glutamate
dehydrogenase is almost completely dissociated and inhibited
(Table I), and there is essentially complete recovery of
malate dehydrogenase activity (Table I, Fig. 2, Experiments A

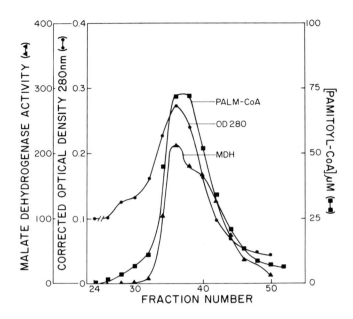

Figure 3.   Sephadex G-200 chromatography of palmitoyl-CoA-
glutamate dehydrogenase-mitochondrial malate dehydrogenase.
In this experiment, [^{14}C] palmitoyl-CoA, 1.3 mM, bovine liver
glutamate dehydrogenase, 61 μM, and heart mitochondrial malate
dehydrogenase, 45 μM, were incubated for 10 min. and applied
to a column of Sephadex G-200, as described in Methods.   The
malate dehydrogenase activity (▲) in the fractions is
expressed in units of change in optical density at 340 nm per
min. per ml of fraction.   The column was calibrated by adding
markers, as described in Methods.   Remaining experimental
details are given in the Methods.

and C, and Fig. 3).   However, malate dehydrogenase is eluted
as a protein with a molecular weight of 1.4 x 10^5, and the
malate dehydrogenase, glutamate dehydrogenase, and palmitoyl-
CoA peaks are all in the same fraction from the column (Fig.
3).   The increase in the apparent molecular weight of malate
dehydrogenase from 7 x 10^4 to 1.4 x 10^5 (Figs. 2 and 3) cannot be due to binding of palmitoyl-CoA alone to malate
dehydrogenase.   This is because in these experiments
palmitoyl-CoA is essentially not bound to malate dehydrogenase
since the ratio of malate dehydrogenase to glutamate dehydrogenase is low, and as mentioned above, palmitoyl-CoA alone can
increase the molecular weight of malate dehydrogenase only to

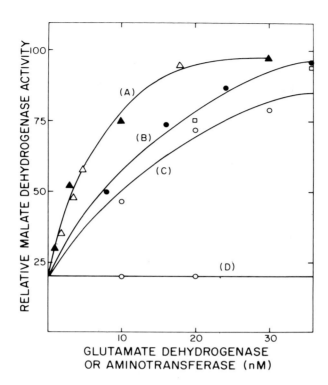

Figure 4. Plot of relative malate dehydrogenase activity
in the presence of palmitoyl-CoA versus the concentration of
glutamate dehydrogenase (Curves A to C) or mitochondrial
aspartate aminotransferase (Curve D). These assays were performed with palmitoyl-CoA (40 μM), heart mitochondrial malate
dehydrogenase (0.6 nM), plus bovine pyridoxal-P glutamate
dehydrogenase (Curve A), native bovine liver glutamate
dehydrogenase (Curve B), rat liver glutamate dehydrogenase
(Curve C), or mitochondrial aspartate aminotransferase
(Curve D). Other experimental conditions are described in
Methods. Similar results were obtained with bovine liver
mitochondrial malate dehydrogenase.

a maximum of 9×10^4. Furthermore, if palmitoyl-CoA was
bound to malate dehydrogenase, there would not be complete
recovery of malate dehydrogenase activity.
     The above results indicate that when palmitoyl-CoA and
both enzymes are incubated, palmitoyl-CoA is bound to glutamate dehydrogenase but not to malate dehydrogenase. However,
malate dehydrogenase is bound to the palmitoyl-CoA-glutamate

dehydrogenase complex, and this prevents palmitoyl-CoA from
inhibiting malate dehydrogenase. Consequently, glutamate
dehydrogenase is inhibited and dissociated, malate dehydrogenase is active and is eluted with palmitoyl-CoA-glutamate
dehydrogenase as a protein with a molecular weight of
1.4×10^5. In the absence of palmitoyl-CoA, glutamate
dehydrogenase has no effect on the elution volume of malate
dehydrogenase (Fig. 2, Experiment D). Therefore, palmitoyl-
CoA is required for significant binding of glutamate dehydrogenase to malate dehydrogenase.

    In kinetic experiments, it was found that the addition of
low levels of glutamate dehydrogenase to palmitoyl-CoA plus
malate dehydrogenase resulted in essentially complete restoration of malate dehydrogenase activity (Fig. 4). This
effect was specific for glutamate dehydrogenase because comparable levels of other proteins, such as serum albumen,
lactate dehydrogenase, or mitochondrial aspartate aminotransferase, had no effect on malate dehydrogenase. The glutamate
dehydrogenase used in these experiments was devoid of malate
dehydrogenase activity in either the presence or absence of
palmitoyl-CoA. Therefore, the observed restoration of malate
dehydrogenase activity was not to contamination of this
enzyme by malate dehydrogenase. It is also quite unlikely
that this effect results from glutamate dehydrogenase forming
a complex with palmitoyl-CoA, and thereby decreasing the concentration of palmitoyl-CoA available to inhibit malate
dehydrogenase. This is because 3 µM levels of palmitoyl-CoA
inhibit malate dehydrogenase about two-fold. Thus, in order
to completely restore malate dehydrogenase activity, the low
30 nM levels of glutamate dehydrogenase used in this experiment would have to form a complex with essentially all of the
40 µM palmitoyl-CoA added or each glutamate dehydrogenase
polypeptide chain would have to form a complex with about
1000 equivalents of palmitoyl-CoA. This seems quite unlikely,
and as mentioned above, would exceed the capacity of glutamate
dehydrogenase for palmitoyl-CoA, which is apparently 25 mols
per mol enzyme polypeptide chain. Furthermore, if $[^{14}C]$
palmitoyl-CoA was incubated with both enzymes (under the conditions of the assays described in Fig. 4) and chromatographed
on Sephadex G-200, it was found that less than 1% of the
palmitoyl-CoA was eluted in fractions expected to contain
glutamate dehydrogenase (molecular weight, 3×10^5 to 5×10^4).
Therefore, under these conditions, 1000 equivalents of
palmitoyl-CoA are not tightly associated with glutamate
dehydrogenase. Thus, these kinetic-gel filtration results
indicate that malate dehydrogenase forms an enzyme-enzyme
complex with palmitoyl-CoA-glutamate dehydrogenase. The
palmitoyl-CoA in this complex is bound to glutamate dehydrogenase and is not bound to malate dehydrogenase. Furthermore,

binding of malate dehydrogenase to palmitoyl-CoA-glutamate dehydrogenase prevents free palmitoyl-CoA from being bound to malate dehydrogenase. This is apparently because palmitoyl-glutamate dehydrogenase has a much greater affinity than free palmitoyl-CoA for malate dehydrogenase. In the absence of palmitoyl-CoA, glutamate dehydrogense has no effect on malate dehydrogenase activity.

B. Physiological Function

During gluconeogenesis, oxalacetate is converted to malate in liver mitochondria (21). In liver, the level of glutamate dehydrogenase is quite high (4,22,23) and is higher than that of malate dehydrogenase (5,23). Therefore, palmitoyl-CoA-glutamate dehydrogenase could protect malate dehydrogenase against inhibition. In our in vitro kinetic experiments, there is significant interaction between these enzymes when the level of palmitoyl-CoA is 1 µM and the levels of the two enzymes are in the range of 1 to 10 nM. This was the case with either heart or liver mitochondrial malate dehydrogenase. These concentrations are considerably lower than the mitochondrial levels of palmitoyl-CoA and these two enzymes in liver (23,24).

Our previous experiments have demonstrated that glutamate dehydrogenase can also form complexes with several mitochondrial aminotransferases (9). This might indicate non-specific binding of glutamate dehydrogenase to several proteins. Indeed, since one glutamate dehydrogenase molecule can associate with another, it is possible that the same forces enable glutamate dehydrogenase to form a complex with other proteins. However, rat liver glutamate dehydrogenase and pyridoxal-P-glutamate dehydrogenase, which do not associate (17,25), also form complexes with malate dehydrogenase in the presence of palmitoyl-CoA (Fig. 4) and with amino-transferases (9,26). Furthermore, the level of specific ligands would determine if glutamate dehydrogenase is bound to malate dehydrogenase or to an aminotransferase. Thus, for example, binding of glutamate dehydrogenase to ornithine aminotransferase is enhanced by ornithine and aspartate (9). Significant binding of glutamate dehydrogenase to malate dehydrogenase requires palmitoyl-CoA. In the presence of palmitoyl-CoA, mitochondrial aspartate aminotransferase does not prevent glutamate dehydrogenase from protecting malate dehydrogenase and does not prevent malate dehydrogenase from being eluted from Sephadex columns with palmitoyl-CoA-glutamate dehydrogenase.

IV. REFERENCES

1. Kawaguchi, A., and Bloch, K., J. Biol. Chem. 251:1406 (1976).
2. Taketa, K., and Pogell, B.M., J. Biol. Chem. 241:720 (1966).
3. Zahler, W.L., Barden, R.E., and Cleland, W.E., Fed. Proc. (Abs.) 26:672 (1976).
4. Fahien, L.A., Strmecki, M., and Smith, S.E., Arch. Biochem. Biophys. 130:449 (1969).
5. Fahien, L.A., and Strmecki, M., Arch. Biochem. Biophys. 130:478 (1969).
6. Fahien, L.A., and Strmecki, M., Arch. Biochem. Biophys. 130:456 (1969).
7. Morino, Y., and Wada, H., Biochem. Biophys. Res. Commun. 13:348 (1963).
8. Martinez-Carrion, M., and Tiemeir, D., Biochemistry 6:1715 (1967).
9. Fahien, L.A., Hsu, S.L., and Kmiotek, E., J. Biol. Chem. 252:1250 (1977).
10. Smith, E.L., Landon, M., Piskiewicz, D., Brattin, J.W. Jr., Langley, T.J., and Melamed, M.E., Proc. Nat. Acad. U.S. 67:724 (1970).
11. Cassman, M., and Schachmann, H.K., Biochemistry 10:1015 (1971).
12. Noyes, B.E., Glatthaar, B.E., Garavelli, J.S., and Bradshaw, R.A., Proc. Nat. Acad. Sci. U.S. 71:1334 (1974).
13. Egan, R.R., and Dalziel, K., Biochem. Biophys. Acta 250:47 (1971).
14. Wimmer, M.J., Mo, T., Sawyers, D.L., and Harrison, J.H., J. Biol. Chem. 250:710 (1975).
15. Thorne, C.J.R., and Kaplan, N.O., J. Biol. Chem. 238: 1861 (1963).
16. Lowry, O.H., Rosebrough, N.J., Farr, A.L., and Randall, R.J., J. Biol. Chem. 193:265 (1951).
17. Anderson, B.M., Anderson, C.P., and Churchich, J.E., Biochemistry 5:2893 (1966).
18. Fairbanks, G., Steck, T.S., and Wallach, D.R.H., Biochemistry 10:2606 (1971).
19. Rasched, I.R., Bohn, A., and Sund, H., Eur. J. Biochem. 74:365 (1977).
20. Shemisa, O.A., Happy, J.H., and Fahien, L.A., J. Biol. Chem. 247:7556 (1972).
21. Lardy, H.A., in "The Harvey Lecture" Series, Vol. 60, p. 261. Academic Press, New York, 1966.
22. Klingenberg, M., Van Hofen, H., and Wenske, G., Biochem. Z. 353:136 (1965).

23. Sottocasa, G.L., Kuylenstierna, B., Ernster, L., and Bergstrand, A., Methods Enzymol. 10:448 (1967).

24. Williamson, J.R., Browning, J.T., and Olson, M.S., in "Advances in Enzyme Regulation" (G. Weber, ed.), Vol. VI, p. 67. Pergamon Press, Oxford, 1968.

25. King, K.S., and Frieden, C., J. Biol. Chem. 245:4391 (1970).

26. Fahien, L.A., and Van Engelen, D., Arch. Biochem. Biophys. 176:298 (1976).

DISCUSSION

P. SRERE: As you know palmitoyl CoA has been shown to bind to citrate synthase. Have you tried the citrate synthase-malate dehydrogenase interaction with palmitoyl CoA.

L. FAHIEN: No, because I just saw your paper a couple of weeks ago on that complex. I know that palmitoyl CoA is bound to citrate synthase but I have never done a control with citrate synthase in this system.

P. SRERE: It binds at about the same level that you find binding to glutamate dehydrogenase.

L. FAHIEN: I find it binds at 0.1 micromolar.

P. SRERE: Well, 25 moles of palmitoyl CoA are bound per mole of citrate synthase.

L. FAHIEN: Oh, the same amount on the enzyme. In those experiments there are micelles of palmitoyl CoA while in kinetic experiments micelles are not present because we are working at a much lower palmitoyl CoA level.

F. LIPMANN: Did you ever try palmitic acid alone?

L. FAHIEN: Yes, palmitate has no effect. The interaction is very specific. Acetyl-CoA has no effect nor does palmitoyl carnitine, or palmitoyl pantetheine. It takes a long chain acyl-CoA.

F. LIPMANN: Do you have a rationalization to this effect?

L. FAHIEN: Well, it turns out that a palmitoyl CoA inhibits malate dehydrogenase only in the direction of converting oxaloacetate to malate. It is a very poor inhibitor of the reverse reaction. Konrad Bloch has proposed (Kawaguchi, A. and Bloch, K., J. Biol. Chem. 251, 1406-1412, 1976) that this is to enable MDH to convert malate to oxaloacetate in the Kreb's cycle and to prevent the reverse reaction. Now, in gluconeogensis of course oxaloacetate is converted to malate and we think that in liver the level of glutamate dehydrogenase would be so high that it would protect this reaction. There are also other very complicated controls that I haven't gone into concerning the effect of ADP and malate on this system.

S. BESSMAN: Have you found any relation between GDH and the α ketoglutarate oxidase complex of the cycle?

L. FAHIEN: We never have looked at them.

S. BESSMAN: There seems to be a very direct relationship because of the toxicity of ammonia which Potter and Recknagel (J. Biol. Chem. 191, 263-275, 1951) first showed. It subtracts the pool of α ketoglutarate.

MICROENVIRONMENTAL ASPECTS

THE INTRALYSOSOMAL pH

Christian de Duve [1]
Shoji Ohkuma
Brian Poole
Paul Tulkens [2]

The Rockefeller University
New York, New York, USA
and
International Institute of Cellular and Molecular Pathology
Brussels, Belgium

Lysosomes are small intracellular pockets completely sur-
rounded by a membrane and containing a variety of hydrolytic
enzymes capable by their co-operative action of breaking
down completely or almost completely all major classes of
biological constituents. Together the lysosomes, which may
number as many as several hundred per cell, make up a specialized space or compartment the main function of which is
to serve as site of intracellular digestive processes. The
vast majority of the hydrolases that are the agents of these
processes have an acid pH optimum. Hence the surmise that
the pH inside lysosomes must be acid (1).

First reached inferentially and based essentially on a
belief in the functional adaptation of lysosomes, this conclusion has been confirmed by a variety of observations made
both "in vivo" and "in vitro". In fact, the existence of
acidic pockets in the cytoplasm has been known for more than
50 years (2, 3), but only recently have these pockets been
identified as lysosomes. Two problems remain unsettled. One
is the exact value of the lysosomal pH; the other the nature
of the mechanism whereby it is maintained.

Studies on isolated lysosomes by Goldman and Rottenberg
(4, 5) and by Reijngoud, Tager and coworkers (6-8), using

---

[1] Supported by NSF grant PCM-76-16657 and by NIH grant
AG-00367.
[2] Chargé de Recherches of the Belgian FNRS.

Copyright © 1978 by Academic Press, Inc.
All right of reproduction in any form reserved.
ISBN 0-12-660550-5

the distribution of ^{14}C-methylamine between lysosomes and
medium as a means of assessing the corresponding proton
gradient, have revealed an intralysosomal pH 1-1.5 units
lower than that of the surrounding medium, and maintained
by fixed negative charges operating through a typical
Donnan equilibrium. In contrast, Mego and coworkers (9, 10)
have concluded from the effect of ATP on intralysosomal
protein degradation that the lysosomal membrane must contain
an ATP-driven proton pump. The existence of such a pump is
disputed by Reijngoud and Tager (8), who point out that
other explanations can account for the findings of Mego et
al., and mention further that both they and Henning (11)
have failed to detect any effect of ATP on the distribution
of ^{14}C-methylamine between isolated lysosomes and medium.
The opposite finding has however been reported recently by
Schneider and Cornell (12) who claim that addition of MgATP,
though not of CaATP, increases the uptake of methylamine by
isolated lysosomes 1.5 to 2-fold. This result does not
entirely fit with the observation that the membrane-bound
ATPase identified by Schneider (13) in purified preparations
of lysosomes as a possible agent of proton transport is
activated equally by magnesium or calcium.

A crucial element which could explain part of the discrepancies between the "in vitro" results is represented by
the permeability of the lysosomal membrane to protons. Free
passage of protons is required for a true Donnan equilibrium, and at the same time would tend to nullify the effects
of a proton pump should such a pump exist. The question
therefore is whether permeability to protons is an intrinsic
property of the lysosomal membrane as it exists in the
intact cell, or an artifact of "in vitro" conditions. It
could be the latter, since the permeability of the lysosomal
membrane to cations is known to be a delicate property,
dependent critically on temperature among other factors. It
is lower at 25° than at 0° (14,15), and could conceivably
be even lower "in vivo", to the point of allowing protons
to be excluded. It is noteworthy in this respect that the
results supporting the existence of a proton pump have been
obtained at 37°. Even at 25° free permeability to protons
may not be an invariable property of the lysosomal membrane.
In their review, Reijngoud and Tager (8) mention one observation suggestive of a restricted permeability to protons.
They found that the potassium ionophore valinomycin
appeared unable to promote a rapid proton-potassium exchange
unless an uncoupler (CCP) was added. In contrast, nigericin
which can effectively exchange K$^+$ for H$^+$ ions, was effective alone.

In conclusion, what the results obtained on isolated lysosomes tell us is that these particles contain an excess of fixed negative charges capable of maintaining a pH differential of some 1 to 1.5 units across a proton-leaky membrane. The possibility does, however, remain open that lysosomes may be endowed with the ability of further lowering their internal pH by means of an energy-dependent mechanism requiring conditions of restricted proton permeability for efficient performance. Such conditions could obtain "in vivo", and perhaps sometimes "in vitro".

Our own interest in this problem has been stimulated by a number of studies carried out both in Brussels and in New York showing that cells take up and concentrate markedly within their lysosomes a variety of weak basic compounds, including chloroquine (16), streptomycin and other aminoglycoside antibiotics (17), daunorubicin and adriamycin (18), morphine (19) and neutral red (20), among others. Although the behavior of each compound is to some extent characteristic, the accumulation process shows certain general features common to all or most of them. Firstly, it is rapid, so much so that endocytosis can be ruled out as a significant mode of penetration, which must take place by permeation. Aminoglycoside antibiotics are an exception; their rate of entry is slow and compatible with either mechanism. A second important property of the uptake process is that it leads to steady state levels which, within certain limits, are directly proportional to outside concentration. The steady state ratio of intralysosomal to external concentration varies from about 30 to as much as 1000 or more, depending on the compound. With substances of sufficient solubility and relatively low toxicity, such as for instance chloroquine or ammonia, the intralysosomal concentration may approach iso-osmolality in the presence of a sufficiently high external concentration. When this happens, uptake may slow down but it does not stop. It is then accompanied by progressive swelling of the lysosomes, eventually leading to intense vacuolation of the cells. The concentration necessary for vacuolation ranges from 10 mM for compounds like NH_3, down to 100 µM for compounds like chloroquine.

These properties have led us to conclude that the intralysosomal accumulation of basic compounds occurs by proton trapping, and is supported by a proton pump. Trapping by pre-existing binding sites cannot be excluded, but cannot alone account for the massive accumulation that is observed with certain compounds. This is ruled out by simple stoichiometric considerations. For instance, fibroblasts exposed to 100 µM chloroquine may take up as much as 150 pmols of

this substance per mg cell protein, or about 5 μmols per mg
lysosomal protein. This would require one binding site for
every 200 daltons of lysosomal protein, not a very plausible
figure. For the same reason, passive proton trapping can
also be ruled out, since it would require a similarly large
number of dissociable groups. Reijngoud and Tager (21)
have measured chloroquine uptake by isolated lysosomes.
At a concentration of 100 μM the isolated lysosomes took
up only one-tenth as much as they take up in vivo (16). To
account for this difference between isolated lysosomes and
those in living cells, we must postulate the existence of
a mechanism capable of lowering the intralysosomal pH one
unit or more below the level maintained by the fixed negative
charges, and of compensating a rapid influx of base by a
commensurate supply of protons.

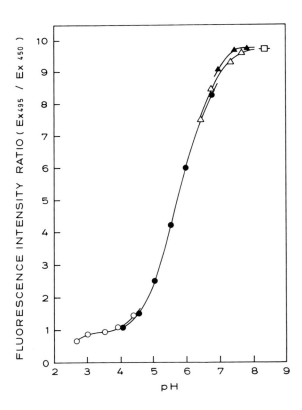

FIGURE 1. Ratio of fluorescence at 519 nm
measured after excitation at 495 and 450 nm.

Recent experiments in New York have provided direct support for this contention. We have developed a method for the measurement of the intralysosomal pH in intact cells, using as sensor fluorescein isothiocyanate attached to dextran. The polysaccharide serves as "lysosomotropic carrier" allowing the probe to be actively endocytized and stored in lysosomes. The intralysosomal pH is derived from the fluorescence excitation spectrum of the captured fluorescein-dextran, in particular from the ratio of signals recorded at excitation wave-lengths of 495 and 450 nm, which is strongly dependent on pH within the range of 4 to 8 (Fig. 1). We have constructed a device allowing rapid fluorescence scanning of living cells attached to a cover slip. Working with mouse peritoneal macrophages bathed by a medium of pH 7.6, we have found a stable intralysosomal pH of about 4.8, which transiently could fall as low as 4.5 under certain conditions. Addition of weak bases to the medium caused a rapid rise of the intralysosomal pH to a new steady state level. Removal of the base caused an equally rapid fall of the intralysosomal pH back to, or sometimes even below, its initial level (Fig. 2). The H^+/K^+ exchange ionophores X537A and nigericin similarly caused the intralysosomal pH to increase rapidly up to about 6.0. A somewhat slower and more moderate increase

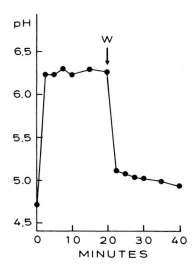

FIGURE 2. Changes in pH induced in macrophage lysosomes by 10 mM methylamine. At the arrow the CH_3NH_2 was removed.

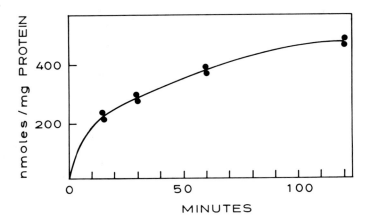

FIGURE 3. Uptake of methylamine by
macrophages from medium containing
10 mM methylamine.

in intralysosomal pH, up to a steady state level of 5.4,
was obtained by a combination of 50 mM 2-deoxy-glucose and
10 mM sodium azide. When added alone, each of these metabolic inhibitors had little effect on the intralysosomal pH.
      These findings provide strong corroborative evidence of
the participation of an energy-dependent process in the
maintenance of intralysosomal acidity. The pH inside the
lysosomes of living cells seems to be considerably lower
than that in isolated lysosomes and it rises when the cells
are deprived of energy from both glycolysis and oxidative
phosphorylation. Fig. 3 shows the time course of methylamine uptake by macrophages. While the pH change caused
by the amine was very rapid (see: Fig. 2), the bulk uptake
is relatively slow and proceeds without further change in
intralysosomal pH. As protons are pumped into the lysosomes
more and more methylamine comes in to neutralize them.
      An important observation is that different weak bases
may differ greatly in their ability to become concentrated
in lysosomes and to cause vacuolation of cells. Interestingly, these differences are not necessarily correlated with
similar differences in the ability of the bases to raise
the intralysosomal pH. The correlation, in fact, seems to
be more of a negative one. Substances that achieve low
steady state concentration ratios tend to have a strong
effect on the intralysosomal pH, and vice versa. These
differences are found between compounds which from their

pK's should give comparable concentration ratios (22), and are best explained by differences in the rates at which the protonated bases are able to leak out of the lysosomes. This variable has not been considered by other authors, who have generally assumed the lysosomal membrane to be completely impermeable to the protonated bases. It has been included in our own theoretical considerations, which have shown that even a low permeability coefficient of the membrane to the protonated form, one-thousandth or less the value for the unprotonated form, may, depending on the pK of the base, have a marked collapsing effect on the lysosomal pH gradient (22). Bases possessing this property tend to act like proton ionophores, and to uncouple the proton pump. In our opinion, they include ammonia, as well as methylamine which has been widely used as a pH probe in studies on isolated lysosomes.

While the case in favor of a lysosomal proton pump now rests on solid experimental support, several important problems remain to be solved. The most important one concerns the nature and mechanism of the pump. As mentioned above, some circumstantial evidence has been reported to indicate the existence of an ATP-driven pump. But the occurrence of a proton-translocating ATPase in the lysosomal membrane remains to be established. Should ATP provide the driving force, the stoichiometry and possible reversibility of the reaction raise interesting questions. If we assume the pH value of 4.5, which is the lowest observed so far, to represent an equilibrium situation, then we may take it that the pump translocates 3, or possibly even 4, protons per ATP molecule hydrolyzed. Furthermore, the possibility then arises that proton-generating processes occurring inside lysosomes may support ATP synthesis. There could be a form of "digestive phosphorylation" since digestion is an acidifying process.

Another unresolved problem concerns the fate of anions. If our views on base accumulation within lysosomes are correct, some anion, possibly chloride, must be secreted together with protons. This could conceivably occur by simple diffusion across a permeable membrane, or by some more complex mechanism.

Finally, the manner in which cells become vacuolated in the presence of high enough concentrations of weak bases requires an explanation. In essence, the mechanism seems to be osmotic. As weak base and the required protons and counter-anions penetrate into the lysosomes, water must accompany them to maintain osmotic equilibrium. Supporting this view is the finding in highly vacuolated cells of an intralysosomal concentration of base in the range of iso-osmolality. This, however, does not tell us how the lysosomal volume increases to accomodate the influx of water. Simple swelling with stretching of the membrane can hardly be involved. The alternative is membrane addition. This could occur without either new synthesis or contribution from other pools simply by fusion of the lysosomes together to form a smaller number of larger particles. Indeed, in fibroblasts exposed to gentamicin, the volume of lysosomes increases and their number decreases, so that the total surface area of the lysosomal membranes increases only slightly (23). In last analysis, the proton pump would provide the driving force for this process, but its mechanism is not clear and must depend upon the existence of some sort of interlysosomal connections.

REFERENCES

1. de Duve, C., and Wattiaux, R., Ann. Rev. Physiol. 28:435 (1966).
2. Rous, P., J. Exp. Med. 41:379 (1924).
3. Rous, P., J. Exp. Med. 41:399 (1924).
4. Goldman, R., and Rottenberg, H., FEBS Letters 33:233 (1973).
5. Goldman, R., in "Lysosomes in Biology and Pathology", vol.5, (J.T. Dingle and R.T. Dean, eds.), p. 309. North Holland Pub. Co., Amsterdam, 1976.
6. Reijngoud, D.J., and Tager, J.M., Biochim. Biophys. Acta 297:174 (1973).
7. Reijngoud, D.J., Oud, P.S., Kas, J., and Tager, J.M., Biochim. Biophys. Acta 448:290 (1976).
8. Reijngoud, D.J., and Tager, J.M., Biochim. Biophys. Acta 472:419 (1977).
9. Mego, J.L., Farb, R.M., and Barnes, J., Biochem. J. 128:763 (1972).
10. Mego, J.L., Biochem. Biophys. Res. Commun. 67:571 (1975).
11. Henning, R., Biochim. Biophys. Acta 401:307 (1975).
12. Schneider, D.J., and Cornell, E., in "Protein turnover and Lysosomal Function" (H.L. Segal, ed.) Academic Press, New York, in press.
13. Schneider, D.J., J. Membr. Biol. 34:247 (1977).
14. Davidson, S.J., and Song, S.W., Biochim. Biophys. Acta 375:274 (1975).
15. Reijngoud, D.J., and Tager, J.M., FEBS Letters 54:76 (1975).
16. Wibo, M., and Poole, B., J. Cell Biol. 63:430 (1974).
17. Tulkens, P., and Trouet, A., Biochem. Pharmacol. 27:415 (1978).

18. Noel, G., Trouet, A., Zenebergh, A., and Tulkens, P., in "Adriamycin Review II", p. 99. European Medikon Press, Ghent, 1975.
19. Liesse, M., Lhoest, G., Trouet, A., and Tulkens, P., Arch. Intern. Physiol. Biochim. 84:638 (1976).
20. Bulychev, A., Trouet, A., and Tulkens, P., Arch. Intern. Physiol. Biochim. 84:1055 (1976).
21. Reijngoud, D.J., and Tager, J.M., FEBS Letters 64:231 (1976).
22. de Duve, C., de Barsy, Th., Poole, B., Trouet, A., Tulkens, P., and Van Hoof, F., Biochem. Pharmacol. 23:2495 (1974).
23. Aubert-Tulkens, G., and Van Hoof, F., Arch. Intern. Physiol. Biochim., in press.

DISCUSSION

R. DAVIS: Have you tried basic amino acids as a way of influencing intralysosomal pH?

C. deDUVE: I thought about that when I heard your paper yesterday, and the answer is no.

S. BEN-OR: Is an electropotential gradient generated?

C. deDUVE: We do not know whether there is a membrane potential. It cannot be measured since lysosomes are too small.

S. BEN-OR: Does DNP short the pH gradient.

C. deDuve: It has not been tried. CCCP does.

S. BEN-OR: How can you be sure that the dextran compound doesn't interfere and change the pH of the lysosomes.

C. deDUVE: We do not know. What is measured here is the pH of lysosomes containing the probe dextran.

R. ESTABROOK: I am sure you have done it, but the binding of many dyes to proteins attenuates the fluorescence emission spectrum. Are you certain that what you are measuring is not the result of specific binding causing the change in fluorescence rather than truly reflecting the pH of the system?

C. deDUVE: In vitro there is relatively little interference by proteins and other additions. What may happen inside the lysosome is of course not known. However, the spectrum that is measured on living cells coincides perfectly with the spectrum found in vitro at a given pH value. It seems not to be deformed therefore. Also, the rapid changes occurring when ammonia and other agents are added are very likely to represent authentic pH changes.

THE MICROENVIRONMENT OF IMMOBILIZED MULTISTEP ENZYME SYSTEMS

Klaus Mosbach

Department of Biochemistry
University of Lund
Lund, Sweden

INTRODUCTION

During the last decade there has been considerable interest in the immobilization of various (bio)molecules such as enzymes, coenzymes or inhibitors to a large number of different supports (= carriers, matrices). The preparations obtained in this manner have found wide use for example in affinity chromatography. Another major area in which immobilized (bio)-molecules have proven to be of great value is that of "immobilized enzymes" which are used in enzyme technology including applications in analysis, medicine and organic chemistry and as model systems. Finally, it should be added that the immobilization technique per se is gaining increased interest as a tool in solving fundamental problems in biochemistry (1).

In this chapter I wish to restrict myself primarily to the use of immobilized enzymes as models for naturally occurring enzyme sequences. The examples to be described I wish to define as "multi-step enzyme systems", thereby reserving the term multi-enzyme complex or multi-functional protein for systems occurring in vivo in order to avoid confusion since these latter terms as normally used, refer to tightly agglomerated complexes occurring in the cell. The immobilization technique, however, enables sequentially acting enzymes, not necessarily naturally aggregated to be co-immobilized artificially, thus forming tightly coupled enzyme systems. In this chapter I will focus only on aspects related to intermediate concentration in enzyme sequences and where the intrinsic catalytic activities of the participating enzymes have not been changed.

Four principal types of immobilized enzyme preparations are usually applied and these are outlined in Fig. 1. For an extensive review on the topic of immobilized enzymes, the reader is referred to volume 44 in the Methods in Enzymology series (2).

In Fig. 2 some of the terminology usually referred to in the context of immobilized enzymes is given as an introduction to the discussion that follows.

Copyright © 1978 by Academic Press, Inc.
All right of reproduction in any form reserved.
ISBN 0-12-660550-5

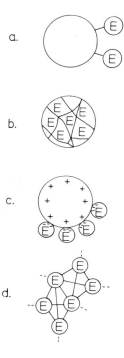

FIGURE 1.   Schematic drawings of the four major types of
            immobilized enzyme preparations. (a) covalent
            binding, (b) entrapment, (c) adsorption and (d)
            crosslinking.

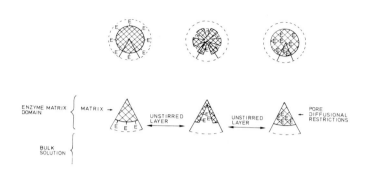

FIGURE 2. Schematic presentation of the types of diffusional
restrictions encountered in immobilized enzyme
preparations: surface-attached enzyme, both surface-attached and entrapped enzyme (e.g. within
the pores of agarose), entrapped enzyme (e.g.
within a polyacrylamide network) (22).

Before we discuss at greater length the use of immobilized
multi-step enzyme sequences as model systems, I wish to mention the type of problems for which those models may have
relevance. These include questions such as how do problems of
diffusion affect cellular metabolism; how will different
proximal arrangement of enzymes affect such systems; what are
the actual concentrations of the metabolites in the intermediate vicinity of the enzymes, i.e. in the microenvironment;
how are pathways competing for common metabolic intermediates
in vivo segregated?
    As is realized by most workers any analysis of metabolism,
which is based on kinetic data obtained from studies of isolated enzymes is bound to have limitations. Most conventional
studies, that could be characterized as "solution enzymology",
are conducted far from the natural milieu and under nonphysiological conditions, e.g., in artificial buffer systems
or at high substrate - low enzyme concentrations (often 10^6
substrate molecules/every enzyme molecule). In addition, upon
isolation, for example of membrane-bound enzymes, the microenvironment may be changed, or the intrinsic properties of
enzymes may be modified.
    Such problems outlined above, I feel, can be tackled for
instance by the use of immobilized enzyme systems. Obviously,
this approach also has its limitations, because both the
structural matrix and the way in which the enzymes are kept
immobilized are usually non-biological. On the other hand, the
virtues of this approach are that these preparations are

easily handled, they can be prepared in such a way that they
are chemically and physically well-defined, and they simplify
the study of the effects of changes in individual parameters.
In contrast, natural systems of enzyme sequences render
interpretation of data (e.g., as to the efficiency of enzyme
systems) highly difficult, because of the inherent complexity
of the system which involve variables that cannot be controlled. Thus, it would be difficult to evaluate the contribution of every possible parameter that might lead to a change
in the catalytic efficiency of such naturally occurring enzyme
sequences.

Indeed, one might even hope that the "immobilization" approach would reveal heretofore unknown effects of biological
relevance, which would be important in natural systems. Finally, it deserves mentioning that in immobilized enzyme systems, high local enzyme concentrations as found in nature,
are easily obtained on the solid-phase and can in this form
be conveniently assayed and studied. In the model systems to
be discussed the following microenvironmental factors that
may influence the overall efficiency of an enzyme sequence
and which would be difficult to evaluate in natural systems,
will be considered: proximity of the enzymes, presence of unstirred layers, other diffusional restrictions, exclusion
effects (structured water).

Some Multi-Step Enzyme Model Systems

Two-step enzyme systems. The first two-step enzyme system
described (3) was prepared by immobilizing two sequentially-
acting enzymes on the same particulate matrix. The system
studied was hexokinase and glucose 6-phosphate dehydrogenase:

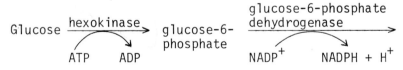

Glucose $\xrightarrow{\text{hexokinase}}$ glucose-6-phosphate $\xrightarrow[\text{dehydrogenase}]{\text{glucose-6-phosphate}}$

ATP   ADP   NADP$^+$ NADPH + H$^+$

6-phosphogluconolactone.

The enzyme activities were assayed using a stirred-batch
procedure (4). First, the overall activity in the coupled reaction was assayed, and then the two separate enzyme activities were determined, starting with the last enzyme step. A
reference system comprising the free enzymes was subsequently
prepared by mixing the same number of enzyme units of each
enzyme per volume of incubation solution as were bound to the
gel. As an additional control, a system consisting of a
mixture of the two enzymes immobilized to separate particles

was studied. It was found that in the initial stage the co-immobilized system was far more efficient, as compared with the soluble enzyme; after a lag phase the two systems operated at identical rates. A generalized picture of this behaviour is depicted in Fig. 3.

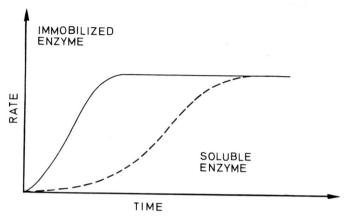

FIGURE 3.   Comparison of the overall rates of consecutive enzymic reactions catalyzed by the co-immobilized enzymes and the enzymes in free solution (from J.M. Engasser and C. Horvath in Applied Bio-chemistry and Engineering, vol. 1, pp. 127-220 (eds. L.B. Wingard, Jr., E. Katchalski-Katzir, and L. Goldstein), Academic Press, New York 1976).

Comparisons were made of the enzymes immobilized by different methods. Cyanogen bromide activation of Sepharose gave products with the enzymes bound on the surface of the particles, as well as within the pores of the matrix. Similar results were obtained by entrapping the enzymes in polyacrylamide or when they were covalently coupled to a copolymer of acrylic acid and acrylamide. The differences in length of the lag phases between the co-immobilized and the free systems have been interpreted as follows: the product from the first enzyme reaction will be present at a higher concentration within the particle than in the bulk solution, so that in the vicinity of the second enzyme a more favourable concentration of the rate-limiting substrate, glucose-6-phosphate,is found than in the bulk of the solution. Thus, the first enzyme reaction generates, within the microenvironment of the enzyme sequence, a high local concentration of intermediate. This is due to a) the fact that the product of the first step, glucose-6-phosphate, has a shorter distance to diffuse to the second enzyme in the co-immobilized system than is the case in the

soluble system, b) pore diffusional restrictions, and c) the
presence of an unstirred layer, which impedes diffusion of the
intermediates into the bulk solution. The reference system,
the soluble system, and the system with the enzymes immobilized to separate particles all operate in a larger effective
volume than the co-immobilized system; hence, the build-up of
the required intermediate-concentration takes a longer time,
which is expressed in a longer lag phase.

   The kinetic behaviour of such two-enzyme systems was confirmed independently by theoretical calculations based on
membrane-bound enzyme systems (5, 6).

   In another study the effect of varying enzyme-activity
ratios on the overall reaction rate was investigated (7).

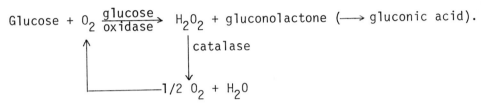

   Three-step enzyme systems. Extension of the previously
described scheme to multi-step enzyme systems, by addition of
additional sequentially-acting enzymes, made it possible to
study the relationships between the length of the lag period
and the efficiency of the overall reaction, on the one hand,
and the number of participating enzymes within the sequence on
the other hand.

   The overall reaction rates of an immobilized three-step
enzyme system (Fig. 4) (8) and that of the corresponding system in free solution were compared. Reaction rates were also
measured for the last two enzymes in the sequence, both in the
immobilized state and in free solution. The efficiency of the
initial stage of the overall reaction for the matrix-bound
three-step enzyme system was higher than that for the soluble
system. A similar trend was observed, although to a lesser
extent, when the two-step enzyme systems were compared. The
results indicate a cumulative efficiency effect as the number
of enzymes participating in the reaction sequence is enlarged.

   It should be stressed that the enzyme molecules in the
sequences studied so far have been randomly distributed in the
immobilized phase, probably resulting in a mosaic pattern of
enzymes throughout the support.

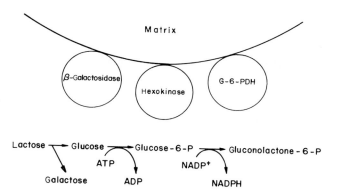

FIGURE 4. Schematic presentation of the matrix-bound three-enzyme system: β-galactosidase-hexokinase-glucose-6-phosphate dehydrogenase (G-6-PDH) with the respective reactants (ref. 8).

An enzyme system containing a thermodynamically unfavourable reaction will now be discussed (9). In the following three-step enzyme system described

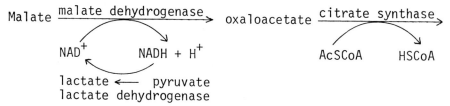

citrate

the malate dehydrogenase-catalyzed step is thermodynamically unfavourable in the direction of oxaloacetate, and hence concentration of the intermediate is not to be expected. Catalysis by malate dehydrogenase creates a constant concentration of oxaloacetate in the microenvironment of the enzyme and a decreasing concentration gradient of oxaloacetate away from its site of production. Differences between the immobilized system for the coupled reaction with malate dehydrogenase and citrate synthase and the corresponding free system are observed (at low concentrations of malate). However, the steady-state rates differ quite markedly between the two enzymes, the immobilized system being up to 100 % more efficient. The statistical mean distance between molecules of malate dehydrogenase and citrate synthase is shorter when the enzymes are

matrix bound than when they are free in solution and may in
the immobilized system lead to a steeper oxaloacetate concentration gradient and a higher mass transfer, making citrate
synthase condense oxaloacetate with acetyl-SCoA more effectively. This removal of oxaloacetate from the unfavourable
equilibrium will in turn result in a higher rate of catalysis
by malate dehydrogenase and hence increase the rate of the
overall reaction. When pyruvate is added to the system
lactate dehydrogenase, also bound to the matrix, starts
catalyzing the oxidation of NADH to NAD$^+$. This increases the
efficiency of the immobilized system compared to the free, by
as much as 400 % in some preparations. In addition to the
effect on oxaloacetate concentration, creation of a favourable
NADH gradient as well as the enrichment of NAD$^+$ in the microenvironment of the enzyme (as compared to the situation in
free solution) takes place also, resulting in an even more
pronounced accelerated conversion of malate to oxaloacetate.

The favourable arrangement of having the reduction and the
oxidation processes of NAD$^+$/NADH in close proximity to each
other facilitates a recycling of the coenzyme between the two
dehydrogenases per se which also contributes to the increase
in the production of citrate.

pH-activity profiles of sequential two-step enzyme systems

To investigate the influence of microenvironmental pH-effects
on the kinetic behaviour of sequentially-acting enzyme systems, studies have been carried out on the pH-activity
profile of a system composed of two enzymes with markedly
separated pH-activity profiles.

The particulate-bound, two-step enzyme system amylo-
glucosidase and glucose oxidase studied was (10):

$$\beta\text{-maltose} + H_2O \xrightarrow{\text{amyloglucosidase}} 2\ \beta\text{-D-glucose}$$

$$\xrightarrow[\nearrow]{\text{glucose oxidase}} 2\ \text{D-gluconolactone} + 2\ H_2O_2$$
$$O_2$$

The two participating individual enzymes have the same pH-
optima in free solution, as well as when immobilized on
Sepharose, of 4.8 and 6.4, respectively (Fig. 5).

A difference of 0.3 pH-units was observed between the pH-
optima for the coupled reactions catalyzed by the immobilized
and the soluble systems. When the ratio of the enzyme activities was varied, differences of up to 0.75 pH-units were observed. This phenomenon may be interpreted as resulting from
enrichment of the products of the first enzyme reaction in the

vicinity of the second enzyme, thereby making the overall system more efficient as compared with the free system.

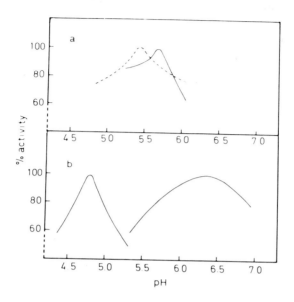

FIGURE 5.   (a) Profiles for the two-step enzyme system, amylo-glucosidase and glucose oxidase, in the coupled reaction: (————) Sepharose-bound (pH optimum 5.7); and (-----) in solution (pH optimum 5.4) (ref. 10).

(b) Profiles for the separate enzyme activities: amyloglucosidase (left, pH optimum 4.8) and glucose oxidase (right, pH optimum 6.4).

Regulation.   One of the most important reasons for the existence of multi-enzyme systems characterized by the close aggregation of the components might have been the necessity to develop better and more efficient means to control metabolic events, which may be accomplished by protein-protein inter-action or microenvironmental effects. The following example of the latter may be considered as model system designed to il-lustrate the inhibitory effects of externally-added substrate on enzymes participating in the sequences.

Inhibition.   A membrane system containing co-immobilized xanthine oxidase and uricase was studied (11).

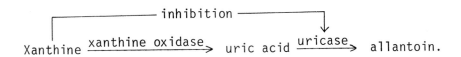

Xanthine $\xrightarrow{\text{xanthine oxidase}}$ uric acid $\xrightarrow{\text{uricase}}$ allantoin.

The system differs from those discussed earlier in that the second enzyme of the sequence, uricase, is inhibited by xanthine, which is substrate for the first enzyme of the sequence. From studies on individual enzymes, it is known that immobilized enzymes are less sensitive to inhibition by competitive inhibitors present in the external solution than are the free enzymes, and, one would therefore expect the immobilized enzyme sequence to be more efficient (= less inhibition) as compared with the soluble enzyme system. Indeed, the enzyme membrane system showed increased activity of the overall reaction. This is explained both by the fact that the immobilized uricase apparently is less inhibited by xanthine, because of diffusional hindrances, and also by the fact that the enzymic action of xanthine oxidase produces uric acid locally in the membrane, thereby creating more optimal substrate concentrations for uricase, while simultaneously reducing the concentration of the competitive inhibitor xanthine.

Exclusion effects. High concentrations of polymers within the living cell may lead to the partial structuring of water surrounding the macromolecules and thus lead to altered environmental conditions for enzyme reactions, as compared to a milieu with no structuring of water (12). To evaluate the effect of exclusion of solutes on an enzyme sequence, the system

p-Nitropheny-β-D-glucoside $\xrightarrow{\beta\text{-glucosidase}}$ glucose

p-nitrophenol

$\xrightarrow[\text{O}_2]{\text{glucose oxidase}}$ gluconolactone + H_2O_2

was studied with the enzymes free in solution as well as in soluble bifunctional enzyme aggregates (13). The kinetic behaviour was examined in pure buffer solutions with increasing concentrations of dissolved polymer, either polyethylene glycol or dextran. It was found that exclusion of substrate molecules as well as enzyme molecules from the space occupied by the hydrated polymer resulted in higher concentrations of re-

actants, thus enhancing the rate of reaction. This positive
effect was, however, counteracted by diffusional restrictions
when very high polymer concentrations were employed. Possible
effects on changes in enzyme conformation resulting from their
interaction with the macromolecules (14) have not been evaluated in this study.

Discussion of the Model Systems

In the immobilized multi-step enzyme systems described
above both diffusional restrictions including the unstirred
layers as well as enzyme proximity (and in the last case exclusion effects), which all lead to intermediate enrichment,
may account for the observed increased overall rates of the
systems. It is likely that in most of these systems diffusional restrictions occur first of all within the pores and
network of the gels. Likewise, the existence of unstirred
layers, the thickness of which is usually in the region of
< 400 μm (15), around these particles hindering " in and out"
diffusion has to be assumed. (It should be added that in the
assays described excess of substrate for the first enzyme in
the sequence is usually supplied to prevent hindered "in-
diffusion"). Finally, we know that we have achieved proximal
arrangement of the enzymes upon and within these matrices.
This evidence is based on calculations of measured enzyme
loading in relation to the support structure although exact
distances are difficult to obtain.

In the following I wish to discuss briefly some of the
studies made to evaluate the contribution of each of these
parameters to the observed overall rate enhancements. In one
study (8) diffusional restrictions occurring within the support
were eliminated by surface-attachment of the enzymes so that
the observed increase in efficiency had to be ascribed only
to proximity and unstirred layer effects.

In another recent study, soluble bi-enzyme conjugates of
malate dehydrogenase and citrate synthase were prepared (16)
in which the enzyme molecules were arranged randomly and studied
in free solution, as well as when immobilized on Sepharose. It
was found that the immobilized conjugates were more efficient
than those in solution, indicating that diffusional restrictions play an important role. On the other hand, somewhat
surprisingly, it was found that the conjugate in free solution
was not more efficient than a reference system comprised of
non-crosslinked enzymes free in solution. Therefore, under
these specific conditions, the proximity effect appears to
provide little advantage.

On extrapolating to in vivo conditions, it appears, that
one factor responsible for obtaining a high catalytic rate in

a loosely aggregated multi-enzyme sequence is not so much proximity per se but rather the fact that the participating aggregated enzymes are arranged in high concentration within a small volume, subject to exclusion effects and restricted diffusion of metabolites: this results in locally high concentrations of intermediates and therefore has kinetic advantages. In this context, I wish to mention that we are at present looking deeper into possible effects through proximity in bi-enzyme aggregates and are attempting to prepare aggregates with the active sites of the enzymes facing one another (in contrast to previously studied "at random" aggregates) to ascertain what possible kinetic advantage may be gained by such an arrangement.

Discussion on the Relevance of Immobilized Multi-Step Enzyme Systems as Biological Models for Naturally-Occurring Systems (Microenvironmental Compartmentation)

Although we know little about the conditions in the interior of the cell it is likely that all the factors mentioned above, including exclusion effects, exist and will affect metabolism. Even the existence of unstirred layers within the cell has been considered likely (17). Therefore, it can be assumed that also in vivo, compartmentation of metabolites in the microenvironment of enzyme aggregates takes place (and affects metabolism) even in loosely associated multi-enzyme systems which are neither segregated by membranes nor are the intermediates bound covalently as in some multi-enzyme complexes.

In this chapter I wish to mention briefly some examples of natural systems where model systems of the kind described herein have thrown some light on metabolic questions.

One example that has led to better understanding of the control of metabolism is the previously discussed model system of malate dehydrogenase/citrate synthase/lactate dehydrogenase (9). It has been said that the concentration of oxaloacetate is primarily responsible for the regulation of the rate of oxidation in the Krebs cycle. One of the problems in understanding this regulatory mechanism was that the apparent free concentration of oxaloacetate in the mitochondrial matrix is so low that the rate of its reaction in the citrate synthetase reaction would not be commensurate with the known rate of the Krebs cycle in mitochondria as estimated from O_2 utilization. If, however, the enzymes of the Krebs cycle are assembled within a matrix in organized structures, it is possible to imagine segregated metabolic pools in which a locally high substrate concentration could be maintained in the region of each enzyme's active site. This could occur in spite of a low (measured or calculated) average concentration of the substrate in the whole mitochondrion. At low malate concentrations the model system containing two sequential enzymes of the Krebs cycle was more efficient than the system of corresponding soluble enzymes, strongly suggesting that clustering of enzymes belonging to the Krebs cycle has a kinetic advantage.

Subsequent studies using mitochondria treated with increasing concentrations of digitonin (18) supported the interpretation derived from these studies of models. The loss of latency of enzymes observed as the inner membrane became permeable to substrates and acceptors, was compatible with the picture of compartmentalization of the enzymes of the Krebs cycle in the mitochondrial matrix. Recently, kinetic results in line with this interpretation have been obtained with a two-enzyme system, aspartate aminotransferase and malate dehydrogenase, which seems to constitute a natural complex (19). In this system no lag phase was observed for the overall activity, nor did any equilibration occur between the intermediate, oxaloacetate, formed and the "bulk" oxaloacetate present, indicating some kind of compartmentalization of the intermediate (20).

Another example illustrating that such "model building" is of biological significance has been demonstrated by studies of the "aromatic complex" of Neurospora crassa, an enzyme system that catalyzes five consecutive reactions in the central pathway leading to the biosynthesis of aromatic amino acids. The overall reaction catalyzed by the complex showed lags (transient times) that were shorter than for a hypothetical unaggregated system (21). It was suggested that, in addition to "channeling" of intermediates of competing pathways, reduction of the transient time is an important consequence of the confinement of intermediates within a physically associated enzyme sequence.

The previously mentioned model enzyme aggregate with juxtaposed active sites could be considered to be another kind of model for a naturally occurring enzyme cluster, i.e. tryptophane synthetase, for which a similar arrangement has been suggested.

At this point I wish to close this section. The reader is referred to a more extensive review on this subject, namely "Immobilized model systems of enzyme sequences" (22) and to a review dealing with compartmentation which includes microenvironmental aspects (23).

The Practical Utilization of Microenvironmental
Effects as Found in Immobilized Multi-Step Enzyme
Systems

There is an obvious parallel in the demands for efficiency
and regulation of metabolism in a living cell and those required for an industrial process or analytical device, where
enzymes or whole cells are often utilized as catalysts. Thus,
the results obtained and understanding gained from studies of
more theoretical nature will also be beneficial to the practical application of immobilized enzymes. In this brief paragraph
I wish to provide some examples in which immobilized, multi-
step enzyme systems of the type $A \xrightarrow{E_1} B \xrightarrow{E_2} C$ have been
utilized for practical purposes.

One of the first questions to be asked in designing an
immobilized enzyme sequence system is whether it will be advantageous to have the individual enzymes bound adjacent to
one another on a matrix, by co-immobilization, as normally
found in the cell or not. As will be seen, in many instances
such co-immobilized systems have a number of advantages; these
will be discussed in some detail below.

High overall activity. As discussed in the previous sections, arrangements of sequentially-acting enzymes on the same
matrix particles can lead to (a) a higher overall rate in the
initial phase of the reaction, if the concentration of the
intermediate is rate-limiting; (b) a "permanent", higher overall steady state rate in systems containing thermodynamically
unfavourable steps; or (c) higher overall rates if one of the
products in the enzyme sequence is recycled. An example is
given in a study carried out with the system glucose oxidase/
catalase (see scheme on page 6).

The objective of this study, at least in part, was to utilize this dual system for the production of gluconic acid (7,
24). As expected, this system, which combines both factors (a)
and (c) above, was shown to be more efficient when used as
dual system (i.e., with both enzymes co-immobilized on the same
matrix particles), as compared to preparations made up of
glucose oxidase and catalase immobilized to separate particles.

Sensitivity. The same properties, inherent in co-immobilized enzyme sequences, that give rise to higher overall rates
in the initial phase may also be utilized in analytical de-
vices. This allows a higher sensitivity at low substrate concentrations. An example is seen with the following reaction
scheme: L-aspartate $\longrightarrow$ oxaloacetate + NH_4^+; oxaloacetate +
$NADH + H^+ \longrightarrow$ malate + NAD^+. In the microassay of L-aspar-

tate, the sensitivity of the co-immobilized enzyme sequence was 10 times higher, as compared with a system with aspartate aminotransferase immobilized and malate dehydrogenase free in solution (25). Similar results were found for the determination of tryptophan using the system, tryptophanase - lactate dehydrogenase (26).

In addition, when operating in flow-systems, losses of intermediates can be reduced by arrangement of the participating enzymes on the same matrix particles. This permits higher flow rates when applied to enzyme reactor systems and higher sensitivity when used in enzyme columns designed for analytical applications. Likewise, in co-immobilized systems the risk of out-diffusion of intermediates is reduced, thereby minimizing the risk of their interaction with contaminating enzymes that may be present in the flow-stream containing the substrates.

From the examples given, it is clear that in many instances a close spatial arrangement of enzymes acting in sequence is advantageous for their practical applications, in analogy to their function in the living cell. However, it should also be mentioned that in some instances binding of the enzymes to separate matrices could be the most suitable choice, for example, if one enzyme in the sequence is particularly more unstable than the others or when the separate enzyme-catalyzed reactions require much different conditions.

Amplification. A sequentially-acting enzyme system can also be utilized to amplify signals. A two-enzyme system has been applied to thermal analysis, increasing the sensitivity, by using a device called an enzyme thermistor to amplify the heat response of the primary reaction. The amplification of the response is achieved by the heat produced by the additional step(s) per se; but, simultaneously, more rapid response and higher sensitivity at low substrate concentrations are obtained. Thus, the heat signals obtained from the reaction of glucose in an enzyme thermistor filled with co-immobilized glucose oxidase-catalase preparations were significantly higher than those obtained with immobilized glucose oxidase alone (27).

Speed of response. In addition to higher sensitivity, a more rapid response can be obtained with co-immobilized enzyme systems because a shorter time is required to reach the critical concentration at which on the system can be measured. Recently, a system discussed earlier, hexokinase - glucose-6-phosphate dehydrogenase, was co-immobilized on nylon tubing. Structuring the enzyme system led to extended linearity and more rapid glucose and ATP analysis in reagentless Technicon flow systems (28).

Enzyme systems involving coenzymes. Many enzyme-catalyzed steps of potential practical interest require the participation of expensive, dissociable coenzymes such as NAD^+. Methods for the reuse of these coenzymes, based on their retention and regeneration, have been studied extensively of late. This subject has been reviewed recently (29) and I want to restrict the discussion to one specific approach.

A special case of coenzyme regeneration is found in preparations where enzyme and coenzyme are immobilized in close proximity. One such preparation is made up of a complex of Sepharose-alcohol dehydrogenase-NAD(H). The immobilization technique was similar to that used in the co-immobilization of enzyme sequences, i.e., CNBr-activated Sepharose was added to a solution containing a binary complex of alcohol dehydrogenase-NAD(H) analog (the latter carrying a terminal NH_2-group suitable for binding, namely N^6-[(6-aminohexyl)carbamoylmethyl -NAD(H)]. Thus, preparations were obtained in which both enzyme and coenzyme are covalently bound to the matrix in such a manner that the coenzyme is located at or near the active site of the enzyme (30). Regeneration could now be accomplished by alcohol dehydrogenase using the coupled oxido-reduction between two alternative substrates, ethanol and lactaldehyde (see Fig. 6), with several thousand-fold coenzyme recycling rates per hour.

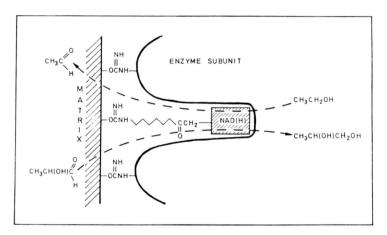

FIGURE 6.   Schematic drawing of an active alcohol dehydrogenase - NAD(H)-Sepharose complex (ref. 30).

Another special way of arranging enzyme and coenzyme in proximity is via the direct covalent coupling of the same NAD-analog onto the enzyme liver alcohol dehydrogenase, so that the normally dissociable NAD coenzyme is now bound as "prosthetic group" to the enzyme (31). This system, when assayed e.g. according to the above coupled oxido-reduction procedure, requires no externally-added coenzyme for activity (31).

CONCLUSION

In closing I wish to emphasize that even though it may be difficult or impossible to design a model system coming very close to the "real thing", model studies of the type described herein have their value. First of all they bear an important message: Whenever an understanding of metabolic sequences is attempted, one should always consider the microenvironment of the participating enzymes as they are influenced by the surrounding membrane (= matrix) or the general cellular milieu itself and/or by the proximity of the enzymes.

In addition, immobilized enzyme preparations permit the study of the influence of one single parameter at a time. Thus, it is conceivable to prepare a series of a particular immobilized two-enzyme system of varying and defined distance between the two different enzymes to obtain information on the influence of enzyme proximity on the overall rate. Another similar systematic study for which model systems appear ideal would be to prepare a series of enzyme supports of gradually changing hydrophobicity and study to what extent a hydrophobic milieu will influence the system (this has been attempted in a preliminary investigation (see ref. 32).

Furthermore, in the course of such and similar investigations related to "solid-phase biochemistry", techniques are developed or conceptual by-products obtained that are of interest for the general area of enzyme complexes. Thus, in our attempts to prepare two-enzyme aggregates with juxtaposed active sites (33) we have made use of ligands similar to those applied in affinity chromatography. I also feel that compounds of this type and other affinity material, in particular coenzyme-bearing, will be useful in the isolation of naturally occurring stable and unstable enzyme complexes. An indication that this is a realistic proposition is seen from the work in which an ATP-analogue immobilized to Sepharose as affinity matrix was successfully employed in the isolation of a cross-linked citrate synthase - malate dehydrogenase aggregate (16). Similarly, recent work using "magnetic" affinity material suggests that this method will allow quick isolation of labile complexes thus avoiding portions of their structure being "nicked off" by proteolytic enzymes which are often present in crude extracts (34). An example of a useful by-product from investigations on exclusion effects in enzyme sequences, discussed previously (13), is the demonstration of a specific interaction between citrate synthase and mitochondrial malate dehydrogenase in the presence of polyethylene glycol (35) as indicated by increased solution turbidity.

In the preparation of immobilized enzyme systems one ought, besides preparing suitable model systems, dare to go even a step further beyond those found in nature. Thus, it should be possible to construct systems comprised of totally new sequences tailored to suit practical needs, in the direction of what may be called "synthetic biochemistry". One example of such artificially changing Nature's system is the previously mentioned coupling of normally dissociable NAD^+-coenzyme, in the form of a suitable analog, to the enzyme horse liver alcohol dehydrogenase; the coenzyme is now bound directly to the enzyme as "prosthetic group" (31). Such a preparation does not require externally added NAD^+ for its activity and the coenzyme can be recycled. Through this permanent and proximal arrangement of the NAD^+ to the enzyme some advantages are obtained. For instance, the concentration of NAD^+, normally present in large excess relative to the enzyme in a free solution situation, can be reduced to equimolarity and yet give the same activity. For example in one experiment it was found that when operating at a coenzyme concentration of 25 nM, the NAD-dehydrogenase system was at least 50 times more efficient than the corresponding reference system.

ACKNOWLEDGMENTS

I wish to thank my co-workers, in particular Drs. B. Mattiasson and A.-C. Koch-Schmidt, for their collaboration in most of the work cited herein coming from this Institute. I am also obliged to Dr. P. Srere who during a sabbatical stay at this Institute and since then has pointed out to us a number of questions related to general metabolism in which model systems of the type described here may have some relevance. Supported by the Swedish Natural Science Research Council.

REFERENCES

1. Mosbach, K., and Andersson, L., in "Pyridine Nucleotide-Dependent Dehydrogenases" (H. Sund, ed.), p.173. Walter de Gruyter & Co., Berlin, New York, 1977.
2. "Immobilized Enzymes", Methods in Enzymology (K. Mosbach, ed.), vol. 44, Academic Press, New York, 1976.
3. Mosbach, K., and Mattiasson, B., Acta Chem. Scand. 24:2093 (1970).
4. Mattiasson, B., and Mosbach, K., in "Methods in Enzymology" (K. Mosbach, ed.), vol. 44, p.335. Academic Press, New York, 1976.
5. Goldman, R., and Katchalski, E., J. Theor. Biol. 32:243 (1971).
6. Gondo, S., Chem. Eng. J. 13:153 (1977).
7. Bouin, J. C., Atallah, M. T., and Hultin, H. O., Biochim. Biophys. Acta 438:23 (1976).
8. Mattiasson, B., and Mosbach, K., Biochim. Biophys. Acta 235:253 (1971).
9. Srere, P. A., Mattiasson, B., and Mosbach, K., Proc. Nat. Acad. Sci. U.S. 70:2534 (1973).
10. Gestrelius, S., Mattiasson, B., and Mosbach, K., Biochim. Biophys. Acta 276:339 (1972).
11. Hervagault, J. F., Joly, G., and Thomas, D., Eur. J. Biochem. 51:19 (1975).
12. Laurent, T. C., Eur. J. Biochem. 21:498 (1971).
13. Mattiasson, B., Johansson, A. C., and Mosbach, K., Eur. J. Biochem. 46:341 (1974).
14. Keleti, T., Batke, J., Ovadi, J., Jancsik, V., and Bartha, F., in "Advances in Enzyme Regulation" (G. Weber, ed.), vol. 15, p.233. Pergamon Press, New York, 1977.
15. Wilson, F. A., and Dietschy, J. M., Biochim. Biophys. Acta 363:112 (1974).
16. Koch-Schmidt, A. C., Mattiasson, B., and Mosbach, K., Eur. J. Biochem. 81:71 (1977).
17. Rosenberg, M., in "Symp. of Int. Soc. Cell Biol." Intracellular Transport (K. B. Warren, ed.), vol. 5, p.45. Academic Press, New York, 1966.
18. Matlib, M. A., and O'Brien, P. J., Arch. Biochem. Biophys. 167:193 (1975).
19. Backman, L., and Johannsson, G., FEBS Lett. 65:39 (1976).
20. Bryce, C., Williams, D., John, R., and Fasella, P., Biochem. J. 153:571 (1976).
21. Welch, G. R., and Gaertner, F. M., Proc. Nat. Acad. Sci. U.S. 72:4218 (1975).

22. Mosbach, K., and Mattiasson, B., "Immobilized" Model Systems of Enzyme Sequences in "Current Topics in Cellular Regulation" (L. B. Horecker and E. R. Stadtman, eds.), Academic Press, New York, in press.
23. Srere, P., and Mosbach, K., Ann. Rev. Microbiol. 28:61 (1974).
24. Hultin, H. O., J. Food Science 39:647 (1974).
25. Ikeda, S., Sumi, Y., and Fukui, S., FEBS Lett. 47:295 (1974).
26. Ikeda, S., and Fukui, S., FEBS Lett. 41:216 (1974).
27. Danielsson, B., Gadd, K., Mattiasson, B., and Mosbach, K., Clin. Chim. Acta 81:163 (1977).
28. Leon, L. P., Sansur, M., Snyder, L. R., and Horvath, C., Clin. Chem. 23, no. 9:1556 (1977).
29. Mosbach, K., in "Advances in Enzymology" (A. Meister, ed.), John Wiley, in press, 1977.
30. Gestrelius, S., Mansson, M. O., and Mosbach, K., Eur. J. Biochem. 57:529 (1975).
31. Mansson, M. O., Larsson, P. O., and Mosbach, K., Eur. J. Biochem. in press.
32. Johansson, A. C., and Mosbach, K., Biochim. Biophys. Acta 370:348 (1974).
33. Koch-Schmidt, A. C., Larsson, P. O., Mattiasson, B., and Mosbach, K., (to be published).
34. Mosbach, K., and Andersson, L., Nature 270:259 (1977).
35. Halper, L. A., and Srere, P. A., Arch. Biochem. Biophys. 184:529 (1977).

EFFECT OF DIFFUSION BARRIERS ON SOLUTE UPTAKE
INTO BIOLOGICAL SYSTEMS

John M. Dietschy[1]

Department of Internal Medicine
University of Texas Southwestern Medical School
Dallas, Texas

I. INTRODUCTION

While the importance of diffusion barriers as major resistances to the movement of solute molecules into living cells
has been recognized for many years (1,2) only relatively recently have the profound effects of these barriers on the kinetics of active and passive transport processes and solute
interactions with enzymes been fully appreciated. In the present discussion six major situations are described where the
interposition of diffusion barriers between the bulk phase of
a perfusate and the sites of interaction with the cell membrane have marked effects on the kinetics of solute uptake. A
number of other effects have been described and are reviewed
in several recent publications (3,4).

II. GENERAL EQUATIONS FOR SOLUTE MOVEMENT ACROSS DIFFUSION BARRIERS AND CELL MEMBRANES

Shown in Figure 1 is the simplest situation that might be
encountered in biologic systems where a cell membrane is perfused with a bulk solution that is well stirred throughout.
Generally, solute molecules may cross this membrane by two
types of transport mechanisms. The first of these is usually
a linear function of the concentration of the solute molecule

[1]Supported by NIH grants HL09610, AM16386 and AM19329.

Copyright © 1978 by Academic Press, Inc.
All right of reproduction in any form reserved.
ISBN 0-12-660550-5

to which the membrane is exposed. The rate of movement (J_d) of the solute molecule from the outside of the cell into the cytosolic compartment is equal to the product of the concentration of the molecule in the bulk solution (C_1) and the passive permeability coefficient (P_d) for that particular solute molecule crossing that particular membrane.

$$J_d = P_d C_1 \qquad\qquad (1)$$

The passive permeability coefficient describes the amount of solute that crosses 1 cm^2 of the cell membrane per unit time per unit concentration of the solute to which the membrane is exposed and so has units such as nmoles/$cm^2 \cdot$sec$\cdot$(nmoles/cm^3) which reduces to the conventional units used for P_d of cm/sec. When this value is multiplied by the concentration term, J_d describes the flux rate with the units of mass of solute moving across 1 cm^2 of membrane per unit time, e.g., nmoles/cm·sec.

The second type of transport that is important in the trans membrane movement of solutes involves the binding and uptake of solute molecules by a finite number of transport sites on the cell membrane. Since this type of "carrier mediated" transport involves the interaction between solute molecules and a finite number of sites, the kinetics of uptake

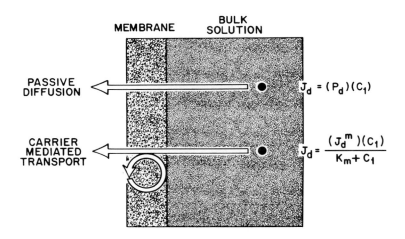

FIGURE 1. Transport of solutes across a cell membrane by passive diffusion or carrier mediated transport in the absence of diffusion barriers.

are usually described by the following relationship

$$J_d = \frac{J_d^m C_1}{K_m + C_1} \qquad (2)$$

where J_d^m is the maximal velocity of transport the system can achieve and K_m defines the concentration of the solute molecule at the aqueous-membrane interface (C_1) at which half the value of J_d^m is achieved. This equation, of course, takes the form of a rectangular hyperbole the configuration of which is defined by the two variables K_m and J_d^m.

Unfortunately, the simple situation illustrated in Figure 1 is probably never encountered in biological systems under either in vitro or in vivo conditions since the concentration of the solute molecule measurable in bulk solution perfusing a particular tissue or cell preparation is usually not the same as the concentration of the solute molecule "seen" by the cell membrane. This is true because there is usually a diffusion barrier, be it simple or complex, interposed be-between the cell surface and the bulk perfusion medium.

The simplest situation shown diagrammatically in Figure 2 involves the movement of a solute molecule from the bulk solution of the perfusate across a single cell membrane into the cytosolic compartment. However interposed between the

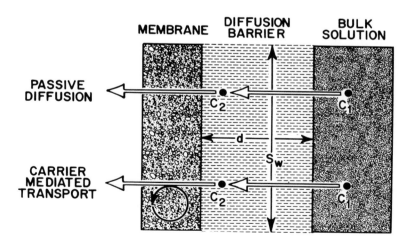

FIGURE 2. The transport of solute molecules across a diffusion barrier and cell membrane by either passive diffusion or carrier mediated transport in the presence of diffusion barriers.

bulk perfusate and the membrane surface are layers of water
which are not subject to the same gross mixing that takes
place in the bulk perfusate and through which diffusion is
the sole means for molecular movement. Obviously, there is
no sharp demarcation between such "unstirred water layers"
and the bulk solution of the perfusate: however, functional
dimensions for these layers can be experimentally measured
and such values are of critical importance in dealing with
unstirred layer effects in any membrane transport system (5-
7). Thus, in this figure C_1 and C_2 represent the concentrations of the solute in the bulk perfusate and at the aqueous-
membrane interface, respectively. S_w denotes the functional
surface area of the unstirred water layer while d equals its
functional thickness and D is the diffusion coefficient for
the specific solute. In this situation the rate of movement
of the solute molecule across the diffusion barrier is dictated by the chemical gradient between C_1 and C_2, the surface
area and thickness of the diffusion barrier and the diffusivity of the solute molecule as shown in the following equation.

$$J_d = (C_1 - C_2)\left(\frac{DS_w}{d}\right) \tag{3}$$

In this situation the rate of solute movement across the
cell membrane will be determined by C_2 rather than C_1. Thus,
the rate of movement of a solute molecule crossing the membrane by passive diffusion will be given by the following expression

$$J_d = P_d C_2 \tag{4}$$

while the rate of uptake of a molecule that is translocated
by a carrier mediated mechanism will be given by the following expression.

$$J_d = \frac{J_d^m C_2}{K_m + C_1} \tag{5}$$

In most experimental circumstances, however, the rate of
movement of a solute across a biologic membrane is related
to the concentration of that molecule in the bulk perfusing
solution. Thus, both equations 4 and 5 must be rewritten to
yield values for J_d in terms of C_1 and not C_2. The value of
C_2 under steady state conditions can be obtained by re-arrang-

ing the terms in equation 3 as shown by the following equation.

$$C_2 = C_1 - \frac{J_d\,d}{DS_w} \tag{6}$$

In this equation the term $J_d d/DS_w$ essentially represents the resistance encountered by the solute in crossing the unstirred water layer: the higher this resistance, the lower the value of C_2. This resistance term is complex, however, and is determined by the physical dimensions of the unstirred water layer (d/S_w), by the diffusivity of the solute molecule in the aqueous phase (D) and by the velocity of solute transport across the system (J_d).

In many physiological situations both *in vivo* and *in vitro* the diffusion barrier overlying a particular tissue consists essentially entirely of an unstirred water layer. This is probably the case, for example, in epithelial membranes such as intestine, gallbladder, choroid plexus and bladder and when isolated cells are studied under *in vitro* conditions. Under both *in vivo* and *in vitro* conditions the unstirred water layers overlying the surface of such epithelial membranes commonly vary in thickness from approximately 100 to 800 μM, depending upon the rate of mixing of the bulk phase, and it is seldom possible to reduce this thickness to less than 75 μM even with the most vigorous mixing that can reasonably be employed under *in vitro* conditions. On the other hand, the thickness of unstirred water layers surrounding individual cells suspended in an incubation medium is probably considerably less than 10 to 20 μM (5-9).

In any event, equations 4 and 5 can be rewritten to give values for J_d as a function of C_1 by substituting the value of C_2 as given in equation 6 into these two expressions. Thus, under the conditions shown diagrammatically in Figure 2 the rate of passive diffusion of a solute molecule from the bulk solution into the cytosolic compartment is given by the following expression.

$$J_d = \frac{P_d\,C_1}{1 + P_d\left(\frac{d}{DS_w}\right)} \tag{7}$$

Similarly, for a solute molecule that is translocated across the cell membrane by a carrier mediated process the rate of uptake is described by the following quadratic expression.

$$J_d = (0.5)\frac{DS_w}{d}\left[C_1+K_m+J_d^m\frac{d}{DS_w}\pm\sqrt{\left(C_1+K_m+J_d^m\left(\frac{d}{DS_w}\right)\right)^2-4\,C_1\,J_d^m\left(\frac{d}{DS_w}\right)}\,\right] \quad (8)$$

Thus, it is apparent from these two latter equations that the rates of uptake of solute molecules into cells may be influenced as much by the resistance of the diffusion barrier, as given by the term (d/DS_w), as by the terms that define the membrane transport processes, i.e., P_d, K_m and J_d^m.

III. EFFECT OF DIFFUSION BARRIERS ON THE CELLULAR UPTAKE OF PASSIVELY ABSORBED SOLUTES

Equation 7 shows the rate of passive solute absorption in the presence of a diffusion barrier between the bulk solu-

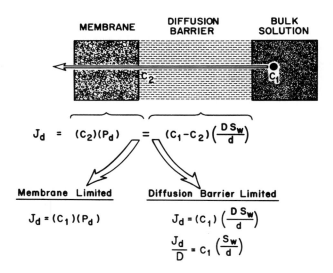

FIGURE 3. The two extreme situations encountered in biological systems during solute movement from the bulk perfusate to the cell interior. The first set of equations describe the rates of movement of the solute across the membrane and diffusion barrier. The left equation applies to the situation when the rate of membrane penetration is totally rate limiting to solute uptake while the right equation is applicable to the situation where the diffusion barrier is totally rate limiting to solute uptake.

tion and the cell membrane. It is apparent from this equation that two extreme situations may be encountered in biological systems: either the cell membrane itself or the unstirred water layer may be overwhelmingly rate limiting to uptake of a particular solute molecule. Stated in a different way in these two extreme situations the major resistance to solute movement into the cell may be either the resistance encountered by the molecule in crossing the cell membrane (which equals $1/P_d$) or the resistance the molecule encounters in crossing the unstirred water layer (which equals d/DS_w).

These two extreme situations and the equations that apply in each of these conditions are shown diagrammatically in Figure 3. Under circumstances where the concentration of the solute molecule inside the cell is set at zero, the overall rate of movement of the molecule from the bulk solution into the cell is determined by both the rate of movement of the molecule across the diffusion barrier (equation 3) and across the cell membrane (equation 4). If the rate of movement of the solute molecule across the diffusion barrier is very rapid relative to its rate of movement across the cell membrane, i.e., if the term DS_w/d is very much larger than P_d, then the resistance of the diffusion barrier is negligible and the rate of molecular penetration through the cell membrane becomes totally rate limiting to cellular uptake. In this extreme situation where solute uptake is totally determined by the membrane resistance the rate of uptake is given by equation 1. In the other extreme situation the rate of movement of a solute molecule may be very much faster through the cell membrane than across the diffusion barrier, i.e., P_d is very much larger than the term DS_w/d. In this situation the rate of solute movement across the diffusion barrier becomes totally rate limiting to cellular uptake, C_2 equals essentially zero and the rate of solute uptake becomes equal to the product of C_1 and DS_w/d. As also shown in Figure 3, in this circumstance where solute uptake into the cell is diffusion limited the quantity J_d/D becomes proportional to C_1 times S_w/d so that in the presence of a given diffusion barrier resistance the rate of uptake of a series of solute molecules is inversely proportional to their free diffusion coefficients.

These two extreme situations as well as the intermediate condition where both the diffusion barrier and membrane resistances influence uptake rates are shown diagrammatically in Figure 4. In this example the rates of cellular uptake of a homologous series of saturated fatty acids are shown in the presence of a diffusion barrier of varying resistance. The logarithm of the value of J_d/D is plotted as a function of fatty acid chain length. Assuming that C_1 for each fatty acid is the same, curve A represents the extreme situation where diffusion barrier resistance is infinitely low and, therefore, negligible. In this situation J_d is principally determined by the passive permeability coefficient for each fatty acid so that the term ln J_d/D increases as an essentially linear function of the fatty acid chain length (the passive permeability coefficients for a homologous series of fatty acids increase as a log linear function of chain length). However, there is significant deviation from this behavior as the diffusion barrier begins to exert a finite resistance. In the first example, curve B, fatty acids with two to eight carbon atoms have such low passive permeability coefficients that membrane permeation is still totally rate limiting and the value of ln J_d/D still falls on the linear portion of the curve (the segment of line B to the left of point x). In contrast, passive permeability coefficients for the longer chain length fatty acids with 18, 20 and 22 carbon atoms are so high that uptake becomes totally diffusion limited. In this situation the term J_d/D reaches a constant and limiting value dictated by S_w/d (the portion of curve B to the right of point y). The portion of curve B between points x and y delineate those fatty acids where the unstirred water layer and cell membrane both contribute in determining the rates of cellular fatty acid uptake. When a

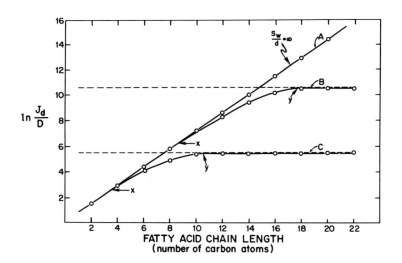

FIGURE 4. Diagrammatic representation of the uptake of a homologous series of saturated fatty acids under circumstances where there is no diffusion barrier resistance (curve A) or where this barrier exerts a modest (curve B) or high (curve C) degree of resistance to molecular diffusion.

diffusion barrier of even greater resistance is introduced in front of the membrane then, as shown by curve C, the diffusion barrier becomes totally rate limiting to cellular uptake for all fatty acids greater than 10 carbon atoms. The important principle illustrated by the data in Figure 4 is that the higher the passive permeability coefficient for a particular solute molecule the more likely the diffusion barriers, rather than the cell membrane, will be rate limiting to monomolecular uptake.

This recognition that either the cell membrane or the diffusion barriers outside of the cell may be rate limiting to uptake of various solute molecules has important implications with respect to the interpretation of temperature effects on the transmembrane movement of solutes. In general, in the past the passive monomolecular diffusion of a solute across the biological membrane has been assumed to have a low Q_{10} value and a correspondingly low activation energy. Furthermore, in some instances an abrupt change in apparent activation energy has been found when the temperature is lowered and this effect has been attributed to a temperature-related phase change in the lipid molecules making up the structure of the cell membrane. Such behavior is illustrated by the "experimental curve" shown in the right panel of Figure 5. At the higher temperatures the slope of the line is shallow corresponding to a change in the rate of

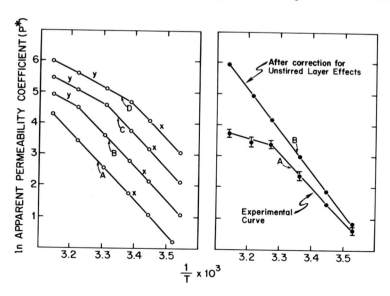

FIGURE 5. Effect of diffusion barriers on apparent activation energies and on apparent transition temperatures.

solute uptake of approximately 1.2 for each 10°C change in
temperature (an activation energy of only about 2800 cal/
mol). As the temperature is lowered, however, a "transition" point is apparently reached below which the line ac-
quires a steeper slope that may correspond to a Q_{10} value
varying from 2.0 to 4.0 and to activation energies varying
from approximately 10,000 to 21,000 cal/mol. However, when
such data are corrected for diffusion barrier effects (curve
B), the "transition" point disappears and a single linear regression curve is produced that has a steep slope corresponding to a high activation energy for the passive penetration
of this solute across the cell membrane (10). Data such as
these suggest that in many instances both the low activation
energies and the apparent transition points reported for
passive solute uptake across biological membranes are artifacts due to failure to recognize that the uptake of the
solute is diffusion limited at physiological temperatures.
Thus, at higher temperatures the Q_{10} value simply reflects
the low activation energy for the diffusion of the solute
through the aqueous environment of the unstirred water layers. As the temperature is decreased, a point is reached
at which penetration through the cell membrane, rather than
through the diffusion barrier, becomes rate limiting and the
apparent activation energy abruptly increases. Thus, the
"transition" point in the right panel of Figure 5 actually
corresponds to the point where the major resistance to molecular uptake of solute shifts from the diffusion barrier to
the cell membrane (10).
       Since the resistance encountered by a solute in cross-
ing the diffusion barrier also is a function of the passive
permeability coefficient of that molecule it follows that
the apparent "transition" temperature seen in a given membrane should vary inversely with the P_d value for a series
of solute molecules. Such a situation is illustrated by the
series of curves shown in the left panel of Figure 5. Curve
A represents the situation encountered for a compound having such a low passive permeability coefficient that the
cell membrane is rate limiting to uptake at all temperatures. As solutes with progressively higher P_d values are
tested, however, an apparent transition point is seen (the
change in slope between the line segments labeled x and y).
This apparent "transition" temperature is not constant, however, but occurs at a progressively lower temperature for
each more permeant solute tested. In each case, correction
for unstirred water layer resistance would eliminate this
transition point and yield curves reflecting the true activation energies for the passive penetration of these solutes
through this particular biological membrane (10). Thus,

these data illustrate a second major point: the presence of significant diffusion barriers outside of a cell membrane leads to underestimation of values for the activation energy of the uptake process and may lead to the erroneous conclusion that phase transitions in the lipid structure of the membrane significantly alters the rate of uptake of solute molecules across the membrane.

IV. EFFECT OF DIFFUSION BARRIERS ON THE KINETICS OF CARRIER MEDIATED TRANSPORT

Often the relationship between the concentration of the solute molecule in the bulk perfusate and the rate of carrier mediated uptake of that solute (or the interaction of the solute with an enzyme) is described in terms of equation 2. This equation takes the form of a rectangular hyperbole that can be defined in terms of two variables, J_d^m and K_m. It is possible by several different mathematical manipulations to convert such hyperbolic curves into a linear form from which direct estimations of K_m and J_d^m can be made. However, in almost all biologic systems a diffusion barrier resistance is interposed between the bulk perfusate and the cell membrane so that equation 8 rather than equation 2 must be utilized to define the relationship between J_d and the concentration of the solute molecule in the bulk phase, C_1. The interposition of these diffusion barriers between the membrane and the bulk perfusate has very important consequences with respect to the kinetics of such carrier mediated processes.

For example, as shown in the left panel of Figure 6, in the absence of the diffusion barrier the relationship between J_d and C_1 is described by equation 2 and takes the form of the rectangular hyperbole shown as curve A. When replotted in the double reciprocal form (right panel) such a curve becomes linear and has an intercept on the vertical axis that equals $1/J_d^m$. However, when a diffusion barrier is present over the transport sites then equation 8 describes the relationship between J_d and C_1 and this equation yields a curve such as example B in the left panel of Figure 6. Since this equation does not take the form of a rectangular hyperbole, plotting these data in the double reciprocal form does not transform curve B into a straight line: rather, as seen in the right panel the curve turns sharply upward as it approaches the vertical axis to intercept at $1/J_d^m$. However, if as is commonly done, the experimental points are used to construct a linear regression curve and this curve is extra-

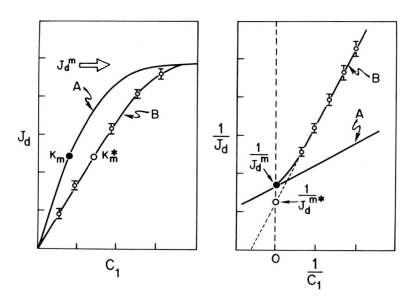

FIGURE 6. Effect of diffusion barriers on the kinetics
of a carrier mediated transport system. Curve A is derived
from equation 2 when no diffusion barrier is present. Curve
B is derived from equation 8 when significant diffusion barrier resistance is present in the experimental system.

polated to the vertical axis (dashed line) then an artifactually high value for J_d^m will be obtained. Thus, if it is experimentally difficult to directly measure the maximal transport rate for a particular transport system (because, for
example, of limited solubility of the solute) then estimation of this value from double reciprocal plots will lead
to an artifactually high value for J_d^m if a diffusion barrier
is interposed between the bulk solution and the transport
sites (11,12).
    Another important consequence of the introduction of
diffusion barriers in front of sites of carrier mediated
solute transport is illustrated by the series of curves in
the left panel of Figure 7. In this figure the resistance
of the diffusion barrier is increased 500 fold in going from
curve A to curve D. As is apparent as the resistance of the
unstirred layer is progressively increased, i.e., as the value of the d/DS_w term is increased in equation 8, the "saturable" appearance of the kinetic curve is lost and the rate
of solute uptake becomes essentially a linear function of
the concentration of the molecule in the bulk phase, C_1.

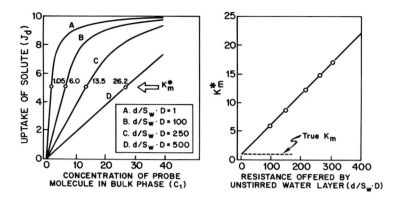

FIGURE 7. The effect of diffusion barriers on the apparent K_m values for a carrier mediated transport system. In this illustration the true K_m value for the transport system was assumed to equal 1.0 concentration units. Curves A, B, C and D illustrate the effects of increasing the diffusion barrier resistance, as given by the term d/S_wD, 500 fold. The curve in the right panel shows the relationship between the apparent K_m value, K_m^*, and the diffusion barrier resistance and is derived from equation 9.

Thus, in the presence of a major diffusion barrier such apparently linear kinetics are to be anticipated and should not be construed as evidence against the possibility that the uptake process involves translocation by a finite number of transport sites on a given membrane.

Thirdly, the presence of significant diffusion barriers leads to gross overestimation of true K_m values for a carrier mediated transport process. This effect also is shown diagrammatically in the left panel of Figure 7 where the true K_m value for the system is assumed to equal 1.0 concentration units. As is apparent, as the resistance of the diffusion barrier is increased over a 500 fold range the apparent K_m value (K_m^*) increases from 1.0 to 26.2 concentration units. In fact, as shown in the right panel of Figure 7, under these circumstances the apparent K_m value increases linearly with the resistance of the overlying diffusion barrier as given by the following equation.

$$K_m^* = K_m + 0.5 \ J_d^m \left(\frac{d}{DS_w} \right) \tag{9}$$

Stated in a different way, if no diffusion barrier were present then this transport system would achieve 80% of the maximal transport rate at a solute concentration of 4 units. In the presence of a high resistance barrier (curve D), the solute would have to be raised to 45 concentration units in the bulk perfusate to attain the same rate of transport.

Finally, in the presence of a significant diffusion resistance the apparent K_m value becomes a dependent variable of the maximal transport velocity. This effect is illustrated by the series of curves shown in Figure 8. As seen in the left panel, under circumstances where the diffusion barrier resistance is low increasing the value of J_d^m 10 fold has only a minimum effect in increasing the apparent K_m value from the true value of 1.0 to 1.2 concentration units. However, a similar increase in J_d^m under circumstances where the diffusion barrier resistance is increased 50 fold (right panel) results in an increase in K_m^* to 9.3 concentration units (12). Thus, as can be seen in equation 9, since the J_d^m term makes up a portion of the total diffusion barrier resistance term, the apparent K_m value for a carrier mediated transport process varies directly with J_d^m.

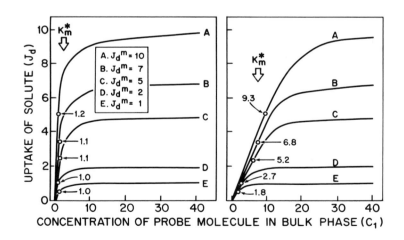

FIGURE 8. The effect of variation in the maximal transport rate of a carrier mediated transport system on the apparent K_m values in the presence of a diffusion barrier of low resistance (left panel) and high resistance (right panel). In this illustration the true K_m for the transport process is set equal to 1.0 concentration units.

V. CONCLUSIONS

In almost all biological systems studied either in vitro or in vivo significant diffusion barriers are interposed between the bulk solution perfusing a given tissue and the cell membranes. Such diffusion barriers may become totally rate limiting to solute uptake, may lead to gross underestimations of passive permeability coefficients and activation energies and may cause marked overestimations of K_m and J_d^m values. Thus, reliable values for these various transport parameters can be obtained only if appropriate corrections are made for diffusion barrier resistance in a particular experimental setting based upon independent experimental measurements of d, S_w and D.

REFERENCES

1. Collander, R., and Barlund, H., Acta. Botanica. Fennica. 11:5 (1932).
2. Dainty, J., Adv. Bot. Res. 1:279 (1963).
3. Dietschy, J.M., Chapter 1 in "Disturbances in Lipid and Lipoprotein Metabolism" (J.M. Dietschy, A.M. Gotto, and J.A. Ontko, eds.), American Physiological Society, Bethesda, 1978.
4. Winne, D. In "Intestinal Permeation" p. 58. Amsterdam-Oxford. Excerpta Medica, 1977.
5. Diamond, J.M., J. Physiol. 183:83 (1966).
6. Westergaard, H., and Dietschy, J.M., J. Clin. Invest. 54:718 (1974).
7. Wilson, F.A., and Dietschy, J.M., Biochim. Biophys. Acta. 363:112 (1974).
8. Sherrill, B.C., and Dietschy, J.M., J. Membrane Biol. 23:367 (1975).
9. Sha'afi, R.I., Rich, G.T., Sidel, V.W., Bossert, W., and Solomon, A.K., J. Gen. Physiol. 50:1377 (1967).
10. Bindslev, N., and Wright, E.M., J. Membrane Biol. 29:265 (1976).
11. Winne, D., Biochim. Biophys. Acta. 298:27 (1973).
12. Thomson, A.B.R., and Dietschy, J.M., J. theor. Biol. 64:277 (1977).

DISCUSSION

S. BESSMAN: I think this is a wonderful presentation because
it is so important to this whole issue. I would like to
point out two different situations where this is critical in
a biological system. We are trying to measure tissue PO_2 with
an ordinary oxygen electrode lying in a solution of water. It
reads nothing until you stir it. Now we see this in our
polarographic work all the time. An unstirred polarographic
system is not worth a darn. It can't read oxygen and yet even
when stirred the diffusion of the gas limits its measurement.
This is a very critical issue when considering the measurement of enzyme activity. The second place which is even more
interesting biologically is the thing that we have forgotten
over and over again and that is, if you raise the blood sugar
of a mammal to over 700 mg per cent then insulin has no effect
on transporting that material across the cell membrane. That
indicates that it is diffusion limited and that over 700 mg
you have enough gradient so that the membrane is no longer
a limiting issue.

J. DIETSCHY: You can study unstirred layer effects very
nicely using a pH electrode if you measure the transient as
a function of the degree of stirring. You can do the same
with the oxygen electrode. That is one of the ways in which
these things can be explored.

R. WELCH: I would like to echo further the importance of the
unstirred layers for in vivo transport within the cell itself.
One aspect which you did not treat in detail and which in-
fluences the diffusion layer is that of electrical effects.
Of course, most (if not all) biological membranes are charged
in some polyelectrolytic fashion. The so-called Gouy-Chapman
electrical double layer [e.g., M. N. Jones, "Biological
Interfaces", Elsevier, New York, 1975] can dramatically
alter the nature of the diffusion layer and can affect the
transport of material into or out of membrane interfaces
[e.g., Shuler, M.L., Aris, R. and Tsuchiya, H. M., J. Theor.
Biol. 35, 67 (1972)]. Moreover, DeSimone [J. Theor. Biol.
68, 225 (1977)] has shown recently that if a membrane interface contains enzymes, the enzymatic activity itself can
"reach out" into the solution and alter diffusion layers.
Also, the whole question of the nature of intracellular water
and how it is structured at membrane interfaces may be very
important to the topic of microenvironmental effects. It
is suggested by some that 10-20% of all the intracellular
water is, indeed, in the form of lattice-like unstirred layers
[Walter, J. A. and Hope, A. B., Prog. Biophys. Mol. Biol.

23, 1 (1971)]. Some electron spin resonance studies suggest
that water-soluble molecules in vivo spend a significant
portion of their time diffusing in two dimensions (i.e.,
along the surface of membranes) [Keith, A. D. and Snipes, W.,
Science, N.Y. **183**, 666 (1974)]. -- Now, I would like to pose
a question concerning the nature of these transport carriers,
or diffusion channels, in the cell membrane. Is it thought
that these entities exist more or less homogeneously throughout the entire outer cell membrane, or are they thought to
exist as localized patches?

J. DIETSCHY: Now, are we talking about carrier mediated
transport systems? Whether these are patches or whether they
are uniformly distributed or not I don't know. For the kinds
of transport systems that most transport physiologists work
with, that is those for amino acids and glucose etc., I don't
believe there is any data at all about that. I invite any
comments from the audience as to whether these are patches
or whether they are uniformly distributed as an array over
the entire cell surface. Many cells are highly polarized,
such as the intestinal cells, where there are certain transport systems on the brush border that are not on the lateral
margin. But I do not know whether they are congregated
together in a given area. I have not seen any data on that.

R. WELCH: My reason for asking is related to the following.
Smeach and Gold [J. Theor. Biol. **51**, 59, 79 (1975)] did a
study using, not a deterministic-type of diffusion equation
like yours, but rather a stochastic master-equation type of
diffusion process. The system was modeled as an enzymatic
process, having K_m and V_{max}. They assumed there was a finite
number of such "molecular channels" throughout the membrane.
The previous authors found that, even though the penetrating
substrate might be present in saturating quantity, there
would be persistent local fluctuations in the supply of product. They argued that, if the transport "channels" were
dispersed completely homogeneously in the membrane envelope,
this would raise very important questions in the overall
economy of cellular metabolism, particularly in a larger
eukaryotic cell (which is not a well-mixed volume).

J. DIETSCHY: Well, I think you are talking about a kind of
facilitated diffusion which is supposed to have saturation
kinetics and which is nonenergy linked and does not transport
against gradients. Concepts I think are changing widely
over the past few years as to what is really going on. The
concept that there are water channels in membranes has now
largely disappeared. There are four kinds of transport,

that in an anatomic sense you have to differentiate. There
is passive diffusion through tight junctions. If you are
dealing with epithelial membrane where you have cells attached
together by junctional complexes there are small molecular
weight polar molecules that clearly diffuse between the
cells. That is one kind, but that is strictly limited by
molecular size or radius. That is important for certain
molecules, but it is relatively unimportant in terms of the
whole spectrum of molecules. Second. There is carrier
mediated, energy linked or active transport. Third there is
facilitated diffusion which appears saturable, carrier mediated but unable to transport against a gradient. Then there
is this vast array of molecules which penetrate directly
through the substance of the membrane. It is now clear that
even small molecular weight passive permeation goes directly
through the lipid membrane. The thermodynamics of this are
fairly well worked out and it has to do with the displacement of chains of the hydrocarbon of the cholesterol molecules. There is an extensive amount of data in all kinds
of membranes about what are the determinants of these
passive permeation rates. The feeling is that this is
really in fact direct penetration through the membrane
and that these membranes behave as polar structures.

J. REEVES: As I understand it, the influence of the unstirred water layer diminishes as the size of the cell diminishes.

J. DIETSCHY: Yes, it probably has to. There are direct
measurements now to support this.

J. REEVES: Many of the earlier experiments with breaks in
the Arrhenius plot were first demonstrated in bacteria.

J. DIETSCHY: Yes, I am not saying that all of these effects
will disappear, but certainly the flat surface epithelial
breaks disappear. But you are perfectly right. Let me say
that in flat sheets of cells and in complex tissues, like
diaphragm of the rat, epidydimal fat pads, any epithelial surface, the unstirred layers are of the order of
50 to 400 micrometers thick, depending upon how much stirring
you have going on in the system. As soon as you look at
the isolated adipocyte or the red cell where there are very
good indirect data, it suggests that the unstirred layers
are less than 10 micrometers. Under those circumstances they
exert relatively little resistance. It is there, but it
increases the conductance term so you can still get an effect.

INTERACTION OF CITRATE SYNTHASE
AND MALATE DEHYDROGENASE[1]

Paul A. Srere
Laura A. Halper
Mary B. Finkelstein

Veterans Administration Hospital
and Department of Biochemistry
University of Texas Health Science Center
Dallas, Texas

I have postulated earlier that the Krebs cycle enzymes exist within the matrix of the mitochondrion as a multienzyme complex next to or on the inner surface of the inner membrane (1,2). The advantage of such an arrangement is obvious in terms of being able to maintain a high flux of substrates through the cycle with a relatively small number of inter- mediate molecules (i.e. a small average compartmental con- centration) whose apparent concentration in the cycle micro- environment would be high. The postulate was advanced based upon calculations of citrate synthase activity compared to cycle flux, consideration of the comparative morphology and enzymology of mitochondria, and calculations of Krebs cycle enzymes' concentrations. Although these considerations centered mainly on data concerning citrate synthase, it is apparent that a similar argument could be made for other enzymes of the cycle. For instance, the flux through the cycle in rat liver is about 1 μmole of C_2 unit oxidized per gram wet weight of tissues per minute and the Vmax of α-ketoglutarate dehydrogenase complex is also 1 μmole per minute per gram wet weight of tissue. Thus either the complex is completely saturated with all its substrates, a situation which seems to me to be unlikely, or a micro- environment exists around this complex.

[1]Supported by grants from the Veterans Administration and the United States Public Health Service.

Copyright © 1978 by Academic Press, Inc.
All right of reproduction in any form reserved.
ISBN 0-12-660550-5

It is known that succinate dehydrogenase is part of the inner membrane and the two keto acid dehydrogenase complexes are partially bound to the inner membrane. The outer Krebs cycle enzymes apparently are easily released from the matrix space with no apparent binding between them. Nonetheless, we have attempted to investigate the possibility of Krebs cycle enzyme complexes in a more systematic way.

First, however, I want to discuss the possibility that the kinetic data on pure citrate synthase (which were used to generate the paradox) are not relevant to the kinetic constants of the enzyme in situ. The objection might be raised that during the purification of the enzyme its activity site was altered to yield an enzyme with different kinetic constants. In order to test this we have examined

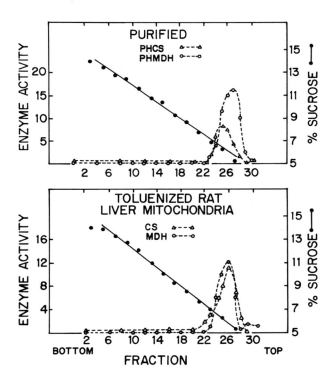

Fig. 1.   5-15% sucrose density gradient ultracentrifugation of (upper) purified pig heart citrate synthase and malate dehydrogenase and (lower) matrix extract of rat liver mitochondria.   SW 50.1 rotor 40,000 rpm, 18° C, 3 hrs in 25 mM Tris-Cl pH 7.4 (Δ··Δ··Δ citrate synthase; o-o-o malate dehydrogenase).

the kinetic constants of citrate synthase of rat liver mitochondria in situ. The results indicated that for oxalacetate there is no change in Km nor is there a change in the apparent Vmax[2]. An increase in the Km for acetyl CoA was found, but this is probably due to a diffusion problem and would in any case exacerbate the original problem.

We and others have observed that in the purification of citrate synthase one of the most difficult contaminating enzyme activities to remove is malate dehydrogenase (3,4). Since a logical Krebs cycle "particle" would include such an interaction, we felt that based on this purification observation, the citrate synthase-malate dehydrogenase system would be a good starting point for trying to demonstrate the existence of a Krebs cycle complex.

Several techniques have been used by us to investigate a possible interaction between citrate synthase and malate dehydrogenase. Commercial preparations of pig heart citrate synthase and pig heart mitochondrial malate dehydrogenase were used in these studies. Our first experiments (with Dr. E. G. Richards) were analytical ultracentrifugations of the enzymes singly, together, in the presence and absence of substrates and at enzyme concentrations which corresponded to their in vivo concentrations. No evidence for an interaction was found as judged from the fact that no species with an increased sedimentation coefficient was observed.

Since it was possible that other components of the mitochondrial matrix were involved in the interaction, we next used concentrated extracts of mitochondrial matrix for our studies. The first technique we employed was sucrose gradient centrifugation of matrix extracts.

Purified marker enzymes were sedimented, singly and together, simultaneously with the matrix extract under a variety of conditions: 5° C and 18° C, 10-40% and 5-20% gradients, 25 mM buffer and isotonic buffer, and 1.5 hrs to 18 hrs centrifugation time. There was no stable demonstrable interaction between CS and MDH (Fig. 1). The enzymatic activities in the matrix sedimented no faster than those of purified CS and MDH, whether sedimented separately or together. If a heavier species of either or both activities existed, either a second, heavier peak of activity would have been shown, or the existence of enzymatic activity in the resuspended pellet would have been found. Under all conditions, the activities of both enzymes were essentially quantitatively recovered in the peaks shown.

[2]Matlib, M.A., Finkelstein, M.B. and Srere, P.A. Unpublished data.

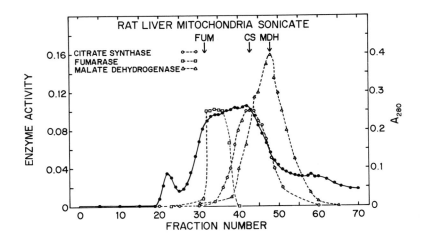

Fig. 2. Biogel P-300 gel filtration of matrix extract
of rat liver mitochondria in 0. 1 M NaCl, 0.05 M potassium
phosphate pH 7.4, 25° C. Arrows indicate elution positions
of purified marker enzymes from the same column under
identical conditions. (o---o, citrate synthase; Δ --Δ, malate
dehydrogenase; □ --□ fumarase; ●--●, A_{280}).

Possible associations of the matrix enzymes were then
examined by gel filtration. Figure 2 shows a representative
elution pattern of mitochondrial matrix extract from Biogel
P-300. The enzyme activities contained in the matrix eluted
at precisely the same volume as did the purified enzymes
filtered on a separate occasion under identical conditions.
No indication of an enzymatically active species in a higher
molecular weight region was evident under any condition of
ionic strength or gel composition studied.

We have also centrifuged inside-out vesicles of mitochondrial inner membrane through a solution of mitochondrial
matrix enzymes[3]. The amount of the enzymes which sedimented
with the vesicles was small and could have been due to
inclusions in the vesicle pellet volume. We have found
about 6% of the citrate synthase sedimenting with the membrane fraction of freeze-thawed mitoplasts[4]. This amount,
which could not be due simply to the water trapped in the
volume of the pellet, is not yet sufficient evidence to
indicate specific binding.

[3]Matlib, M.A. and Srere, P.A. Unpublished results.
[4]Henslee, J. and Srere, P.A. Unpublished results

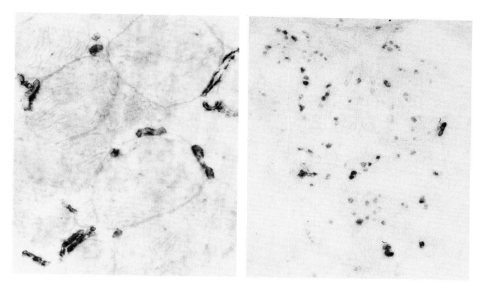

Fig. 3. (Left) Control showing heavy deposits in sar-
coplasmic reticulum. Note lack of reaction in mitochondria
(x 25,000). (Right) Experimental showing reaction products
of citrate synthase activity in the mitochondrial cristae
(x 38,750). Both unstained.

We have also carried out a series of studies on the
histological examination of mitochondria to see whether or
not citrate synthase activity was located on the inner surface of inner membranes of the mitochondria. Using a method
specific for SH groups we were able to show an oxalacetate-
dependent appearance of precipitate on the inner surface of
the inner membrane (Fig. 3) (5). In a series of experiments
using ferritin labeled citrate synthase antibody, non-specific interaction with the plastic embedding material made
definite location of the enzyme difficult. These experiments will be repeated with non-embedded frozen sections
of mitochondria.

The recent work of Bryce et al. (6) showed that the
coupled enzyme system of mitochondrial transaminase and
mitochondrial malate dehydrogenase behaved kinetically as
if the oxalacetate was passed directly from the transaminase
to malate dehydrogenase, yet no physical evidence of their
interaction could be demonstrated. The techniques used were
gel filtration and sucrose gradient centrifugation similar
to the ones reported above. At about the same time Backman
and Johannson (7) reported that when the partitioning of

mitochondrial transaminase and mitochondrial malate dehydrogenase were examined by counter current distribution in
a biphasic mixture of H_2O, dextran and carboxymethyl polyethylene glycol, a definite interaction could be demonstrated. If either enzyme were substituted for with its
cytosolic isozyme, no interaction could be detected. This
gave a physical basis for the observation of Bryce et al.
(6). Interaction between the two enzymes apparently was
weak in aqueous media but could be physically demonstrated
in a medium that more closely resembled "cell sap" as
earlier postulated by Ogston (8).

     Following this lead, we chose to examine the physical
relationship between citrate synthase and mitochondrial
malate dehydrogenase. Our assay system was to follow
the precipitation of an enzyme in polyethylene glycol as
influenced by the presence of other proteins. Under these
conditions, the addition of increasing amounts of mitochondrial malate dehydrogenase to a fixed amount of citrate
synthase results in a nearly linear increase in the
optical density of the solution (Table I). That this
effect represents an interaction between the two enzymes
is shown by the analysis of enzyme activities which are
found in the precipitate (Table II). Similar results are
obtained if the concentration of malate dehydrogenase is
fixed and the concentration of citrate synthase is varied
(Table III). The specificity of this interaction is
indicated by the fact that no precipitate forms when
mitochondrial malate dehydrogenase is replaced by cytosolic
malate dehydrogenase or bovine serum albumin (Table II).

TABLE I.   The Effect of Addition of Mitochondrial Malate
           Dehydrogenase to a Constant Concentration
                   of Citrate Synthase[a]

Concentration of malate dehydrogenase (mg/ml)	O.D. at 650 nm
0.00	0.020
0.10	0.085
0.20	0.230
0.40	0.400

[a]Samples contained 0.2 mg/ml citrate synthase, 2.0 μmoles
of potassium phosphate buffer, pH 7.0, and 14% polyethylene glycol (w/v) in a total volume of 0.4 ml.
Optical density measurments were taken after the
samples had been incubated at 10° C for one hour.

TABLE II.   Precipitation of Enzymes from Polyethylene Glycol Solution[a]

m-MDH	c-MDH	BSA	CS		m-MDH	c-MDH	CS
80	--	--	--		3[d]	-	-
--	80	--	--		-	3[d]	-
--	--	--	40		-	-	4[d]
80	--	--	40		26	-	13
--	80	--	40		-	0	2[d]
--	--	80	40		-	-	5[d]

Protein[b] present in sample (µg) — Protein[c] present in pellet (µg)

[a] Samples were incubated as described in Table I, then were centrifuged at 10° C at 20,000 x g

[b] Protein concentrations were determined by fluorescamine assay.

[c] The amount of precipitated protein was determined by enzymatic assay.

[d] This small amount of protein may represent some contamination of the pellet with the supernatant solution.

TABLE III.   The Effect of Addition of Citrate Synthase to a Constant Concentration of Mitochondrial Malate Dehydrogenase[a]

Concentration of citrate synthase (mg/ml)	O.D. at 650 nm
0.00	0.010
0.10	0.140
0.20	0.320
0.40	0.580

[a] Samples contained 0.2 mg/ml mitochondrial malate dehydrogenase. 2.0 µmoles of potassium phosphate buffer, pH 7.0, and 14% polyethylene glycol (w/v) in a total volume of 0.4 ml.   Incubation conditions were as given in Table I.

Experiments with eight other enzymes showed no specific
interaction with either enzymes, although citrate synthase
from *Escherichia coli* could replace the pig heart enzyme in
the interaction with pig heart mitochondrial malate dehydrogenase. These data only suggest that a complex between
citrate synthase and malate dehydrogenase may exist in the
mitochondrion. Specificity of interaction has been shown
in vitro however, and further experiments with other Krebs
cycle enzymes are in progress.

REFERENCES

1. Srere, P.A.   (1972) in "Energy Metabolism and the
    Regulation of Metabolic Processes in Mitochondria"
    (M. Mehlman and R.W. Hanson, eds.), pp 79-91, Academic
    Press, New York.
2. Srere, P.A. (1976), in "Gluconeogenesis: Its Regulation
    in Mammalian Species" (R.W. Hanson and W.A. Mehlman,
    eds) pp 153-161, John Wiley and Sons, New York.
3. Srere, P.A. and G.W. Kosicke, (1961). J. Biol. Chem.
    236,2557.
4. Loffler, G. and O. Wieland. (1963). Biochem. Z. 336,447.
5. Matlib, M.A., W.A. Shannon, Jr., and P.A. Srere, An
    attempt at the cytochemical localization of citrate
    synthase in rat heart muscle. 34th Annual Proceedings
    of Electron Microscopy Society of America, Miami Beach,
    Fla. 1976. (G.W. Bailey, ed).
6. Bryce, C.F.A., C.C. Williams, R.A. John, and P. Fasella,
    (1976) Biochem. J. 153,571-577.
7. Backman, I. and G. Johannson. (1976). FEBS Lett 65,39-43.
8. Ogston, A.G. (1962). Arch. Biochem. Biophys. Suppl.
    pp 39-51.

DISCUSSION

M. JONES: Do the kinetic constants change for the enzyme complex in the precipitate?

P. SRERE: You can't measure the kinetics of the precipitate. As soon as you change the concentration of the enzymes they start going back into solution and you can't get a measure of kinetics with a mixture of soluble enzyme and precipitated enzymes.

M. JONES: There might be a change or a tendency to change.

P. SRERE: There are some changes because we know from earlier experiments that polyethylene glycol has an effect, but it doesn't change more than 20% for the soluble enzyme. We don't know what could happen with the precipitate.

S. BESSMAN: If we look at the evolutionary significance of this kind of a thing, organ systems did develop in this way or they resulted in this. The question is what was the advantage? Was the advantage to be gained from an increase in rate or was it in conservation of substrate. I think this is the key to understand these compartments. We have to think about it not in terms of how fast we can make it go but whether it gets lost. I think it would be very interesting if you could repeat your experiments on kinetics of the reaction with the swollen mitochondria to see if you could insert between OAA and malate a dilution of one of the intermediates. In other words, is there a very excellent tightly coupled sequence of events; it should have nothing to do with the rate of the reaction of any one of them, but you should not lose substrate. I think that would be a very interesting experiment.

P. SRERE: That would be similar to the non-dilution seen by Fasella and his coworkers in the transaminase MDH system. This is an experiment we have talked about for five years, but because of technical problems we have just not done it yet.

J. WILLIAMSON: As you well know, if the mitochondrial oxalacetate concentration is really as low as you suppose, then there is still a problem with the aspartate aminotransferase equilibrium. My present leanings are to take the 20-50 micromolar measured oxalacetate in the mitochondrial matrix (see Siess, E. A. et al. Biochem. J. 166, 225-235, 1977) as reflecting something close to reality. This figure needs to be decreased by the amount that is bound, which is

presently an unknown quantity. Even with a free oxalacetate
concentration in the range of 2 to 5 micromolar, both the
citrate synthase and aspartate aminotransferase reactions
in the mitochondria can be envisioned as proceeding without
too much difficulty. The problem is then with malate dehydrogenase, which appears to be 2 to 3 orders off equilibrium (Tischler, M. E. et al. Arch. Biochem. Biophys. 184,
222-236, 1977). If equilibrium is assumed, as in your calculations, the calculated oxalacetate concentration is
about 100 times less than the measured. The meaning of this
observation is at present obscure, but might be related
to the fact that the oxalacetate-NAD^+ complex inhibits
malate dehydrogenase (Kaplan, N. O. in Enzymes and
Metabolic Pathways, Whelan, W. J. and Schultz, J., eds.,
North Holland, Vol. 1, pp. 84-97, 1970).

P. SRERE: I know of no freeze clamp measurements of liver
that shows 20 to 100 micromolar oxalacetate. Veech has
never seen it.

J. WILLIAMSON: Let's go then to what are the facts. Using
the digitonin cell fractionation technique (Zuurendonk, P.
I. and Tager, J. M., Biochim. Biophys. Acta. 333, 393-399,
1976) for rapid separation of mitochondria from isolated hepatocytes, Siess et al (reference given above) assayed a
mitochondrial oxalacetate content of about 5 nmol/g dry wt.
of liver cells and a total cell content of 22 nmol/g dry wt.
This latter value agrees well with our published values for
the oxalacetate content of liver (Williamson, J. R. et al.
J. Biol. Chem. 244, 5055-5064, 1969) and with those reported
by Eschenbrenner, E. and Guynn, R. W. (Anal. Biochem. 72,
220-229, 1976). Using an alternative method of cell disruption, Tischler, M. E. et al. (Arch. Biochem. Biophys. 184,
222-236, 1977) in our laboratory measured mitochondrial
oxalacetate concentrations of about 200 μM with isolated
hepatocytes. The direct fluorometric assay we used would tend
to overestimate the true value, which may account partly for
the fact that our values for the mitochondrial oxalacetate
concentration are higher than those of Siess et al.

P. SRERE: Then the redox potential (NAD/NADH) in the mitochondria can't be 7.

J. WILLIAMSON: The higher oxalacetate concentration means
the malate dehydrogenase can't be in equilibrium, but this
value fits very nicely with near-equilibrium of aspartate
aminotransferase.

P. SRERE: Well, if the malate dehydrogenase is not in equilibrium then you have other people to answer to.

L. FAHIEN: Paul, I have a few comments. I am sure you are aware of the work of E. Consiglio, S. Varrone, and I. Covelli (Eur. J. Biochem. 17, 408 1970) where they chromatographed a very high level of mitochondrial malate dehydrogenase on Sephedex G-100 and got two peaks: a minor peak in the void volume followed by a peak of native malate dehydrogenase. The first peak contained a great deal of protein but very little malate dehydrogenase activity. This protein was not entirely malate dehydrogenase because it contained tryptophan. They also did more extensive protein chemistry with antibodies and all that. I think that it would be worthwhile determining if that second protein might be citrate synthase. Are you familar with that?

P. SRERE: No I haven't seen that.

L. FAHIEN: The other thing is do you think you would get a complex if you would add substrates to your gels or gradients.

P. SRERE: We have tried that and substrates had no effect.

L. FAHIEN: With acetylCoA, DPNH and other substrates?

P. SRERE: We have tried, with Dr. Richards, differential ultracentrifugation with malate dehydrogenase and citrate synthase at mitochondrial concentrations with or without substrates. They each appear at their individual sedimentation place without any interaction that we could see.

L. FAHIEN: The second point is that malate dehydrogenase forms complexes with perhaps three different enzymes, glutamate dehydrogenase citrate synthase and aspartate aminotransferase. Can this be correlated with the work of Waksman which indicates that malate dehydrogenase and aspartate aminotransferase migrate together through the inner mitochondrial membrane?

P. SRERE: I never believed that. We have never seen it. Dr. Matlib has done the toluene experiments and all the controls are mitochondria not treated with toluene and you never see any leakage of the matrix enzymes into the outside medium unless you start treating them with excess toluene.

I would like Dr. Veech to comment on the matter of liver oxalacetate concentration because it is a crucial point that

John Williamson has made. We have no problem if the free
oxalacetate is 20 to 100 micromolar, it is just that most of
the measurements that I have seen, and I use your original
measurements John as my reference, give lower values.

J. WILLIAMSON: The provision is that the total amount that
can be measured analytically is split between the bound and
free, therefore the free certainly will be less than the
total measured.

R. VEECH: In response to Dr. Williamson's comments that he
finds the oxalacetate concentration to be 100 μM in his
so-called "mitochondrial fractions" after application of rapid
separation methods to isolated hepatocytes, I would offer the
opinion that this is an impossible value to exist in vivo. It
probably represents a methodological artefact of the type I
tried to illustrate in my discussion of the reported gradients for di- and tri-carboxyclic acids using these separation methods. That is to say, the oxalacetate content reported to exist in mitochondria would be higher than has
been found in whole freeze-clamped liver.

There are essentially four commonly used methods to determine
oxalacetate in tissue. The spectrophotometric method of
Hohorst and Reim (in Methods of Enzymatic Analysis, 1963, ed.
by H. U. Bergmeyer, pp. 335-339, Academic Press, New York)
lacks sensitivity and precision due to the large amounts
of tissue extract required and the low levels of oxalacetate. The fluorometric assays (Goldberg, N. D., Passonneau,
J. V., and Lowry, O. H., J. Biol. Chem. 241, 3997-4003),
while suitable for brain, cannot readily be applied to
liver because of the higher background fluorescence of liver
extracts. This background fluorescence cannot be reduced
with Florisil in the case of oxalacetate due to the accelerated decarboxylation of oxalacetate which such treatment
induces. The silver precipitation method (Weiland, O., and
Loffler, G., in Methods of Enzymatic Analysis, ed. by H. U.
Bergmeyer, Vol. 3, pp. 1611-1615, 1974), while both accurate
and suitable for use in liver, is very time-consuming, requires expensive radioactive acetyl CoA and is therefore
not widely used. The most sensitive and accurate method
would appear to be that of enzymatic cycling (Eschenbrenner,
E., and Guynn, R. W., Anal. Biochem. 72, 220-229, 1976) where
the sensitivity and accuracy are great and the background
fluorescence not of major significance. In normal well-fed
liver the total oxalacetate content (Eschenbrenner et al.,
1976) was reported to be 5.1 $\pm$ 0.6 nmoles/g wet weight
(N = 6) using the enzymatic cycling method. This value agrees

well with the previous reports of G. Loffler and O. Weiland
(Biochem. Z. 336, 447–454, 1963) who found oxalacetate of
5.9 ± 2.4 nmoles/g wet weight using the silver precipitation
method. These values also agree with original spectrophotometric assays of oxalacetate (Hohorst, H. J., Kreutz,
F. H., and Bucher, Th., Biochem. Z. 332, 18–46, 1959).
However, these later values must be viewed as only approxi-
mations because of the limitations of spectrophotometric
assays at this level performed on a Zeiss PMQ II spectrophotometer. The values are however slightly higher than
4.05 nmoles/g wet weight previously reported by Williamson,
J. R., and Corky, B. E. (Methods in Enzymology, Vol. XIII,
pp. 434–513, 1969) using direct fluorometric techniques which,
however, are of limited value for the reasons already cited.
The same laboratory reported oxalacetate values of 6.3 – 2.5
nmoles/gm wet weight in perfused liver (Williamson, J. R.,
Scholz, R., and Browning, E. T., J. Biol. Chem. 244, 4617–
4627, 1969) which are within the in vivo range. Even in
isolated hepatocytes the oxalacetate ranges between 4.05
and 6.2 nmoles/g wet weight of cells (Zuurendonk, P. F.,
Akerboom, T. P. M., and Tager, J. M., in Use of Isolated
Liver Cells and Kidney Tubules in Metabolic Studies (Tager,
J. M., Soling, H. D., and Williamson, J. R., eds.), pp. 17–
27, North Holland, Amsterdam, 1976). If one considers that
mitochondria comprise only 10% of liver cell space, a value
of 100 nmoles/g wet weight would mean that a measured cell
content of 10 nmoles/g wet weight would be expected if cell
contents were measured and no oxalacetate existed in the
cytoplasm. If mitochondria occupy 17% of the cell volume
a value of 17 nmoles/g wet weight of cells would be measured.
Clearly such values are outside the range of any previously
reported values. The value of 100 μM mitochondrial oxalacetate suggested by Dr. Williamson therefore seems extremely unlikely to me based on any previous in vivo value.
Rather, I would suggest that the extremely high value resulted from some artefact induced by the attempted cell
fractionation procedure which is similar to the case of
citrate and isocitrate measurements under similar circumstances (see Veech, this volume, pgs. 17–61).

Simply on analytical grounds, therefore, I think such a proposal should be viewed with some skepticism. If such an
oxalacetate concentration were to exist in mitochondria,
a number of problems -- even more difficult than the one
alluded to by Dr. Srere -- would result. Not only would
malate dehydrogenase reaction be likely to run opposite to the
direction of Krebs cycle flux, but one would also expect
succinic dehydrogenase to be severely inhibited by that level

of oxalacetate.   I therefore believe that, for the present,
Dr. Srere's conundrum of a possible micro-environment within
mitochondrial matrix is the least offensive possibility.

J. WILLIAMSON: I disagree with you.   The discussion about
oxalacetate measurements and concentrations seems circular.
Clearly any method of assay can be used improperly.   What
impresses me is the agreement of values between different
competent laboratories rather than the disagreement.   The
conclusion reached in our study (Tischler et al., 1977)
that mitochondrial malate dehydrogenase is not at near-
equilibrium is in agreement with other studies by Heath,
D. F. (Biochem. J. 110, 313-335, 1968), Zuurendonk, P. F.
et al. (in Use of Isolated Liver Cells and Kidney Tubules
in Metabolic Studies. J. M.Tager, H. D. Soling and J. R.
Williamson, eds., North Holland, Amsterdam, pp. 17-27, 1976).
Siess et al. FEBS Lett. 69, 265-271, 1976) and Williamson,
et al. (in Energy Metabolism and the Regulation of Metabolic
Processes in Mitochondria.   M. A. Mehlman and R. W. Hanson,
eds., Academic Press, New York, pp. 185-210).

J. LOWENSTEIN: There is a large difference in oxalacetate
content of starved liver and fed liver namely, 0.018 and 0.11
μmol per g dry weight, respectively (Brunengraber et al. (1973)
J. Biol. Chem. 248, 2656-2669).   In the starved liver the
rate of operation of the citric acid cycle is relatively low,
with much ketogenesis going on.   In the fed liver it is
operating at maximum rates.   I don't know what the calculated
values for the oxalacetate content would be in the fed
liver, but they will have to be much higher than what you
have quoted here.

P. SRERE: I think the value that I am using (1 micromole per
minute per gram) is a low value.   Professor Krebs would know.
One micromole C2 oxidized per gram per liver per minute is
not a high value for the tissue.

H. KREBS: The assumed QO_2 value (1 μmole/min/g wet wt)
underestimates even the "resting: state.   When liver cells
perform gluconeogenesis and urea synthesis the rate can be
at least four times as high.

PATCHES AND POCKETS
THE MICROENVIRONMENTS OF A MEMBRANE BOUND HEMEPROTEIN[1]

Julian A. Peterson[2]
David H. O'Keeffe[3]
Jurgen Werringloer
Richard E. Ebel[4]
Ronald W. Estabrook

Department of Biochemistry
The University of Texas Health Science Center at Dallas
Dallas, Texas

I. INTRODUCTION

There are many different organizational levels in biological systems. So far in this symposium we have considered practically all of the varieties which can be imagined but in my discussion I would like to consider two additional forms. The title "Patches and Pockets" was chosen after careful consideration because of its appropriate descriptive value for the organization of the hepatic drug oxidizing system involving cytochrome P-450 which is localized in the endoplasmic reticulum (1-3).

[1]Supported by NIH Research Grants GM19036 and GM16488 and Research Grant I-405 from the Robert A. Welch Research Foundation.
[2]Recipient of a USPHS Research Career Development Award GM30962.
[3]Recipient of a Postdoctoral Fellowship from the Robert A. Welch Research Foundation.
[4]Present address: Department of Biochemistry and Nutrition, Virginia Polytechnic and State University, Blacksburg, Virginia.

Copyright © 1978 by Academic Press, Inc.
All right of reproduction in any form reserved.
ISBN 0-12-660550-5

434   *Julian A. Peterson et al.*

II. PATCHES

The cytochromes P-450 are iron-protoporphyrin
IX-containing hemeproteins (4) which catalyze the reaction
shown in Equation 1 which is referred to as a monooxygenation
or mixed-function oxidation (5, 6). The substrate which is

1) $AH + 2H^+ + O_2 + 2e^- \longrightarrow AOH + H_2O$

oxidized (AH) can be one of a large variety of lipophilic
compounds which are found in nature or which have been
created by man. Thus this enzyme system is usually thought
of as serving to detoxicate the pollutants which we ingest.
However, in the case of the polycyclic aromatic hydrocarbons,
this enzyme appears to activate them so that they become
carcinogenic. The common feature of this class of oxidative
enzymes is that they use dioxygen (O_2) with one of the oxygen
atoms being incorporated into the organic compound and the
other in water. The two electrons which are required for
this reaction are derived from reduced pyridine nucleotides,
and are transferred to cytochrome P-450, in the case of
hepatic microsomal drug oxidation, via a flavoprotein
reductase (NADPH-cytochrome P-450 reductase). Based upon
purification and reconstitution studies of the drug oxidation
reaction, it was recognized a number of years ago that the
minimal requirements in addition to the flavoprotein
reductase include a source of electrons (NADPH), cytochrome
P-450, and phospholipid (dilaurylphosphatidylcholine) (7, 8).
The stoichiometry of the enzyme components bound to the
microsomal membrane fraction has been established for a
number of different preparations and is shown in Table I.
The ratio of cytochrome P-450 molecules to flavoprotein
reductase molecules is quite large and certainly in all cases
studied in excess of ten (9, 10).
In considering the kinetics of interaction between these
electron transfer proteins, the fact that they are bound to a
membrane creates a complex situation. Instead of being able
to diffuse through solution in three dimensions the motion of
the proteins in a membrane, or bound to its surface, is
usually thought of as being limited to two dimensions.
Studies on the nature of diffusion of small organic molecules
like phospholipids and steroids as well as proteins in
membranes have shown that their rate of translational motion
at $37^O C$ is quite large (11, 12). In the limiting case of a
membrane which is highly viscous, the diffusion of proteins
may be prevented altogether. Natural membranes are quite
heterogeneous in their lipid and protein composition and

TABLE 1

Concentration of Microsomal Electron Transfer Components

	P-450	FMN	FAD	RATIO
	nmoles/mg protein			P-450/FMN
RATS (9)				
control	0.71	0.075	0.15	9.5
phenobarbital				
pretreatment	2.1	0.08	0.13	26.3
MICE (10)				
C57BL/6J	0.51	0.021	0.094	24.3
DBA/2J	0.53	0.013	0.090	40.8

Since the NADPH specific flavoprotein, cytochrome P-450 reductase has an equimolar amount of FMN and FAD, the amount of this enzyme present in the microsomal membrane is usually assumed to be equal to the FMN content.

distribution (13, 14). Certain regions or <u>patches</u> are considered to be enriched in a given class of lipids and/or proteins and thus may not possess the same properties as the bulk membrane (15). Into such a complex membrane environment are inserted the enzymes of drug oxidation.

The components of the microsomal drug oxidizing system have been purified to homogeneity and their physical properties are beginning to be understood (16, 17). The molecular architecture of the flavoprotein reductase is such that it has a hydrophilic head and a lipophilic tail which is readily cleaved by proteolysis (18, 19). Those forms of the flavoprotein reductase which have had the hydrophobic portion cleaved are inactive in the reduction of cytochrome P-450 but are still functional in transferring electrons from NADPH to the alternate electron acceptors cytochrome c or potassium ferricyanide. Thus, even though the prosthetic groups (FAD, FMN) of the active site of the reductase are found in the hydrophilic head, the hydrophobic tail seems to be required to cause the proteins to assume the appropriate orientation with regard to one another for electron transfer to cytochrome P-450 to occur. Cytochrome P-450 is very difficult to remove from the microsomal membrane and can only be removed in an active form in the presence of detergents and therefore it is considered to be an integral protein of the membrane. The interaction between these proteins can be readily studied during the course of electron transfer from the NADPH-dependent flavoprotein reductase to cytochrome P-450 (20). The carbon monoxide complex of ferrous

cytochrome P-450 has an absorbance maximum at 450 nm. In the
presence of an atmosphere of carbon monoxide, the half-time
of formation of the complex is less than 5 ms and the
kinetics of reduction of cytochrome P-450 by the flavoprotein
reductase can be measured by following the appearance of the
absorbance band at 450 nm in a stopped-flow spectrophotometer
(21). As can be seen in Figs. 1 and 2, the time course of
reduction of cytochrome P-450 is biphasic. The reaction
kinetics can be resolved by a nonlinear estimation procedure
into two concurrent first order processes (20, 22). This

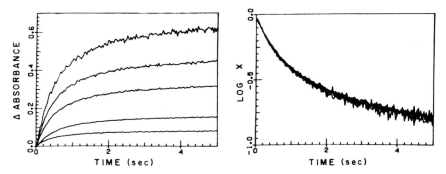

FIGURE 1(left). Time course of NADPH-cytochrome P-450
reductase catalyzed reduction of microsomal cytochrome P-450
from phenobarbital pretreated rats in the presence of 1 mM
hexobarbital using 0.46, 0.92, 1.85, 2.78, and 3.70 mg/ml of
microsomal protein.
FIGURE 2(right). First order plots of cytochrome P-450
reduction using the data from Fig. 1.

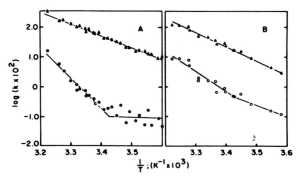

FIGURE 3. Arrhenius plots of NADPH-cytochrome P-450
reductase activity (▲, fast-phase; ○, slow-phase) in
microsomes prepared from phenobarbital pretreated rats: A, 1
mM hexobarbital; B, 2 mM ethylmorphine.

numerical analysis procedure has permitted the determination of the rate constants for both the fast and slow phases as well as the amount of cytochrome P-450 reduced in each phase.

Since this enzyme system is bound to a membrane, the reduction of cytochrome P-450 has been studied as a function of temperature to determine if the fluidity of the membrane affects the interaction of the flavoprotein reductase and cytochrome P-450 (20). As can be seen in Fig. 3, lowering the temperature of the reaction mixture from 37° to 4°C caused a significant change in both the rate constants for reduction of cytochrome P-450 but there was no break in the Arrhenius plot for the fast phase rate constant. There was a break in the plot of the slow phase rate constant; however, this change in activation energy was unusual for a membrane bound enzyme in that at temperatures below the break the activation energy in many instances approaches zero. In the case of most membrane bound enzymes, the ΔH or slope becomes very large below the break point indicating the large amount of energy required for interaction of proteins in the membrane below this point. Most investigators interpret break points of this type as indicating changes in fluidity of the lipids of the membrane either at or near the enzyme being studied (23). An additional interesting observation with regard to cytochrome P-450 reduction at the lower temperatures (less than 22°C) is that the amount of cytochrome reduced in the fast phase was always at least 50 to 60% of the total. This represents approximately 10 to 12 cytochrome P-450 molecules per molecule of flavoprotein reductase (20). The simplest interpretation of these data is that translational motion of the flavoprotein reductase with respect to cytochrome P-450 is not required for reduction of the cytochromes P-450 in the fast phase at the lower temperatures.

Any model which is proposed to explain the nature of the interaction between cytochrome P-450 and its flavoprotein reductase, at the level of the organization of these enzymes on the membrane surface, must take into account the following observations: 1) at low temperature, where translational motion is probably restricted, approximately 10 to 12 cytochrome P-450 molecules are reduced per flavoprotein reductase molecule in a fast first order process; 2) the slow phase of reduction of the remaining cytochrome P-450 molecules probably requires translational motion at higher temperatures but may represent electron tunneling at lower temperatures in the cases where the activation energy is near zero; 3) the fast phase of reduction at higher temperatures may involve 75 to 80% of the total cytochrome P-450; 4) the effect of exogenous substrates on the kinetics of reduction

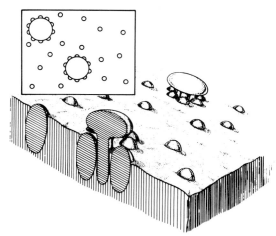

FIGURE 4. Model for the interaction of cytochrome P-450 and NADPH-dependent cytochrome P-450 reductase on the microsomal membrane. The inset is a representation of the model with the view perpendicular to the plane of the membrane.

at room temperature may be a function of their effect on the fluidity of membrane lipids because at $37^{\circ}C$ the substrates do not have a readily discernible effect on the kinetics of cytochrome P-450 reduction.

Our conception of the simplest model which will fit the currently available data is shown in Fig. 4 (20, 24). There are clusters or <u>patches</u> of approximately 10 to 12 cytochrome P-450 molecules arranged around a central flavoprotein reductase molecule which protrudes from the membrane as a consequence of its amphiphatic properties. Reduction of these cytochrome P-450 molecules in the <u>patch</u> is envisioned to take place in a random first order process which does not require translational motion of either of the proteins involved. The remaining cytochrome P-450 molecules, which are reduced in the slow phase, are pictured here as being randomly distributed. These additional cytochrome molecules are reduced even at lower temperatures where translational motion may be hindered. At higher temperatures, where rapid diffusional motion of the membrane components is expected, the reduction of cytochrome P-450 still involves two phases. Close examination of the Arrhenius plot for the fast phase of reduction does not reveal any breaks or discontinuities in the line. Thus, even though the viscosity of the membrane or of those lipids in the immediate environment of a flavoprotein reductase-cytochrome P-450 <u>patch</u> may change abruptly at some transition temperature which clearly affects the reduction of cytochrome P-450 in the slow phase, no comparable effect on the fast phase is observed. The effect which is observed is that the fraction of the cytochrome P-450 reduced in the fast phase increases to 75 to 80% of the total. Conceivably at 37° some of the cytochrome P-450 molecules clustered around a flavoprotein reductase are replaced via a diffusion process by other cytochrome P-450 molecules thus increasing the proportion reduced in the fast phase. However, the basic mechanism whereby the cytochrome is reduced is unchanged since there is no break in the Arrhenius plot.

Implications for the understanding of the metabolic control of cytochrome P-450 arise as a consequence of our hypothesis. For example, a puzzling observation has been made regarding drug metabolism in new-born animals (25). The level of drug metabolism is very low yet the amounts of the drug metabolizing enzymes are almost the same as in a fully competent adult. One of the explanations given for this observation is the absence of an unknown component "X" presumably required for drug metabolism. On the other hand, we would like to propose that the activity of overall drug metabolism may be inhibited because the flavoprotein reductase and cytochrome P-450 molecules are restricted in their interaction. Another example of this type of control could occur if certain classes of cytochrome P-450 were limited in their access to a flavoprotein reductase molecules. Thus, the potential activity of this drug metabolizing system could be modified by changing the fluidity of the membrane without altering the total amount of enzymes present. Thus a new form of metabolic control is envisioned involving segregation of some the cytochrome P-450 molecules from their electron donor enzyme as a function of the membrane lipid composition and/or distribution.

Obviously this generalized hypothesis, in our attempts at simplicity, has neglected what is potentially a crucial step: the mechanism of introduction of the second electron which is required to complete the catalytic cycle of cytochrome P-450. Evidence that cytochrome b_5 may participate in the donation of the second electron has appeared in the literature (26, 27). However, the nature of the cytochrome b_5 (or other electron donor enzymes) interaction with the <u>patches</u> composed of NADPH-flavoprotein reductase and cytochrome P-450 molecules remains to be elucidated.

III. POCKETS

Let us turn now to a second organizational level in
studying the mechanism of action of this fascinating
monooxygenase. The variety of substrates metabolized by
hepatic microsomal cytochrome P-450 is so large that the
usual concept of substrate specificity characteristically
thought to be associated with enzyme action seems to have
lost all meaning. In order to accommodate the enzymatic
properties of cytochrome P-450 into the general theme of
substrate specificity, it has been proposed that cytochromes
P-450 are induced in specific response to each compound or
drug. This type of induction has been likened to the well –
known antigen-antibody response of the immune system. Thus
the presence of a particular drug or agent would cause the
induction of a specific cytochrome P-450 which would bind and
metabolize only that drug or agent. The second possibility
is that induction results in only a limited number of
different cytochromes P-450. Each of these cytochrome P-450
classes would then oxidize a specific class (type) of
compound. The latter explanation seems to account for most
of the data related to substrate induction of and binding to
cytochromes P-450. As techniques have been perfected for
purification of hepatic microsomal cytochrome P-450, it has
become clear that the number of different forms which can be
induced is small. Thus an understanding of control of
substrate specificity of this enzyme system will represent a
major advance in our knowledge of enzyme action.

Instead of focusing on a small group of chemicals and
mammalian cytochromes P-450, we have felt that more can be
learned about substrate specificity by examining a broad
range of compounds using both the mammalian and bacterial
cytochromes. The soluble bacterial cytochrome P-450$_{cam}$ has a
rather rigid substrate specificity for the 5-exo
hydroxylation of d-camphor (28,29) which is contrasted with
the hepatic microsomal cytochromes P-450 discussed above.
Consequently we were somewhat surprised to rediscover in the
literature that mammals also metabolize camphor and that the
position of attack by the hepatic enzyme system is the 5-exo
hydrogen (30). In retrospect, we should not have been
surprised because of the amount of camphor which is used for
relief of upper respiratory congestion in the United States
today. We were somewhat puzzled by the seeming contradiction
of the specificity of this mammalian hydroxylation reaction
because it did not agree with our previously held notion. If
mammalian cytochromes P-450 are in fact so promiscuous, why
is camphor oxidized at only the 5-exo position? Might there

be some unique features about the structures of camphor and the iron protoporphyrin XI prosthetic group which may control the position of hydroxylation and enable us to better understand the metabolism of other compounds? After examining a large number of two dimensional projections of the structures of some compounds which are metabolized, we realized that we must examine three dimensional structures instead. Being dreamers we began to construct molecular models of heme rings and various substrates of cytochrome P-450 to see if we could discover anything unique about them (31). The outgrowth of this flight of fancy is the second section of our presentation in which we discuss some of the factors which control substrate specificity and also describe the hydrophobic pocket which constitutes the active site of cytochrome P-450.

In thinking about the active site of cytochrome P-450 several structural points which must be considered are illustrated in Fig. 5. This figure is a photograph of a stick model of protoporphyrin IX, with an iron ion chelated at the center. The aromatic character of heme, which cannot be illustrated here, results in its flat disc-like shape and it is considered to be extremely hydrophobic. As a consequence of the reactivity and the electrophilic character of the proposed "active oxygen", the assumption is made that

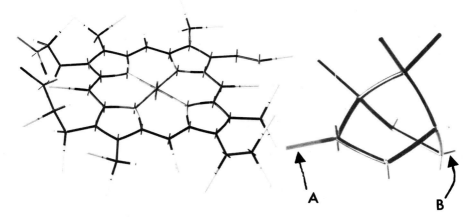

FIGURE 5. Molecular models of iron-protoporphyrin IX (left) and d-camphor (right). The heme ring is oriented so that the propionate side chains are to the left and the iron ion is in the center. The camphor molecule is oriented so that the carbonyl group protrudes to the left and is indicated by the arrow at A while the 5-position is indicated by the arrow at B.

the substrate binding site is going to be in the immediate vicinity of and on the same side of the heme ring as dioxygen binds. Competitive binding of ligands of the heme iron and substrates of cytochrome P-450 have shown that O_2, CO, and NO (32, 33) as well as substrates (34) all bind on the same side of the heme ring. Also the two propionate residues which are side chains on the periphery of the porphyrin ring are very polar and probably oriented to solvent.

In examining the structure of d-camphor, also shown in Fig. 5, several features become apparent. The molecule is rigid, roughly spherical in shape, and contains a polar carbonyl group on the side opposite the 5-exo position. It is well known from the study of the partitioning of small organic molecules such as camphor, at an aqueous – organic solvent interface, that the presence of a polar group such as a carbonyl group will result in a specific orientation of the molecule with the carbonyl group directed toward the aqueous layer.

Now that we have discussed some of the special features of the heme ring and our test organic compound camphor, what is known about the substrate binding site of cytochrome P-450? Studies on substrate free ferric cytochrome P-450$_{cam}$ have shown that bulk solvent protons rapidly exchange with protons linked to an atom in the inner coordination sphere of the hemin iron. This has been interpreted to indicate that in the absence of substrate, water is a ligand of the hemin iron (35). However, upon the addition of substrate to the enzyme, the ability of the paramagnetic hemin iron to relax solvent protons is almost completely abolished. Thus, the immediate environment of the hemin in the presence of substrate is very hydrophobic.

With this evidence, we can begin to construct a hypothetical substrate binding site (pocket) into which can be inserted a variety of organic molecules. In Fig. 6, we have illustrated for simplicity the pocket containing camphor. The points raised in the previous discussion have been considered: 1) the carbonyl group of camphor is positioned over the propionate side chains; and 2) the more curved bulky side of camphor is oriented away from the flat disc-shaped heme ring. When this is done it can be seen that the 5-exo hydrogen of camphor is positioned over the iron. Thus, we have described an active site for this hemeprotein which meets the structural limitations and requirements. The obvious question is whether there is any reality in such a hypothesis. We can offer only the following isolated observations which can now be explained by this proposed active site (pocket). A number of years ago in the study of substrate specificity in steroid metabolism by cytochrome

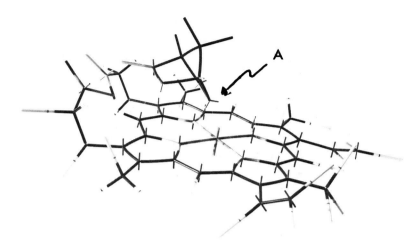

FIGURE 6. Molecular model of the pocket around the active site of cytochrome P-450. The 5-exo position of camphor is indicated by the arrow at A. The orientation of the models is very similar to that in Fig. 5.

P-450 a curious relationship between the position hydroxylated and the position of a polar functional group was recognized (36, 37). The distance between this polar group and the position oxidized is about 5 A which is the same as the distance between the carbonyl oxygen of camphor and the 5-exo hydrogen. Both d- and l-camphor are oxidized by cytochrome P-450 in the same position relative to the carbonyl group (28), thereby meeting the structural requirements discussed above. The position which is oxidized in a number of drugs seems to fit our hypothesis, but in the case of these compounds the molecular structure is not sufficiently rigid to limit the positions oxidized.

In examining structures of a very important class of substrates of cytochrome P-450, the polycyclic aromatic hydrocarbons, we were initially puzzled as to how our proposal could explain their binding and multiple sites of oxidation. The metabolism of these compounds is extremely complex but the first position oxidized appears to be an almost random attack of the molecule with a position of initial oxygen insertion being electron rich (38). Certain products of this oxidation are epoxides which are enzymatically hydrated by epoxide hydrase (39). The oxidative metabolism of the polycyclic aromatic hydrocarbons does not end with just a single oxygenation but they are further oxidized. A typical polycyclic aromatic hydrocarbon, benzo(a)pyrene, is flat, very hydrophobic, and does not possess a polar functional group which could serve to orient it at a water - solvent interface as described above. According to our hypothesis, these types of compounds would enter the active site of cytochrome P-450 and assume a position parallel to the plane of the heme ring. However, the possibility does exist that 𝜋-𝜋 interactions between the porphyrin ring and the polycyclic aromatic hydrocarbon may serve to orient these molecules prior to oxygen activation and insertion. As we discussed earlier, activated oxygen is electrophilic and it would attack the closest position with the highest electron density to form an epoxide. The diol derivatives which are the products of epoxide hydrase action on epoxides, have polar and non-polar regions. The polar end could orient the molecule in the active site of cytochrome P-450 for subsequent metabolism. It will be interesting to see if the position of the second oxidative attack follows the 5 A rule for oxidative metabolism which we have discussed.

In summary, the membrane into which cytochrome P-450 is embedded plays an extremely important role in establishing the microenvironment for the metabolism of these hydrophobic organic compounds. The membrane serves first to provide support for the assembly of this multienzyme complex and results in patches of flavoprotein reductase and cytochrome P-450 on the membrane. Secondly the lipophilic nature of the membrane lipids serves to concentrate the hydrophobic substrates of cytochrome P-450. These substrates can then be transferred to the hydrophobic pocket in the environs the hemin iron of cytochrome P-450 where they are oxidized to give water soluble products which can then be further metabolized or excreted.

REFERENCES

1. Strittmatter, L.F. and Ball, E. G., Proc. Nat'l. Acad. Sci. (U.S.A.) 38:19 (1952).
2. Omura, T., Sato, R., Cooper, D. Y., Rosenthal, O., and Estabrook, R. W., Fed. Proc. 24:1181 (1965).
3. Kamin, H., Masters, B. S. S., Gibson, Q. H., and Williams, C. H., Fed. Proc. 24:1164 (1965).
4. Omura, T. and Sato, R., J. Biol. Chem. 239:2370 (1964).
5. Hayaishi, O., Proc, Int. Union Biochem. 33:31 (1964).
6. Mason, H. S., Adv. Enzymol. 19:79 (1957).
7. Lu, A. Y. H., Junk, K. W., and Coon, M. J., J. Biol.

Chem. 244:3714 (1969).

8. Strobel, H. W., Lu, A. Y. H., Heidema, J., and Coon, M. J., J. Biol. Chem. 245:4851 (1970).

9. Estabrook, R. W., Franklin, M. R., Cohen, B., Shigamatzu, A., and Hildebrandt, A. G., Metabolism 20:187 (1971).

10. Blumer, J. L. and Mieyal, J. J., J. Biol. Chem. 253:1159 (1978).

11. Marsh, D., Essays in Biochem. 11:139 (1975).

12. Cherry, R. J., in "Biological Membranes", Vol. 3, (D. Chapman and D. F. H. Wallach, eds.), p. 47. Academic Press, London, 1976.

13. Coleman, R., Biochim. Biophys. Acta 300:1 (1973).

14. DePierre, J. W. and Ernster, L., Annu. Rev. Biochem. 46:201 (1977).

15. Kleemann, W., Grant, C. W. M., and McConnell, H. M., J. Supramol. Struct. 2:609 (1974).

16. Haugen, D. A. and Coon, M. J., J. Biol. Chem. 251:7929 (1976).

17. Yashukochi, Y., and Masters, B. S. S., J. Biol. Chem. 251:5337 (1976).

18. Masters, B. S. S., Williams, C. H., and Kamin, H., Methods Enzymol. 10:565 (1967).

19. Modirzadeh, J. and Kamin, H., Biochim. Biophys. Acta 99:205 (1965).

20. Peterson, J. A., Ebel, R. E., O'Keeffe, D. H., Matsubara, T., and Estabrook, R. W., J. Biol. Chem. 251:4010 (1976).

21. Peterson, J. A., Ebel, R. E., and O'Keeffe, D. H., Methods Enzymol. 51:221 (1978).

22. Matsubara, T., Baron, J., Peterson, L. L., and Peterson, J. A., Arch. Biochem. Biophys. 172:463 (1976).

23. Wisnieski, B. J., Huang, Y. O., and Fox, C. F., J. Supramol. Struct. 2:593 (1974).

24. Estabrook, R. W., Werringloer, J., Masters, B. S. S., Jonen, H., Matsubara, T., Ebel, R., O'Keeffe, D., and Peterson, J. A., in "The Structural Basis of Membrane Function" (Y. Hatefi and L. Djavadi-Ohaniance, eds.), p. 429. Academic Press, New York, 1976.

25. Dallner, G., Siekevitz, P., and Palade, G. E., Biochem. Biophys. Res. Commun. 20:135 (1965).

26. Hildebrandt, A. and Estabrook, R. W., Arch. Biochem. Biophys. 143:66 (1971).

27. Cohen, B. S. and Estabrook, R. W., Arch. Biochem. Biophys. 143:37 (1971).

28. Hedgaard, J. and Gunsalus, I. C., J. Biol. Chem. 240:4038 (1965).

29. Katagiri, M., Ganguli, B. N., and Gunsalus, I. C., J.

Biol. Chem. 243:3543 (1968).

30. Reinartz, F. and Zanke, W., Ber. 67:548 (1934).

31. Estabrook, R. W., Baron, J., Peterson, J. A., and Ishimura, Y., in "Biological Hydroxylation Mechanisms" (G. S. Boyd and R. M. S. Smellie, eds.), p. 159. Academic Press, New York, 1972.

32. Peterson, J. A., Ishimura, Y., and Griffin, B. W., Arch. Biochem. Biophys. 149:197 (1972).

33. O'Keeffe, D. H., Ebel, R. E., and Peterson, J. A., J. Biol. Chem. 253:in press (1978).

34. Peterson, J. A. and Griffin, B. W., Arch. Biochem. Biophys. 151:427 (1972).

35. Griffin, B. W. and Peterson, J. A., J. Biol. Chem. 250:6445 (1975).

36. Estabrook, R. W., Martinez-Zedillo, G., Young, S., Peterson, J. A., and McCarthy, J., J. Steroid Biochem. 6:419 (1975).

37. Gustafsson, J.-A., Ingelman-Sundberg, M., and Stenberg, A., J. Steroid Biochem. 6:643 (1975).

38. Estabrook, R. W., Werringloer, J., Capdevila, J., and Prough, R. A., in "Polycyclic Hydrocarbons and Cancer", Vol 1 (P. D. P. Tso and H. V. Gelboin, eds.), p. 281. Academic Press, New York, (1978).

39. Oesch, F., Xenobiotica 3:305 (1973).

DISCUSSION

R. WELCH: Could you elaborate on the orientation effect
of a hydrocarbon and P-450?

R. ESTABROOK: That is a complex interaction. You are faced
with the problem that you have a big molecule, highly hydrophobic, which gets preferentially hydroxylated at certain sites. What is it that dictates how that molecule
enters into within about 10 angstrom of the heme plane in
a specific orientation so that oxygen is inserted at those
specific sites. One can do spectrophotometric measurements
to see that such an interaction is occurring and that has
been done and been published. One can then only do theoretical model building or calculations as to what the nature
of the orientation is. Now, we have attempted to answer
this question by using various steroid molecules which also
interact nearly stoichiometrically and which have the advantage in that one can obtain a vast diversity of steroids.
In this instance it appears, at least with the steroid molecules where you get site specific introduction of oxygen,
that steering groups such as keto groups in the 3 and 17
position are absolute requirements for substrates orientation. With polycyclic hydrocarbons where there are no
steering groups, I don't have any simple answer. We are
working on it and we are trying to evaluate what forces are
responsible for directing the site of hydroxylation.

R. WELCH: Is it correct that the hydrocarbon diffuses
into the lipid phase and then it undergoes diffusional
rotation.

R. ESTABROOK: This is apparently a very fast reaction and
it depends on whether it rotates after it gets in or
whether it goes in a specific way. Many investigators
often talk about a hydrophobic environment. I don't know
what the hydrophobic environment is, but I thought in
terms of microenvironments we should mention it.

Index

A
B
C 8
D 9
E 0
F 1
G 2
H 3
I 4
J 5